The Complete Neck Pain Toolkit

A Practical Guide to Finding Your Unique Solution

Jeffery J. Rowe, MD

Rowe Publishing Company

Copyright

The Complete Neck Pain Toolkit: A Practical Guide to Finding Your Unique Solution

Images and Artwork: Rowe Publishing Company
Illustrations: Rowe Publishing Company
Cover Design: Rowe Publishing Company

Printed in The United States of America

First   **edition**   **2023**

Content

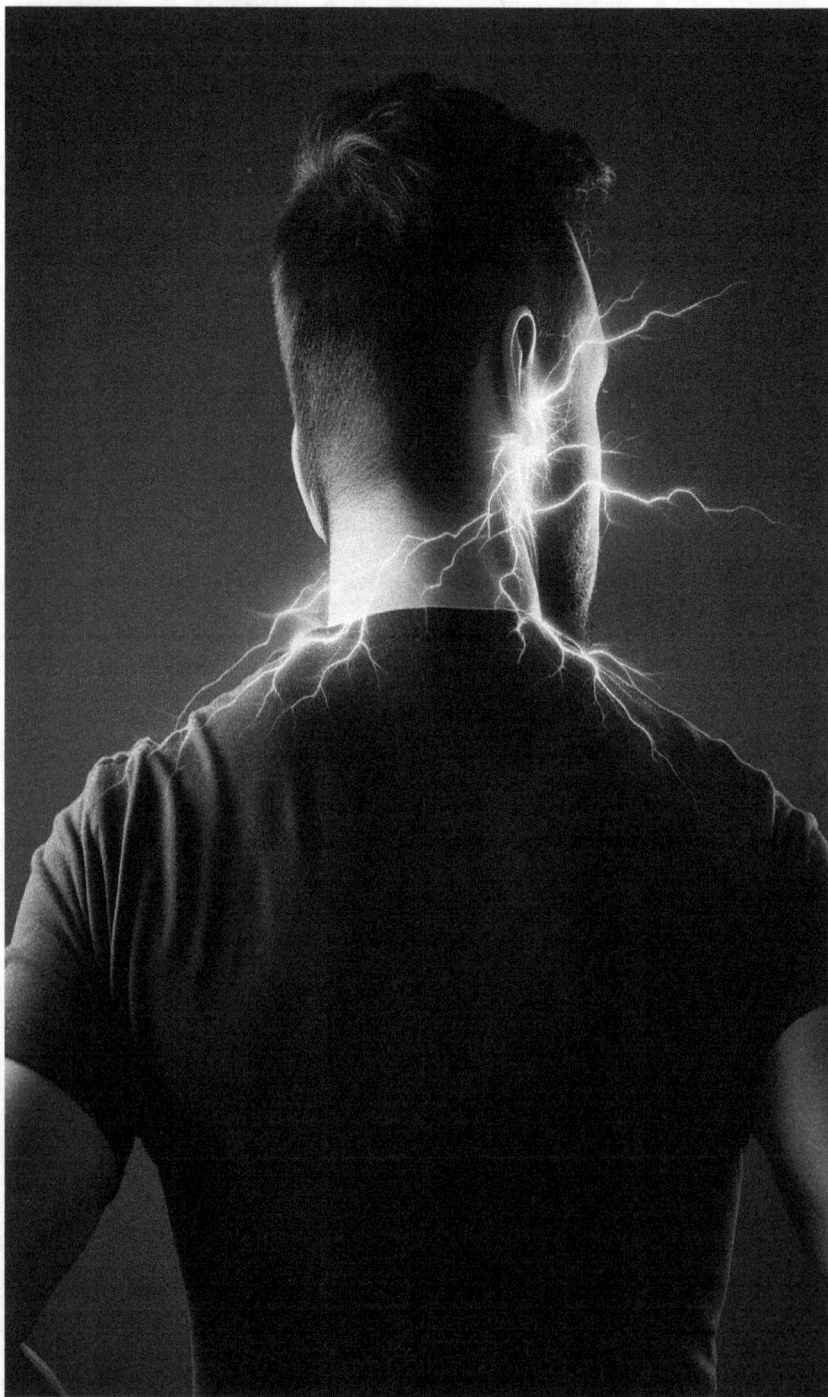

Foreword

The Complete Neck Pain Toolkit

Neck pain is a prevalent issue affecting millions of people worldwide, significantly impacting their quality of life and daily functioning. This comprehensive book has been meticulously crafted to serve as an invaluable resource for patients or anyone interested in understanding and effectively managing neck pain.

The book begins by laying the foundation for understanding the complex anatomy of the neck and the various causes and symptoms of neck pain, emphasizing the importance of accurate diagnosis in order to identify the root cause and implement targeted treatment strategies.

Readers are guided through a range of conservative, non-invasive treatment approaches, including physical therapy, rehabilitation, medication management, alternative and complementary therapies, cervical traction, and orthotic devices. The book also delves into more advanced interventional pain management techniques such as epidural steroid injections, nerve blocks, and radiofrequency ablation, as well as neuromodulation options like spinal cord stimulation, dorsal root ganglion stimulation, and peripheral nerve stimulation.

Recognizing the importance of addressing daily habits and routines, this book also discusses posture, ergonomics, exercise, manual therapy, lifestyle modifications, stress management, and nutrition, providing comprehensive insight into the multifaceted aspects of neck pain management. For those requiring surgical intervention, the book presents an overview of cervical disc replacement, cervical fusion surgery, and minimally invasive spine surgery, as well as post-surgical care and recovery strategies.

This resource not only provides guidance for managing existing neck pain but also emphasizes preventive strategies to avoid future issues, outlining proactive measures that can be taken to promote a healthy, pain-free neck. Furthermore, the book examines the role of technology in neck pain management, including wearables, telemedicine, and remote monitoring solutions.

Finally, the book explores the future of neck pain treatment, highlighting emerging therapies and innovations in pain management that hold promise for improving the lives of individuals suffering from neck pain.

This comprehensive guide is a testament to the dedication and expertise of its author, providing readers with a wealth of knowledge to empower them in their journey to understand, treat, and manage neck pain effectively. The combination of practical advice, evidence-based approaches, and forward-looking insights make this book an indispensable resource for anyone navigating the complex world of neck pain treatment and management.

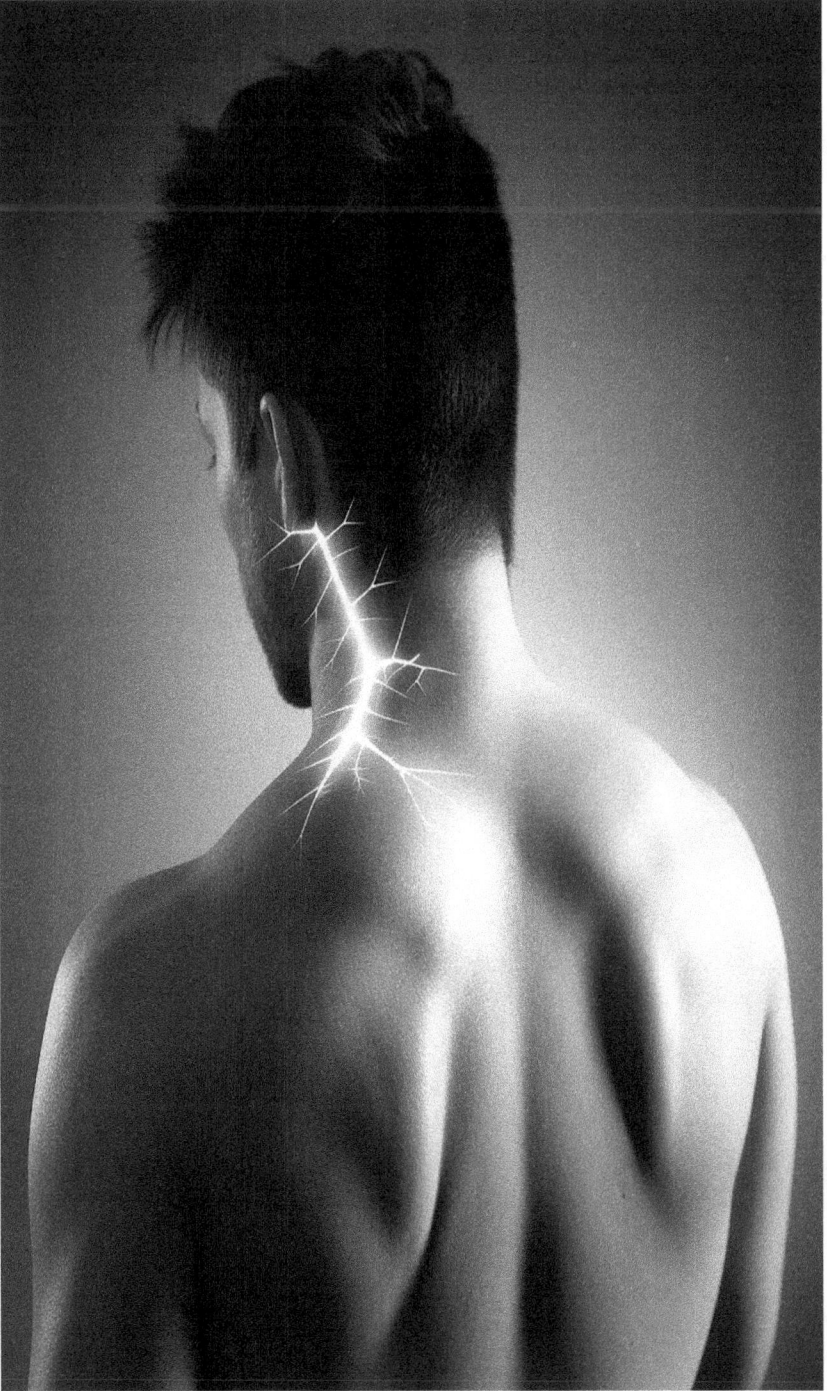

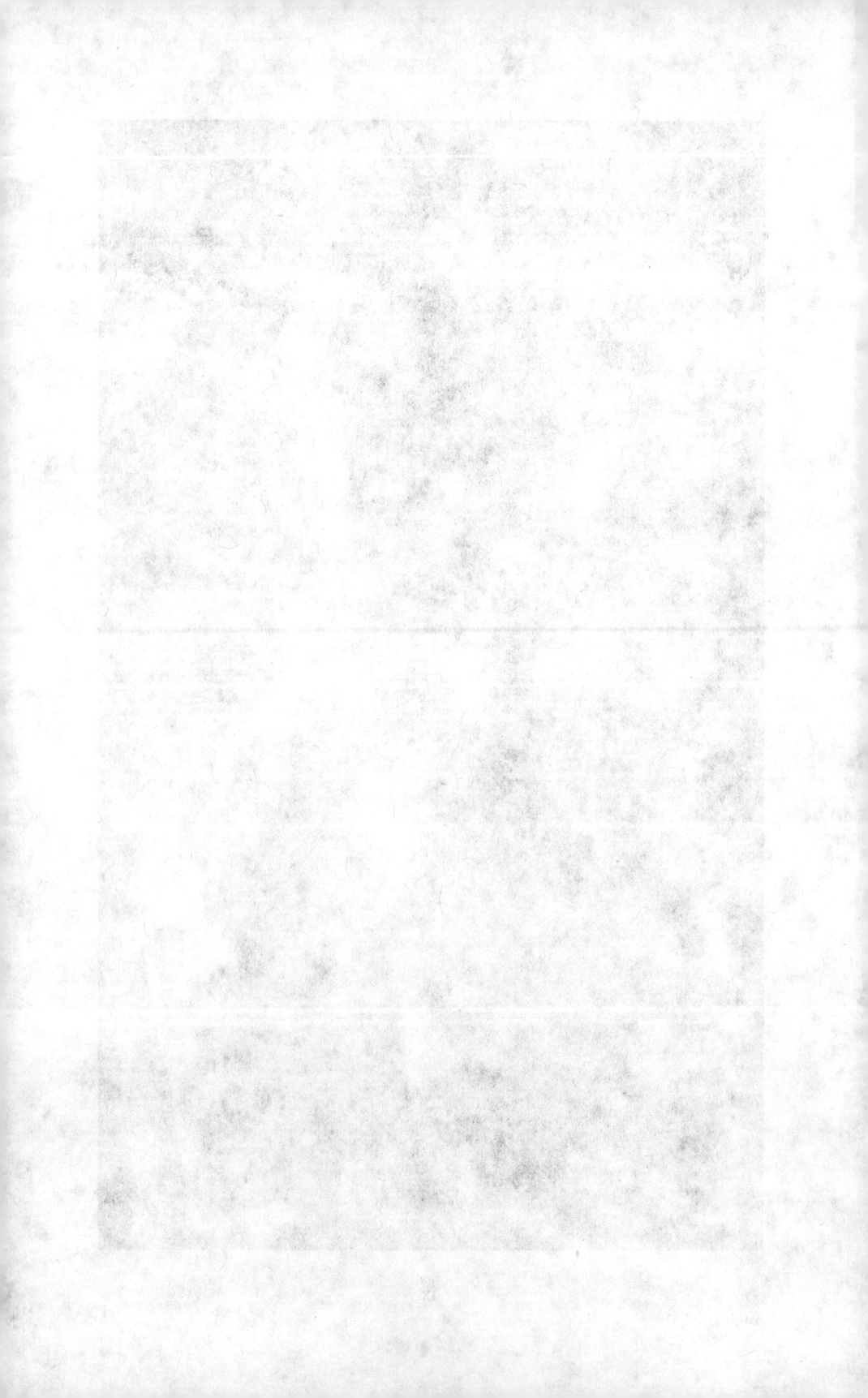

Chapter 1

Understanding Neck Pain

The Anatomy, Causes, and Symptoms of Neck Pain

The neck, or cervical spine, is a highly intricate structure that serves to support the head, facilitate its wide range of movement, and connect it to the rest of the body. The cervical spine's complexity lies in the numerous bones, muscles, ligaments, nerves, and blood vessels that comprise it, each playing a crucial role in maintaining the neck's overall function and stability.

At the core of the cervical spine are seven vertebrae, labeled C1 to C7. The first two vertebrae, the atlas (C1) and the axis (C2), form a distinctive joint known as the atlantoaxial joint. This joint is responsible for the significant range of motion exhibited by the head, allowing for actions such as nodding and rotation. The remaining vertebrae are connected to one another through facet joints, which facilitate smooth, coordinated movements of the neck.

Intervertebral discs separate the cervical vertebrae and are essential for the spine's flexibility and shock-absorbing capabilities. Each disc comprises a gel-like substance called the nucleus pulposus, which is surrounded by a robust fibrous ring known as the annulus fibrosus. This structure enables the discs to withstand the pressures exerted by the vertebrae during movement, preventing them from grinding against each other and causing damage.

The spinal cord, a crucial component of the central nervous system, is housed within the vertebral canal formed by the cervical vertebrae. At each vertebral level, nerve roots exit the spinal cord and branch out into the body, transmitting sensory information from the skin, muscles, and organs to the brain, as well as relaying motor commands from the brain to the muscles for movement.

The cervical spine is stabilized and supported by an intricate network of muscles and ligaments. The deep neck muscles, such as the longus colli and longus capitis, help maintain proper alignment and posture. The superficial muscles, including the sternocleidomastoid and trapezius, contribute to the wide range of motion exhibited by the neck. Ligaments, such as the anterior and posterior longitudinal ligaments, the ligamentum flavum, and the interspinous and supraspinous ligaments, further reinforce the cervical spine's stability.

In addition to the bones, muscles, and ligaments, the neck houses essential blood vessels that supply the brain and other vital structures. The carotid arteries, located on either side of the neck, are responsible for delivering oxygen-rich blood to the brain, while the jugular veins return oxygen-depleted blood from the head back to the heart. Other critical blood vessels, including the vertebral arteries and the thyrocervical trunk, also contribute to the circulation in the neck region.

The anatomy of the neck is a highly intricate and interconnected system of bones, muscles, ligaments, nerves, and blood vessels that work together to support the head and connect it to the rest of the body. Understanding the complexity of the cervical spine is crucial for diagnosing and treating neck pain and related conditions, as well as for maintaining overall health and function.

Neck pain can arise from a multitude of factors, encompassing both acute injuries and chronic underlying conditions. One of the most common causes of neck pain is muscle strain, which typically occurs when the neck muscles are overused or overstretched. This can happen as a result of maintaining poor posture for extended periods, such as when working at a computer or using a smartphone, which can lead to a forward head posture that places excessive stress on the muscles and ligaments of the neck. Prolonged sitting or standing in a slouched or hunched position can also contribute to neck muscle strain.

In addition to poor posture, sleeping in an awkward position that doesn't support the natural alignment of the cervical spine can cause muscle strain and discomfort. Using a pillow that is too high or too low, or sleeping on your stomach with your head turned to one side, can put undue stress on the neck muscles and lead to pain upon waking.

Furthermore, engaging in activities that require repetitive neck movements, such as certain sports or occupations, can also lead to muscle strain. For example, swimmers who use improper technique while executing strokes may experience neck strain due to excessive neck rotation. Similarly, individuals who frequently perform overhead tasks, such as painters or warehouse workers, may overuse their neck muscles, leading to strain and discomfort.

Muscle strain is often accompanied by inflammation and spasms, which can further exacerbate neck pain. The pain associated with muscle strain is usually localized to the affected area and can be exacerbated by specific neck movements or positions. In most cases, muscle strain is a self-limiting condition that can be effectively managed with conservative treatment approaches, such as rest, ice, and gentle stretching exercises. However, if neck pain persists despite these interventions or is accompanied by other symptoms such as numbness, tingling, or weakness, it is essential to consult a healthcare provider to rule out more serious underlying causes.

Muscle strain, commonly known as a pulled muscle, occurs when the neck muscles are overused or overstretched, causing tears in the muscle fibers. The neck contains a multitude of muscles responsible for supporting the head and allowing for a wide range of movement. These muscles include the sternocleidomastoid, scalenes, and various deep neck muscles

3

such as the longus colli and longus capitis. Strains can occur in any of these muscles and may result from various factors.

Poor posture is a significant contributor to neck muscle strain. Prolonged periods of sitting with the head and neck in a forward position, often referred to as "forward head posture," can place excessive strain on the neck muscles. This posture is commonly seen in individuals who spend long hours working at a computer or using electronic devices, as well as those who frequently drive or engage in other activities that require maintaining a forward gaze. Over time, the muscles become fatigued and more susceptible to injury. Correcting posture by maintaining proper spinal alignment and taking regular breaks to change positions can help prevent neck muscle strain related to poor posture.

Sleeping in an awkward position can also lead to neck muscle strain. Using a pillow that is too high or too low, or sleeping on the stomach with the head turned to one side, can force the neck into unnatural positions for extended periods. This may result in muscle strain upon waking or exacerbate existing neck pain. To minimize the risk of neck strain during sleep, it is recommended to use a supportive pillow that maintains the natural curvature of the cervical spine and to sleep on one's back or side.

Repetitive neck movements, particularly those that involve twisting, bending, or extending the neck, can strain the neck muscles over time. Activities such as swimming, dancing, or manual labor that require repeated neck movements can lead to muscle fatigue and subsequent strain. In some cases, muscle strain can be acute, resulting from a sudden movement or forceful impact, as seen in contact sports or accidents. To prevent neck muscle strain related to repetitive movements, it is essential to incorporate regular rest breaks, practice proper technique, and engage in conditioning exercises to strengthen the neck muscles and improve flexibility.

Neck muscle strain is a common cause of neck pain that can result from various factors, including poor posture, sleeping in awkward positions, and engaging in activities requiring repetitive neck movements. By addressing these factors and incorporating preventative measures, individuals can reduce the risk of neck muscle strain and associated pain.

Cervical degenerative disc disease is a common age-related condition that affects the intervertebral discs in the neck. These discs are composed of a gel-like nucleus pulposus surrounded by a tough, fibrous annulus fibrosus. Their primary functions are to provide cushioning between the vertebrae, absorb shock, and allow for flexibility in the cervical spine.

As we age, the intervertebral discs undergo a natural process of degeneration. The water content of the nucleus pulposus gradually decreases, causing the discs to lose their hydration and elasticity. This loss of hydration makes the discs more susceptible to damage from everyday wear and tear. Additionally, the annulus fibrosus can develop small tears over time, which may further compromise the structural integrity of the disc.

The degeneration of the intervertebral discs can lead to several structural changes in the cervical spine. One such change is a reduction in disc height, which can alter the alignment and biomechanics of the spine, increasing the load on the surrounding structures, such as the facet joints and ligaments. This increased pressure can contribute to the development of osteoarthritis, as the cartilage in the facet joints wears down and the bones begin to rub against each other, causing inflammation, pain, and stiffness.

Moreover, the degeneration of the discs can cause the annulus fibrosus to bulge outward or develop small tears, which may result in a condition called cervical disc herniation. This occurs when the nucleus pulposus protrudes through the weakened annulus fibrosus and compresses nearby nerve roots or the spinal cord. Cervical disc herniation can cause pain, numbness, and weakness in the neck, shoulders, arms, and hands, depending on the affected nerve roots.

Cervical degenerative disc disease can manifest in various ways, with some individuals experiencing chronic neck pain and stiffness, while others may have no symptoms at all. The severity of the symptoms can depend on several factors, including the extent of the disc degeneration, the presence of additional spinal conditions, and individual pain tolerance.

Diagnosis of cervical degenerative disc disease typically involves a thorough medical history, physical examination, and imaging studies such as X-rays, magnetic resonance imaging (MRI), or computed tomography

(CT) scans. These tests can help healthcare providers identify changes in the cervical spine, such as reduced disc height or the presence of osteophytes (bone spurs), which can indicate disc degeneration and its potential impact on surrounding structures.

Treatment for cervical degenerative disc disease usually focuses on managing pain and improving function. Conservative approaches, such as physical therapy, medication management, and lifestyle modifications, are often the first line of treatment. In some cases, more invasive interventions, such as injections or surgery, may be necessary to alleviate symptoms and restore spinal stability.

A cervical herniated disc, also known as a slipped or ruptured disc, is a common cause of neck pain and neurological symptoms. It occurs when the nucleus pulposus, the gel-like substance at the center of the intervertebral disc, bulges or leaks through the annulus fibrosus, the tough fibrous outer layer of the disc. The annulus fibrosus can weaken due to age-related degeneration, traumatic injury, or repetitive stress, making it more susceptible to tears and rupture.

When a herniated disc compresses nearby nerve roots or the spinal cord, it can cause a range of symptoms, including pain, numbness, and weakness in the neck and extremities. The specific symptoms experienced by an individual will depend on the location and severity of the disc herniation, as well as which nerve roots are affected. For example, a herniated disc at the C5-C6 level may cause symptoms in the shoulders, arms, and hands, while a herniated disc at the C6-C7 level may affect the triceps and the fingers.

Pain caused by a cervical herniated disc can be localized to the neck, or it may radiate along the affected nerve root, resulting in radicular pain. This pain can be sharp, burning, or electric in nature and may worsen with certain neck movements or positions. In addition to pain, individuals with a cervical herniated disc may experience other sensory disturbances such as numbness, tingling, or a sensation of pins and needles in the affected areas. Muscle weakness and reflex changes may also occur due to nerve compression, potentially affecting the individual's ability to perform daily activities.

Diagnosis of a cervical herniated disc typically begins with a comprehensive medical history and physical examination, during which the healthcare provider will assess the patient's symptoms, neck mobility, and neurological function. Imaging studies, such as magnetic resonance imaging (MRI) or computed tomography (CT) scans, are often used to confirm the diagnosis and evaluate the severity and location of the disc herniation. In some cases, electromyography (EMG) or nerve conduction studies may also be performed to assess the function of the affected nerves.

Treatment for a cervical herniated disc depends on the severity of the symptoms and the individual's overall health. Conservative treatments, such as rest, physical therapy, medication management, and cervical traction, are often the first line of treatment for individuals with mild to moderate symptoms. In cases where conservative treatments fail to provide relief, or when neurological symptoms progress, more invasive treatments such as epidural steroid injections or surgical intervention may be considered. Surgical options for a cervical herniated disc include anterior cervical discectomy and fusion (ACDF), cervical disc replacement, or posterior cervical decompression, depending on the specific circumstances and the patient's overall health.

Cervical radiculopathy is a condition that occurs when the nerve roots in the cervical spine become compressed or irritated, leading to various neurological symptoms. The nerve roots are essential components of the nervous system, as they transmit sensory and motor information between the spinal cord and the rest of the body. When these nerve roots are compromised, the resulting symptoms can be quite debilitating and impact a person's daily functioning and quality of life.

The most common cause of cervical radiculopathy is degeneration of the cervical spine, which can occur as a natural part of the aging process. Over time, the intervertebral discs lose their hydration and elasticity, which can lead to reduced disc height and increased pressure on the surrounding structures. As a result, the nerve roots may become compressed by bone spurs (osteophytes) or herniated discs that protrude into the spinal canal or intervertebral foramen (the opening through which the nerve roots exit the spinal column).

Less common causes of cervical radiculopathy include spinal stenosis, which is a narrowing of the spinal canal that can put pressure on the spinal cord and nerve roots; spondylolisthesis, a condition in which one vertebra slips forward over another; and various inflammatory conditions, such as rheumatoid arthritis or ankylosing spondylitis, which can cause swelling and pressure on the nerve roots.

The symptoms of cervical radiculopathy can vary depending on the specific nerve root affected and the severity of the compression or irritation. Pain is often the most prominent symptom and can be felt in the neck, shoulders, arms, or hands. This pain is typically described as sharp, burning, or shooting and may be exacerbated by certain neck movements or postures. In addition to pain, individuals with cervical radiculopathy may experience numbness, tingling, or a "pins and needles" sensation in the affected areas, which is indicative of sensory nerve involvement.

Motor nerve involvement can lead to muscle weakness in the neck, shoulders, arms, or hands, making it difficult for individuals to perform daily tasks that require strength and coordination. In severe cases, cervical radiculopathy can also cause a reduction in reflexes, which may be detected during a clinical examination.

Diagnosing cervical radiculopathy typically involves a thorough medical history, physical examination, and imaging studies, such as X-rays, magnetic resonance imaging (MRI), or computed tomography (CT) scans, to assess the cervical spine and identify the cause of the nerve root compression or irritation. In some cases, nerve conduction studies and electromyography (EMG) may be used to further evaluate the function of the affected nerve roots and determine the extent of the damage.

Treatment for cervical radiculopathy is often multidisciplinary and aims to alleviate the symptoms, address the underlying cause, and prevent further nerve damage. Depending on the severity and cause of the condition, conservative treatments such as pain medications, physical therapy, and activity modification may be effective in relieving symptoms. In more severe cases or when conservative treatments fail to provide relief, surgical intervention may be considered to decompress the affected nerve roots and restore spinal stability.

Cervical spondylosis, often referred to as osteoarthritis of the neck, is a degenerative condition that affects the joints and intervertebral discs in the cervical spine. This condition occurs as a result of the natural aging process, with wear and tear on the cartilage and bones of the neck causing structural changes over time. While cervical spondylosis is common in older adults, it can also develop in younger individuals due to factors such as genetics, occupation, or a history of neck injury.

The degeneration associated with cervical spondylosis involves multiple processes. The intervertebral discs lose hydration and become less flexible, reducing their ability to act as shock absorbers and leading to decreased disc height. The loss of disc height can cause increased pressure on the facet joints, the small joints located at the back of the spine that help stabilize the vertebrae and facilitate movement. The increased pressure on the facet joints can lead to the formation of osteophytes, or bone spurs, which can cause pain and further restrict movement.

Additionally, the degeneration of the cervical spine can result in the development of spinal stenosis, a narrowing of the spinal canal that can compress the spinal cord and nerve roots. This compression can cause pain, numbness, and weakness in the neck, shoulders, arms, and hands, a condition known as cervical radiculopathy or myelopathy, depending on whether the nerve roots or the spinal cord itself are affected.

The symptoms of cervical spondylosis can vary depending on the severity of the degeneration and the structures involved. Common symptoms include chronic neck pain that may worsen with movement, stiffness, limited range of motion, and muscle weakness. In some cases, individuals with cervical spondylosis may also experience headaches, dizziness, and balance issues.

Diagnosing cervical spondylosis typically involves a comprehensive medical history, physical examination, and imaging studies such as X-rays, MRI, or CT scans. These tests can help the healthcare provider assess the extent of the degeneration and identify any associated complications, such as spinal stenosis or nerve compression.

Treatment for cervical spondylosis often begins with conservative approaches, including medication for pain relief and inflammation reduction, physical therapy to improve strength and flexibility, and lifestyle modifications to reduce strain on the neck. In some cases, more invasive treatments may be necessary, such as epidural steroid injections to alleviate inflammation and pain, or surgery to address structural abnormalities, decompress the spinal cord and nerve roots, or stabilize the cervical spine. The choice of treatment depends on the severity of the condition, the patient's overall health, and the specific symptoms and complications associated with the cervical spondylosis.

Cervical stenosis is a condition characterized by the narrowing of the spinal canal in the neck, which can lead to compression of the spinal cord or nerve roots. This compression can cause a range of symptoms, including pain, numbness, and weakness in the neck, shoulders, arms, and legs. Cervical stenosis can result from various factors, with age-related changes and congenital abnormalities being the most common causes.

As we age, degenerative changes can occur in the cervical spine, leading to the development of cervical stenosis. These age-related changes include the growth of bone spurs (osteophytes), thickening of ligaments, and degeneration of the intervertebral discs. Osteophytes can form as a result of osteoarthritis, which is the wear and tear of the joints over time. These bony growths can encroach upon the spinal canal, narrowing the space available for the spinal cord and nerve roots. Similarly, the thickening of ligaments, particularly the ligamentum flavum, can contribute to the narrowing of the spinal canal. Degeneration of the intervertebral discs can also cause a loss of disc height, leading to a reduction in the space between the vertebrae and potential compression of the spinal cord or nerve roots.

In addition to age-related changes, congenital abnormalities can play a role in the development of cervical stenosis. Some individuals may be born with a naturally narrow spinal canal, making them more susceptible to spinal cord or nerve root compression. Other congenital factors that can contribute to cervical stenosis include skeletal dysplasia, which affects the formation and growth of bones, and abnormalities in the alignment of the vertebrae, such as scoliosis or kyphosis.

Diagnosis of cervical stenosis typically involves a comprehensive medical history and physical examination, followed by imaging studies such as X-rays, computed tomography (CT) scans, or magnetic resonance imaging (MRI). These imaging studies allow healthcare providers to visualize the anatomy of the cervical spine and identify any structural abnormalities that may be causing the stenosis.

Treatment for cervical stenosis varies depending on the severity of the condition and the specific symptoms experienced by the patient. Conservative treatments, such as physical therapy, medication management, and activity modification, may be recommended for mild cases of cervical stenosis. In more severe cases or when conservative treatments are ineffective, surgical intervention may be necessary to decompress the spinal cord or nerve roots and restore normal function. Surgical options for cervical stenosis include laminectomy, laminoplasty, or cervical fusion, depending on the specific cause and location of the stenosis.

Cervical stenosis is a condition that results from the narrowing of the spinal canal in the neck, leading to compression of the spinal cord or nerve roots. Age-related changes and congenital abnormalities are common causes of cervical stenosis, and appropriate diagnosis and treatment are essential for managing symptoms and preventing further complications.

Whiplash is a neck injury that results from the rapid acceleration and deceleration of the head and neck, often experienced in car accidents, contact sports, or other situations involving sudden and forceful impacts. This abrupt motion can cause the neck muscles, ligaments, and other soft tissues to stretch or tear, leading to pain, stiffness, and other symptoms.

The severity of a whiplash injury can vary greatly, depending on factors such as the force of the impact, the position of the head and neck during the event, and individual differences in anatomy and tissue resilience. Whiplash injuries are classified into different grades based on their severity, ranging from Grade I (mild) to Grade IV (severe), with more severe grades involving damage to the intervertebral discs, facet joints, or spinal nerves.

Symptoms of whiplash can manifest immediately following the injury or may develop gradually over several hours or days. Common symptoms include neck pain, stiffness, reduced range of motion, headache, dizziness, fatigue, and tenderness in the neck and shoulder muscles. In some cases, individuals may also experience symptoms such as difficulty concentrating, memory problems, irritability, or sleep disturbances.

Diagnosing whiplash typically involves a thorough medical history, a physical examination, and, in some cases, imaging studies such as X-rays, computed tomography (CT) scans, or magnetic resonance imaging (MRI) to rule out more severe injuries or underlying conditions. During the physical examination, the healthcare provider will assess the patient's neck posture, range of motion, and sensitivity to touch, as well as evaluate for any neurological symptoms that may indicate nerve damage.

Treatment for whiplash focuses on managing pain, reducing inflammation, and restoring function to the affected muscles and joints. Initial treatment may include rest, ice, compression, and elevation (RICE) to alleviate pain and swelling, followed by a gradual return to activity as tolerated. Pain relief medications, such as nonsteroidal anti-inflammatory drugs (NSAIDs) or muscle relaxants, may be prescribed to manage pain and muscle spasms. Additionally, physical therapy, including exercises to improve flexibility, strength, and posture, can be helpful in promoting recovery and preventing chronic neck pain.

In most cases, individuals with whiplash injuries can expect to make a full recovery within several weeks to months, depending on the severity of the injury and the effectiveness of the treatment plan. However, some individuals may continue to experience persistent neck pain or other symptoms, which may require further evaluation and treatment to address any underlying issues contributing to the ongoing discomfort.

Tension headaches are the most common type of headache, affecting a large portion of the population at some point in their lives. These headaches are often associated with tightness and tension in the neck muscles, which can contribute to pain in the head, neck, and shoulders. Understanding the relationship between tension headaches and neck pain is essential for accurately diagnosing and effectively managing these interconnected issues.

Tension headaches typically present as a constant, dull, pressing, or band-like pain on both sides of the head, often extending into the neck and shoulders. The pain can vary in intensity and duration, ranging from mild discomfort lasting a few hours to more severe pain that can persist for several days. In some cases, tension headaches can become chronic, occurring frequently over an extended period.

The precise cause of tension headaches is not fully understood, but they are believed to result from a combination of factors, including muscle tension, stress, and imbalances in pain-regulating chemicals in the brain. Neck muscle tension, in particular, is thought to play a significant role in the development of tension headaches. Tightness in the neck muscles can be caused by various factors, such as poor posture, sedentary lifestyle, stress, anxiety, and fatigue. When the neck muscles become tight or tense, they can put pressure on the surrounding structures, including nerves and blood vessels, leading to pain and discomfort in the head and neck.

To accurately diagnose tension headaches and their relationship to neck pain, healthcare providers will conduct a thorough assessment, including a detailed medical history, a physical examination, and, if necessary, imaging studies or laboratory tests. This assessment will help to rule out other potential causes of head and neck pain, such as migraines, cluster headaches, or underlying structural abnormalities in the cervical spine.

Once tension headaches and their association with neck pain have been identified, an appropriate treatment plan can be developed. This plan may include a combination of pharmacological and non-pharmacological interventions, such as pain-relieving medications, muscle relaxants, relaxation techniques, stress management, physical therapy, and posture correction. Addressing the underlying causes of neck muscle tension, such as poor posture or high levels of stress, is essential for effectively managing tension headaches and preventing their recurrence.

Tension headaches are a common cause of head and neck pain, often resulting from tightness and tension in the neck muscles. By understanding the relationship between these issues and addressing the underlying causes of muscle tension, healthcare providers can help patients manage tension headaches and improve their overall quality of life.

In rare cases, neck pain can be caused by various infections that involve the structures of the neck or the central nervous system. These infections can lead to inflammation, tissue damage, and compression of the surrounding structures, resulting in pain and other neurological symptoms.

13

Some notable infections that can cause neck pain include meningitis, cervical lymphadenitis, and spinal epidural abscess.

Meningitis is an infection of the meninges, the protective membranes that surround the brain and spinal cord. It can be caused by bacteria, viruses, fungi, or other microorganisms. Meningitis often presents with symptoms such as severe headache, fever, and a stiff neck. The neck pain and stiffness associated with meningitis are typically caused by inflammation of the meninges and the resulting pressure on the cervical spine and surrounding tissues. Prompt diagnosis and treatment of meningitis are crucial, as the condition can be life-threatening, particularly when caused by bacterial infections. Treatment may involve antibiotics for bacterial meningitis, antiviral medications for viral meningitis, or antifungal medications for fungal meningitis, along with supportive care to manage symptoms and reduce the risk of complications.

Cervical lymphadenitis is an infection of the lymph nodes in the neck, often caused by bacteria such as Staphylococcus or Streptococcus species. This condition typically presents with swollen, tender lymph nodes in the neck, which can cause pain and stiffness, as well as fever, fatigue, and other systemic symptoms. Treatment for cervical lymphadenitis typically involves antibiotics to target the underlying infection, along with pain relief and anti-inflammatory medications to manage symptoms. In some cases, surgical drainage of the affected lymph nodes may be necessary if an abscess forms or the infection does not respond to antibiotic therapy.

Spinal epidural abscess is a rare but serious infection that occurs within the epidural space, the area surrounding the spinal cord and nerve roots. This condition can be caused by bacteria or fungi, and often results from the spread of infection from another site in the body, such as the skin, bloodstream, or urinary tract. Spinal epidural abscess can cause severe neck pain, as well as fever, weakness, numbness, or paralysis, depending on the location and severity of the infection. Prompt diagnosis and treatment are essential to prevent permanent neurological damage or life-threatening complications. Treatment options for spinal epidural abscess include intravenous antibiotics or antifungal medications, as well as surgical drainage of the abscess to relieve pressure on the spinal cord and nerve roots.

14

Although infections are a less common cause of neck pain compared to musculoskeletal issues and degenerative conditions, they should not be overlooked, particularly when neck pain is accompanied by fever, systemic symptoms, or neurological deficits. Early recognition and appropriate treatment of these infections can help prevent serious complications and alleviate neck pain.

Tumors affecting the cervical spine or surrounding structures, although relatively rare, can be a cause of neck pain and various neurological symptoms. These tumors can be classified as benign or malignant and may originate from the spinal structures themselves (primary tumors) or spread from other parts of the body (secondary or metastatic tumors).

Benign tumors, while typically non-cancerous and slow-growing, can still cause significant symptoms due to their size, location, and potential to compress or displace nearby structures. Some examples of benign tumors that can affect the cervical spine include osteochondromas, hemangiomas, and schwannomas. Osteochondromas are the most common type of benign bone tumors, forming cartilage-capped bony growths that can cause pain and reduced range of motion. Hemangiomas are benign vascular tumors arising from blood vessels, which can occur in the vertebral bodies and potentially lead to spinal instability or compression of neural structures. Schwannomas are tumors arising from the Schwann cells that surround nerve fibers, and when they occur in the cervical spine, they can compress the spinal cord or nerve roots, causing pain and neurological deficits.

Malignant tumors, on the other hand, are cancerous and often more aggressive, with the potential to invade surrounding tissues and spread to other parts of the body. Primary malignant tumors of the cervical spine are relatively rare, with examples including osteosarcomas, chondrosarcomas, and Ewing's sarcomas. These tumors can cause bone destruction, spinal instability, and compression of the spinal cord or nerve roots, leading to pain and various neurological symptoms. Secondary or metastatic tumors are more common than primary tumors in the cervical spine, as cancer cells from other regions of the body, such as the lungs, breast, or prostate, can spread through the bloodstream and invade the spine. These metastatic tumors can weaken the vertebrae, leading to fractures, instability, and compression of neural structures, resulting in pain and neurological deficits.

The diagnosis of spinal tumors typically involves a combination of medical history, physical examination, and imaging studies, such as X-rays, CT scans, and MRI. In some cases, a biopsy may be required to confirm the diagnosis and determine the tumor type. Treatment options for spinal tumors depend on the type, size, location, and aggressiveness of the tumor, as well as the patient's overall health and preferences. Treatment strategies may include a combination of surgery, radiation therapy, chemotherapy, targeted therapy, or immunotherapy, with the goal of removing or controlling the tumor while preserving spinal function and minimizing side effects. In some cases, palliative care may be recommended to help manage pain and improve the patient's quality of life.

Rheumatoid arthritis (RA) is a chronic autoimmune disorder that primarily affects the synovial joints, causing inflammation and destruction of joint structures. In the cervical spine, this inflammation can lead to chronic pain, stiffness, and instability, significantly impacting the patient's quality of life.

RA typically affects the joints symmetrically, and its involvement in the cervical spine is relatively common. The most commonly affected cervical joints in RA are the atlantoaxial joint (formed by the first and second cervical vertebrae, C1 and C2) and the subaxial cervical spine (from C3 to C7). The inflammation and subsequent destruction of these joints can lead to joint laxity, subluxation (partial dislocation), and even spinal cord compression in severe cases.

Patients with RA-related neck pain may experience a range of symptoms, such as localized pain and stiffness in the neck, as well as headaches and occipital pain. They may also have difficulty turning their head or maintaining a comfortable neck posture. In more severe cases, patients may exhibit neurological symptoms due to spinal cord or nerve root compression, including numbness, tingling, or weakness in the arms and hands, as well as balance and coordination problems.

Diagnosing RA-related neck pain typically involves a comprehensive medical history and physical examination, including an assessment of the patient's overall joint health and function. Imaging studies, such as X-rays, magnetic resonance imaging (MRI), or computed tomography (CT) scans, may be necessary to evaluate the extent of joint damage in the cervical spine and assess the risk of spinal cord compression. Blood tests for rheumatoid factor (RF) and anti-citrullinated protein antibodies (ACPAs) can also help confirm the diagnosis of RA and its involvement in the cervical spine.

Treatment for RA-related neck pain focuses on managing the underlying autoimmune disorder, as well as addressing the specific symptoms and complications arising from cervical spine involvement. Medications such as nonsteroidal anti-inflammatory drugs (NSAIDs), corticosteroids, and disease-modifying antirheumatic drugs (DMARDs) can help reduce inflammation, alleviate pain, and slow down the progression of joint damage. Physical therapy and occupational therapy can assist patients in maintaining mobility, improving posture, and learning strategies to minimize neck strain.

In cases where conservative treatments are insufficient, surgical intervention may be necessary to address instability, subluxation, or spinal cord compression. Procedures such as cervical fusion or decompression can help stabilize the spine, relieve pressure on the spinal cord or nerve roots, and alleviate pain. However, surgery carries inherent risks and should be considered carefully in consultation with the patient's healthcare team.

Overall, managing neck pain related to rheumatoid arthritis requires a comprehensive approach that addresses the underlying autoimmune disorder, as well as the specific complications arising from cervical spine involvement. By working closely with their healthcare providers, patients can develop a tailored treatment plan to manage their neck pain and maintain their overall spinal health.

Fibromyalgia is a complex chronic pain disorder characterized by widespread musculoskeletal pain, fatigue, and heightened sensitivity to touch. Although the exact cause of fibromyalgia remains unclear, it is believed to involve a combination of genetic, environmental, and psychological factors. Researchers have suggested that fibromyalgia may be the result of abnormal pain processing in the central nervous system, leading to a heightened perception of pain and an exaggerated response to stimuli that would not typically be painful.

Neck pain is a common symptom in individuals with fibromyalgia, as the disorder tends to affect the body symmetrically and often involves the muscles and soft tissues of the neck, shoulders, and upper back. The neck pain experienced by fibromyalgia patients is typically described as a dull, aching discomfort that may be accompanied by stiffness, muscle spasms, and tenderness to touch. Additionally, fibromyalgia patients often report headaches, which can further exacerbate neck pain and discomfort.

One possible explanation for the prevalence of neck pain in fibromyalgia patients is the presence of tender points or trigger points in the neck and shoulder muscles. Tender points are specific areas of the body where light pressure elicits pain, while trigger points are localized areas of muscle tightness that can refer pain to other areas when pressed. Both tender points and trigger points can be found in the trapezius, sternocleidomastoid, and levator scapulae muscles, among others, which are all involved in the support and movement of the neck.

Diagnosing fibromyalgia can be challenging, as there are no definitive tests or imaging studies that can confirm the disorder. Instead, healthcare providers must rely on a thorough patient history and physical examination to identify the characteristic symptoms of fibromyalgia and rule out other potential causes of the patient's pain. The American College of Rheumatology has established diagnostic criteria for fibromyalgia, which include the presence of widespread pain for at least three months and a specific number of tender points on physical examination.

Treatment for fibromyalgia typically involves a multidisciplinary approach, combining pharmacological and non-pharmacological interventions to address the various symptoms of the disorder. In the case of fibromyalgia-related neck pain, treatment options may include medications such as analgesics, nonsteroidal anti-inflammatory drugs (NSAIDs), and muscle relaxants to help alleviate pain and inflammation. Non-pharmacological therapies, such as physical therapy, massage, and chiropractic care, may also be beneficial in improving neck pain by addressing muscle imbalances, promoting relaxation, and improving posture.

Cognitive-behavioral therapy (CBT) and other psychological interventions can be helpful in addressing the emotional and cognitive aspects of fibromyalgia, as well as teaching patients effective coping strategies for managing their pain. Finally, lifestyle modifications, such as maintaining a regular sleep schedule, engaging in low-impact exercise, and practicing stress management techniques, can play a crucial role in improving overall functioning and quality of life for individuals with fibromyalgia and associated neck pain.

The presentation of neck pain is highly variable, as it depends on the underlying cause and the specific structures involved. One common symptom associated with neck pain is localized or radiating pain. This pain can originate in the cervical spine and spread to the shoulders, upper back, arms, or even the head. Depending on the nature and severity of the condition, the pain may range from a dull, persistent ache to a sharp or stabbing sensation that can be debilitating.

Localized neck pain typically occurs when there is an issue directly affecting the cervical spine, such as muscle strains, ligament sprains, or joint inflammation. In these cases, the pain is concentrated in the neck region and may worsen with movement or certain positions. Conversely, radiating pain often results from irritation or compression of the cervical nerve roots or the spinal cord. This type of pain can extend beyond the neck, following the path of the affected nerve, and may be accompanied by other neurological symptoms such as numbness, tingling, or weakness in the arms or hands.

The intensity and quality of neck pain can also fluctuate based on various factors, such as the individual's pain tolerance, the duration of the condition, and the presence of any complicating factors like muscle spasms or inflammation. For some individuals, neck pain may be a mild annoyance that is easily managed with conservative treatments like rest, ice, or over-the-counter pain relievers. For others, the pain may be severe and disabling, requiring more intensive interventions such as physical therapy, prescription medications, or even surgery.

It is essential to recognize that the experience of neck pain is highly subjective and can vary significantly from person to person. Consequently, healthcare providers must carefully assess each patient's unique presentation and consider the various potential causes to develop an appropriate and effective treatment plan. By understanding the range of possible symptoms and their underlying mechanisms, patients and healthcare providers can work together to address neck pain and improve overall quality of life.

Stiffness is a common symptom of neck pain that can manifest as limited range of motion, difficulty turning the head, or problems bending the neck. This symptom can arise from various factors, including muscle tightness, joint inflammation, and structural abnormalities. Understanding the potential causes of stiffness can help healthcare providers identify the underlying issue and develop an appropriate treatment plan.

Muscle tightness is one of the primary reasons for neck stiffness. Prolonged poor posture, repetitive neck movements, or muscle strain can lead to muscle imbalances, tightness, and weakness in the neck and shoulder region. As a result, the affected muscles may have a reduced ability to relax and stretch, limiting the neck's range of motion. Furthermore, muscle tightness can cause pain, which may lead to a protective reflex in which the body instinctively limits movement to prevent further discomfort. Treatment for muscle tightness often includes physical therapy, stretching exercises, and massage therapy to help restore muscle balance and flexibility.

Joint inflammation is another possible cause of neck stiffness. Conditions like cervical spondylosis, rheumatoid arthritis, or facet joint syndrome can lead to inflammation and swelling in the joints of the cervical spine. The resulting inflammation may cause pain and stiffness by reducing the joint's range of motion and restricting the neck's mobility. To address joint inflammation, healthcare providers may recommend anti-inflammatory medications, physical therapy, or other conservative treatments to help alleviate symptoms and improve joint function.

Structural abnormalities in the cervical spine can also contribute to neck stiffness. These abnormalities can include cervical disc degeneration, herniated discs, spinal stenosis, or congenital issues such as ankylosing spondylitis. In cases where structural abnormalities are the primary cause of stiffness, the range of motion may be limited due to mechanical factors, such as disc bulges or bone spurs impinging on the spinal cord or nerve roots. The resulting compression or irritation of neural structures can cause pain and stiffness, as well as other neurological symptoms. In such cases, treatment may involve a combination of conservative therapies, medication management, or surgical intervention, depending on the severity of the condition and the patient's individual needs.

Neck stiffness is a multifaceted symptom that can arise from muscle tightness, joint inflammation, or structural abnormalities in the cervical spine. Accurately identifying the cause of stiffness is essential for developing an appropriate treatment plan that addresses the underlying issue and helps improve the patient's neck mobility and overall quality of life.

Muscle spasms in the neck, also known as cervical muscle spasms, are involuntary contractions or tightening of the muscles that support and move the cervical spine. These spasms can result in pain, stiffness, and restricted neck movement, and may occur suddenly or develop gradually over time. There are several factors that can contribute to the development of neck muscle spasms, and understanding these triggers can help in effectively managing and preventing this painful condition.

In many cases, muscle spasms in the neck occur as a protective response to an underlying injury, such as a strain, sprain, or damage to the cervical spine structures like the intervertebral discs, facet joints, or ligaments. When the body detects an injury, it may initiate a spasm in the surrounding muscles to limit movement and prevent further damage. This protective mechanism, while helpful in some instances, can also lead to additional pain and discomfort.

Poor posture, particularly when using electronic devices or working at a desk for extended periods, can place excessive strain on the neck muscles, leading to muscle fatigue, tension, and eventual spasms. Similarly, physical activities that involve repetitive neck movements or holding the head in an awkward position can also contribute to the development of muscle spasms. Moreover, emotional stress and anxiety can cause muscle tension in the neck and shoulder region, increasing the likelihood of spasms.

Dehydration and electrolyte imbalances, particularly deficiencies in minerals such as potassium, magnesium, and calcium, can affect muscle function and contribute to muscle spasms. Ensuring proper hydration and maintaining a balanced diet can help prevent these issues and promote overall muscle health.

In some cases, muscle spasms in the neck may be related to underlying medical conditions, such as fibromyalgia, rheumatoid arthritis, or cervical dystonia. These conditions can cause increased muscle tension, inflammation, or abnormal muscle contractions, resulting in spasms and associated symptoms.

Diagnosing the cause of neck muscle spasms typically involves a comprehensive assessment, including a medical history, physical examination, and, if necessary, imaging studies or laboratory tests. Treatment for neck muscle spasms will depend on the underlying cause and may include a combination of conservative measures, such as rest, ice or heat therapy, over-the-counter pain relievers, muscle relaxants, and physical therapy. In some cases, more targeted treatments, such as nerve blocks or botulinum toxin injections, may be recommended for persistent or severe spasms.

Neck muscle spasms are a common and often painful condition that can result from a variety of factors, including injury, poor posture, stress, and underlying medical conditions. By understanding the triggers and mechanisms of muscle spasms, patients and healthcare providers can work together to develop effective treatment plans and prevention strategies to promote long-term neck health and comfort.

Numbness and tingling are common symptoms associated with neck pain, often resulting from compression or irritation of the cervical nerve roots or the spinal cord. These sensory disturbances can manifest in various ways, affecting the neck, shoulders, arms, or hands, depending on the specific nerves involved.

The cervical nerve roots exit the spinal cord through small openings called foramina between the vertebrae. These nerves transmit sensory information from the skin, muscles, and other tissues to the brain and relay motor commands from the brain to the muscles. When a cervical nerve root becomes compressed or irritated, it can disrupt these signals, leading to altered sensation in the areas of the body served by that nerve. This disruption can cause a range of symptoms, including numbness, tingling, or burning sensations, as well as pain or weakness.

There are several factors that can contribute to cervical nerve root compression or irritation. One of the most common is a herniated disc, in which the nucleus pulposus of an intervertebral disc bulges or leaks through the annulus fibrosus, impinging on the adjacent nerve root. Cervical spondylosis, or osteoarthritis of the neck, can also lead to nerve compression as degenerative changes in the joints and discs cause narrowing of the foramina through which the nerve roots exit the spinal canal. Other causes of cervical nerve root compression or irritation include spinal stenosis, foraminal stenosis, bone spurs, spinal tumors, or inflammation due to conditions such as rheumatoid arthritis.

In addition to nerve root compression, numbness and tingling can also result from direct compression or damage to the spinal cord itself. This can occur in cases of severe cervical stenosis, where the narrowing of the spinal canal places pressure on the spinal cord. Spinal cord compression can lead to a condition called cervical myelopathy, which is characterized by a range of neurological symptoms, including numbness, tingling, pain, weakness, and difficulty with balance and coordination.

The evaluation and management of numbness and tingling in the context of neck pain require a thorough assessment by a healthcare professional. This assessment may include a detailed medical history, physical examination, and diagnostic imaging studies to identify the specific cause of the sensory disturbances and guide the development of an appropriate treatment plan. Depending on the underlying cause, treatment options may include conservative measures such as physical therapy, medication, and lifestyle modifications, or more invasive interventions such as injections or surgery. In any case, addressing the root cause of the nerve compression or irritation is essential to alleviating the associated numbness and tingling and improving the patient's overall function and quality of life.

Weakness related to cervical spine dysfunction can manifest in several ways due to the involvement of nerve roots or the spinal cord. When damage or compression occurs to these critical structures, it can have a direct impact on the muscles in the neck, shoulders, arms, or hands.

23

Understanding the various causes and mechanisms of muscle weakness in these regions is essential for effective diagnosis and treatment.

One common cause of muscle weakness is cervical radiculopathy, which occurs when nerve roots that exit the spinal cord at the cervical spine level become compressed or irritated. The nerve roots in the cervical spine are responsible for transmitting motor and sensory signals to and from the muscles in the neck, shoulders, arms, and hands. When these nerve roots are compromised, the signals become disrupted, leading to muscle weakness in the corresponding region.

Cervical spondylotic myelopathy (CSM) is another potential cause of muscle weakness. This condition occurs when degenerative changes in the cervical spine, such as osteoarthritis, disc herniation, or spinal stenosis, lead to compression of the spinal cord itself. As the spinal cord is responsible for transmitting signals between the brain and the rest of the body, compression can disrupt these signals, causing muscle weakness in the upper extremities. In severe cases, CSM can also lead to problems with coordination and fine motor skills, as well as gait disturbances and difficulty with balance.

In addition to these common causes, muscle weakness can result from a variety of other factors related to the cervical spine. These may include acute injuries, such as whiplash or direct trauma to the spinal cord, or chronic conditions, such as rheumatoid arthritis, tumors, or infections. In some cases, muscle weakness may also be a secondary symptom, resulting from pain or stiffness in the neck that makes it difficult to use the affected muscles effectively.

Diagnosing the cause of muscle weakness in the context of neck pain typically involves a thorough physical examination, including assessment of muscle strength, reflexes, and sensation in the upper extremities. In some cases, imaging studies, such as X-rays, MRI, or CT scans, may be necessary to visualize the cervical spine and identify potential sources of nerve root or spinal cord compression. Additional diagnostic tests, such as electromyography (EMG) or nerve conduction studies, can help to further evaluate the function of the affected nerves and muscles and pinpoint the underlying cause of the weakness.

By understanding the various mechanisms by which cervical spine dysfunction can lead to muscle weakness in the neck, shoulders, arms, or hands, healthcare providers can more effectively diagnose and treat the underlying cause, helping to restore function and alleviate pain for their patients.

Headaches are a common symptom that can accompany neck pain, and they may share similar underlying causes or be directly related to dysfunction in the cervical spine. Two primary types of headaches associated with neck pain are tension headaches and cervicogenic headaches.

Tension headaches are the most common type of headache and are often characterized by a dull, aching pain that feels like a tight band around the head or pressure at the temples or back of the head and neck. These headaches are typically caused by muscle tension or stress, which can originate from poor posture, muscle strain, or emotional factors. When neck muscles are strained or tense, they can contribute to tension headaches by causing referred pain to the head. Maintaining proper posture, engaging in relaxation techniques, and addressing muscle imbalances can help alleviate tension headaches and associated neck pain.

Cervicogenic headaches, on the other hand, are secondary headaches that stem from a primary issue in the cervical spine or surrounding structures. These headaches are usually characterized by a unilateral, dull ache that starts at the base of the skull or upper neck and radiates toward the forehead or around the head. Cervicogenic headaches can be caused by various factors, including cervical joint dysfunction, nerve compression, muscle tightness, or injuries such as whiplash.

Diagnosing cervicogenic headaches can be challenging, as their symptoms often overlap with other types of headaches, such as migraines or tension headaches. A thorough examination of the cervical spine, as well as a detailed medical history and assessment of the patient's symptoms, can help healthcare providers identify cervicogenic headaches and develop appropriate treatment plans. Treatment for cervicogenic headaches typically involves addressing the underlying cause of the dysfunction in the cervical spine. This may include physical therapy, manual therapy, postural corrections, medication management, or, in some cases, interventional procedures or surgery.

Headaches are a common symptom that can accompany neck pain, particularly tension headaches and cervicogenic headaches. Both types of headaches can be related to dysfunction in the cervical spine, with tension headaches often resulting from muscle tension or strain, and cervicogenic headaches arising from issues with the cervical joints, nerves, or surrounding structures. A thorough assessment and accurate diagnosis are essential for developing appropriate treatment strategies to address both neck pain and associated headaches.

In some cases, neck pain may be associated with dizziness, vertigo, or balance problems. These symptoms can arise when the cervical spine or surrounding structures affect the vestibular system, which plays a critical role in maintaining balance and spatial orientation. The vestibular system comprises the inner ear, the vestibulocochlear nerve, and the brainstem, all of which work together to process sensory information related to balance, movement, and spatial orientation. When the cervical spine or its related structures disrupt the normal functioning of the vestibular system, patients may experience dizziness, vertigo, or balance issues alongside neck pain.

One possible cause of dizziness and balance problems related to neck pain is cervicogenic dizziness, a controversial and not universally recognized condition. Cervicogenic dizziness is thought to arise from dysfunction in the cervical spine, particularly the upper cervical segments, causing a disturbance in the proprioceptive input from the neck. Proprioception is the sense of body position and movement, and when disrupted, it can lead to a mismatch between the information coming from the vestibular, visual, and proprioceptive systems, resulting in dizziness and balance issues.

Another potential cause of dizziness and balance problems in patients with neck pain is vertebral artery insufficiency. The vertebral arteries pass through small openings in the cervical vertebrae, supplying blood to the brainstem and the cerebellum, which are critical components of the vestibular system. Compression or damage to the vertebral arteries, as seen in cervical spondylosis, herniated discs, or traumatic injuries, can reduce

26

blood flow to these areas of the brain, leading to dizziness, vertigo, or balance problems.

Additionally, muscle tension and tightness in the neck can contribute to dizziness and balance issues. When neck muscles are tense, they can put pressure on the nerves and blood vessels in the cervical region, potentially affecting the vestibular system's function.

Diagnosing the cause of dizziness and balance problems in patients with neck pain can be challenging, as these symptoms can be multifactorial and overlap with other conditions such as benign paroxysmal positional vertigo (BPPV), Meniere's disease, or vestibular migraines. A thorough assessment, including a detailed medical history, physical examination, and, in some cases, imaging or vestibular testing, is necessary to identify the underlying cause and develop an appropriate treatment plan.

Treatment for dizziness and balance issues related to neck pain will depend on the specific cause and may include physical therapy, targeted exercises, medication, or manual therapy. In some cases, addressing the underlying neck pain through conservative or surgical interventions may also help alleviate dizziness and balance problems.

In rare cases, neck pain and cervical spine dysfunction can be associated with visual disturbances, tinnitus, or other auditory symptoms. These symptoms may be related to the complex interplay between the cervical spine, the nervous system, and the vascular structures that supply the head and neck.

Visual disturbances related to neck pain can manifest in various ways, including blurred vision, double vision, or a reduction in the visual field. One possible explanation for these symptoms is the mechanical compression or irritation of the nerves or blood vessels in the neck. For instance, cervical spine misalignments or muscle tension may lead to compression of the vertebral artery, which supplies blood to the brain and the eyes. This could result in reduced blood flow, causing temporary visual disturbances. Additionally, irritation or compression of the cervical nerve roots or the sympathetic nervous system can lead to changes in pupillary function or ocular blood flow, potentially contributing to visual symptoms.

Tinnitus, a ringing or buzzing sensation in the ears, can also be linked to neck pain or cervical spine dysfunction. Although the exact mechanisms underlying this association are not fully understood, several theories have been proposed. One hypothesis is that muscle tension or imbalances in the neck can cause changes in the tension of the tensor tympani muscle in the middle ear, leading to tinnitus. Another possibility is that dysfunction in the cervical spine can affect the nerve pathways responsible for auditory processing, either through direct nerve compression or through alterations in the central nervous system's perception of auditory signals.

Other auditory symptoms that may be associated with neck pain include hyperacusis (increased sensitivity to sound), distortion of sounds, or difficulty localizing sound sources. These symptoms could be related to changes in the tension of the middle ear muscles, alterations in the auditory nerve pathways, or central nervous system dysfunction resulting from cervical spine issues.

It is important to note that the association between neck pain, visual disturbances, and auditory symptoms is relatively rare, and these symptoms can have numerous other causes. As such, it is crucial for patients experiencing these symptoms to consult with their healthcare provider for a thorough evaluation and accurate diagnosis. In some cases, addressing the underlying cervical spine dysfunction through appropriate treatment may help alleviate these visual and auditory symptoms, although the exact relationship between neck pain and these symptoms remains an area of ongoing research.

Diagnosing the cause of neck pain requires a comprehensive assessment to accurately identify the source of the discomfort and determine the most appropriate treatment plan. The diagnostic process typically begins with a detailed medical history, followed by a physical examination and, if necessary, imaging or laboratory tests.

During the medical history portion of the assessment, the healthcare provider will ask the patient questions about their symptoms, including the onset, duration, and severity of the pain. They will also inquire about any recent injuries or accidents that may have caused the neck pain, such as a fall or a motor vehicle accident. Additionally, the healthcare provider will gather information on underlying medical conditions that could contribute to the pain, such as a history of arthritis, disc degeneration, or previous neck surgery. Lifestyle factors, such as occupation, exercise habits, and daily activities, are also considered, as these can play a role in the development and exacerbation of neck pain. For instance, individuals with sedentary jobs or those who regularly engage in activities that place strain on the neck may be more prone to developing neck pain.

The healthcare provider will use this information to guide the physical examination, during which they will assess the patient's neck posture, range of motion, strength, reflexes, and sensitivity to touch. They may perform specific tests, such as the Spurling test or the neck distraction test, to help determine if the pain is related to nerve root compression or other structural abnormalities in the cervical spine. The provider will also evaluate the patient for signs of nerve root or spinal cord compression, such as muscle weakness, numbness, or altered reflexes. This comprehensive physical examination helps to identify the most likely cause of the neck pain and informs the next steps in the diagnostic process.

In some cases, the healthcare provider may order imaging studies to further investigate the cause of the neck pain. These studies may include X-rays, which can reveal abnormalities in the alignment of the cervical spine, degenerative changes in the vertebrae, or the presence of fractures. Magnetic resonance imaging (MRI) is often used to visualize soft tissues, such as the intervertebral discs, spinal cord, and nerve roots, and can help identify disc herniation, spinal stenosis, or inflammation in the cervical spine. Computed tomography (CT) scans can provide detailed images of the bones and joints, aiding in the diagnosis of fractures, bone spurs, or other structural abnormalities.

Laboratory tests may also be ordered to rule out infection, inflammation, or other systemic causes of neck pain. Blood tests can provide information on markers of inflammation, such as C-reactive protein and erythrocyte sedimentation rate, or specific antibodies related to autoimmune disorders like rheumatoid arthritis. In rare cases, a healthcare provider may order a cerebrospinal fluid analysis if they suspect an infection, such as meningitis, or another central nervous system disorder.

Depending on the suspected cause of the neck pain, the healthcare provider may order additional tests, such as nerve conduction studies, electromyography (EMG), or diagnostic injections to help identify the source of the pain. Nerve conduction studies and EMG can provide valuable information about the function of the nerves and muscles, helping to pinpoint nerve damage or muscle dysfunction. Diagnostic injections, such as nerve blocks or epidural steroid injections, can temporarily relieve pain and help determine the specific structure or nerve responsible for the discomfort.

Overall, the diagnostic process for neck pain involves a thorough assessment, including a detailed medical history, a comprehensive physical examination, and, when necessary, imaging and laboratory tests. By accurately identifying the cause of neck pain, healthcare providers can develop targeted treatment plans that address the underlying issue and promote long-term spinal health.

During the physical examination, the healthcare provider will assess various aspects of the patient's neck and upper body to identify potential causes of neck pain and dysfunction. The examination typically begins with an evaluation of the patient's neck posture, as poor posture can contribute to muscle strain, joint stress, and nerve compression. The provider will observe the patient's head and neck alignment in relation to the shoulders and upper back, both in a static position and during movement.

Next, the healthcare provider will assess the patient's neck range of motion by asking them to perform a series of movements, such as flexion (bending the head forward), extension (bending the head backward), lateral flexion (tilting the head to the side), and rotation (turning the head to the left and right). The provider will note any limitations, pain, or discomfort during these movements, which can help identify specific structures that may be contributing to the neck pain.

The examination will also include an assessment of the patient's neck strength, particularly in the muscles that support and stabilize the cervical spine. The healthcare provider will ask the patient to perform various resisted movements, such as pressing their head against the provider's hand in different directions, to evaluate the function of the neck muscles. Muscle weakness or imbalance can contribute to neck pain and dysfunction.

Another important aspect of the physical examination is the assessment of the patient's reflexes and sensitivity to touch. The healthcare provider will use a reflex hammer to elicit tendon reflexes in the upper extremities, such as the biceps, triceps, and brachioradialis reflexes, to evaluate the function of the cervical nerve roots. Additionally, the provider will gently tap or press on specific areas of the neck, shoulders, and arms to determine if the patient experiences tenderness, numbness, or pain, which can help localize the source of the neck pain or identify potential nerve involvement.

Lastly, the healthcare provider will specifically evaluate the patient for signs of nerve root or spinal cord compression, as these can cause serious neurological symptoms and may require urgent intervention. Signs of nerve root compression include muscle weakness, numbness, or altered reflexes in the distribution of the affected nerve root. In cases of spinal cord compression, the patient may present with more widespread or bilateral neurological symptoms, such as difficulty with balance, coordination, or fine motor tasks, as well as possible changes in bowel or bladder function.

By carefully and methodically assessing the patient's neck posture, range of motion, strength, reflexes, and sensitivity to touch, the healthcare provider can gather valuable information about the underlying cause of the neck pain and inform their diagnostic and treatment decisions.

Imaging studies play a crucial role in diagnosing and evaluating the underlying causes of neck pain. These tests provide healthcare providers with valuable information about the structure and integrity of the cervical spine and surrounding tissues, enabling them to identify abnormalities, assess the severity of the condition, and determine the most appropriate course of treatment.

X-rays are a common imaging modality used to evaluate neck pain. They use a small amount of ionizing radiation to produce images of the bones and joints in the cervical spine. X-rays can help detect fractures, dislocations, bone spurs, or degenerative changes such as arthritis or disc degeneration. However, they are limited in their ability to visualize soft tissues like muscles, ligaments, and nerves, which may also contribute to neck pain.

Magnetic resonance imaging (MRI) is a more advanced imaging technique that uses a powerful magnetic field and radio waves to create detailed images of the soft tissues and bones in the neck. MRI is particularly useful for visualizing the intervertebral discs, spinal cord, nerve roots, and other soft tissue structures that may be involved in neck pain. It can help identify disc herniation, spinal stenosis, tumors, infections, or inflammation, providing healthcare providers with valuable information to guide treatment decisions. However, MRI is more expensive and time-consuming than X-rays and may not be necessary for all patients with neck pain.

Computed tomography (CT) scans use a series of X-ray images taken from different angles to create detailed cross-sectional images of the cervical spine. CT scans can provide a more detailed view of the bones and joints than conventional X-rays and are particularly useful for identifying fractures, dislocations, or other bony abnormalities. They can also help visualize certain soft tissue structures, such as the spinal canal and intervertebral foramen, which are critical for understanding conditions like spinal stenosis or nerve root compression. However, like X-rays, CT scans use ionizing radiation, and their ability to visualize soft tissues is limited compared to MRI.

Ultrasound is a non-invasive imaging technique that uses high-frequency sound waves to produce images of soft tissue structures in the neck. Although ultrasound is not typically the first choice for evaluating neck pain, it can be a useful tool for assessing certain conditions, such as muscle strains, tendonitis, or enlarged lymph nodes. Ultrasound can also be used to guide certain diagnostic or therapeutic procedures, such as injections or biopsies.

Imaging studies are an essential component of the diagnostic process for neck pain, providing healthcare providers with valuable information about the structure and function of the cervical spine and surrounding tissues. By selecting the most appropriate imaging modality based on the patient's symptoms, medical history, and suspected cause of pain, healthcare providers can gain valuable insights into the underlying pathology and develop an effective treatment plan tailored to the patient's needs.

Laboratory tests can be an essential component of the diagnostic process for neck pain, as they help healthcare providers rule out or confirm certain underlying systemic causes. While imaging studies provide valuable information about the structural components of the cervical spine, laboratory tests offer insights into the biochemical and physiological aspects of the patient's condition.

Blood tests are commonly used to detect markers of infection, inflammation, or autoimmune disorders that may contribute to neck pain. For instance, a complete blood count (CBC) can be ordered to assess the patient's overall health and to identify signs of infection or anemia, which may be relevant in cases of neck pain accompanied by fever or fatigue. The erythrocyte sedimentation rate (ESR) and C-reactive protein (CRP) tests may be used to evaluate the presence of inflammation in the body, which could indicate conditions such as rheumatoid arthritis or polymyalgia rheumatica.

In cases where an autoimmune disorder is suspected, tests for specific autoantibodies may be ordered. For example, the rheumatoid factor (RF) and anti-cyclic citrullinated peptide (anti-CCP) tests can help diagnose rheumatoid arthritis, while antinuclear antibody (ANA) testing can be useful for identifying a range of autoimmune conditions, including lupus and Sjögren's syndrome.

Other laboratory studies may be indicated based on the patient's specific symptoms or risk factors. For example, a healthcare provider may order tests to evaluate thyroid function, as both hypothyroidism and hyperthyroidism can cause neck pain and stiffness. Similarly, tests for vitamin D levels may be conducted to assess the patient's bone health and potential risk for osteoporosis, which could contribute to cervical spine degeneration.

In some cases, additional diagnostic procedures may be required to identify the source of infection, particularly if there is a suspicion of a spinal epidural abscess, meningitis, or discitis. In such instances, a lumbar puncture (also known as a spinal tap) may be performed to collect cerebrospinal fluid (CSF) for analysis. The CSF can be tested for the presence of bacteria, viruses, or fungi that may be causing the infection.

Overall, laboratory tests play a crucial role in the comprehensive evaluation of neck pain by providing valuable information about the patient's overall health, as well as specific indicators of infection, inflammation, and systemic disorders. By incorporating these tests into the diagnostic process, healthcare providers can gain a more complete understanding of the patient's condition and develop a targeted treatment plan to address the underlying cause of the neck pain.

In certain cases, when standard diagnostic methods are insufficient to pinpoint the source of neck pain, healthcare providers may resort to additional diagnostic procedures. These tests can provide more detailed information about the function and integrity of the nerves and muscles in the neck, helping to identify the precise cause of the pain.

Nerve conduction studies (NCS) are non-invasive tests that evaluate the speed and strength of electrical signals traveling through nerves. By applying small electrical stimuli to the skin overlying the nerves in the neck and upper extremities, healthcare providers can measure the response of the nerves and assess their overall function. NCS can be particularly helpful in diagnosing cervical radiculopathy, as they can detect nerve damage or compression caused by herniated discs, stenosis, or other structural abnormalities in the cervical spine.

Electromyography (EMG) is a diagnostic test that measures the electrical activity of muscles at rest and during contraction. This test involves inserting fine needles, called electrodes, into the muscles of the neck, shoulders, and arms to record the muscle's electrical activity. EMG can help identify muscle weakness or dysfunction resulting from nerve damage, muscle diseases, or other neurological disorders. When combined with NCS, EMG can provide a comprehensive picture of the nerve and muscle function in the cervical region, assisting healthcare providers in determining the cause of neck pain.

Diagnostic injections, such as facet joint injections or selective nerve root blocks, can also be useful in identifying the source of neck pain. These procedures involve injecting a local anesthetic, and sometimes a corticosteroid, into specific structures or nerves within the cervical spine. If the injection provides significant pain relief, it can help confirm the targeted structure as the primary source of the neck pain. For instance, a facet joint injection can help determine if the pain originates from the facet joints, while a selective nerve root block can help identify the specific nerve root responsible for the pain. These diagnostic injections can also provide therapeutic benefits by reducing inflammation and pain in the affected area.

By utilizing these additional diagnostic procedures when necessary, healthcare providers can enhance their understanding of the underlying cause of neck pain and develop a more targeted and effective treatment plan.

Understanding the complex anatomy, diverse causes, and varied symptoms of neck pain is crucial for accurately diagnosing and effectively treating this common condition. A comprehensive understanding of the cervical spine's structures, including the vertebrae, intervertebral discs, ligaments, muscles, and nerves, allows healthcare providers to better identify the source of pain and discomfort. This knowledge also helps patients recognize the importance of maintaining a healthy cervical spine and taking proactive measures to prevent neck pain.

With a thorough assessment, healthcare providers can identify the underlying cause of neck pain and develop an appropriate treatment plan tailored to the individual patient's needs. This personalized approach is essential to ensure that each patient receives targeted care addressing their specific condition, whether it be muscular, degenerative, or neurological in origin. By recognizing the importance of the cervical spine in maintaining overall health and function, patients and healthcare providers can work together to address neck pain and improve the patient's quality of life.

In the following chapters, we will delve deeper into the various treatment options and protocols for neck pain. These will encompass conservative approaches such as lifestyle modifications, physical therapy, and medication management, as well as alternative and complementary therapies like acupuncture, chiropractic care, and massage therapy. Furthermore, we will discuss surgical interventions for cases where conservative treatments are ineffective or when the patient's condition necessitates more invasive procedures. By understanding the range of available treatments and their potential benefits and risks, patients and healthcare providers can make informed decisions about the best course of action for managing neck pain and promoting long-term spinal health.

The chapters will also emphasize the importance of preventive strategies, including proper ergonomics, exercise, and stress management. By incorporating these practices into their daily lives, patients can reduce the risk of developing neck pain or prevent its recurrence. It is essential to recognize that maintaining a healthy cervical spine requires a multi-faceted approach, and both patients and healthcare providers must actively participate in implementing these strategies.

In conclusion, a comprehensive understanding of the cervical spine's anatomy, causes of neck pain, and associated symptoms is crucial for accurate diagnosis and effective treatment. By exploring various treatment options and protocols, as well as preventive measures, healthcare providers and patients can collaboratively address neck pain and work towards improved spinal health and overall well-being.

Chapter 2

The Importance of Accurate Diagnosis

Identifying the Root Cause for Targeted Treatment

The accurate diagnosis of neck pain is essential for providing effective and targeted treatment to patients. Neck pain, a common condition that affects a large proportion of the population, can have various underlying causes. These causes can range from simple muscle strains to more complex issues like degenerative conditions, nerve compression, and trauma. By identifying the root cause, healthcare providers can tailor treatment options that address the underlying issue, minimize the risk of recurrence, and promote long-term relief for patients.

Muscle strain is one of the most common causes of neck pain, often resulting from overuse, poor posture, or sleeping in an awkward position. When the neck muscles are strained or overworked, they can become inflamed and painful, leading to reduced mobility and discomfort. Identifying muscle strain as the root cause of neck pain allows healthcare providers to recommend appropriate treatments, such as rest, ice, heat, gentle stretching, and over-the-counter pain relievers.

Poor posture can also contribute significantly to neck pain. The prolonged use of electronic devices, sitting at a desk for extended periods, and other lifestyle factors can lead to improper alignment of the cervical spine, placing excessive strain on the neck muscles and ligaments. Identifying poor posture as the underlying cause of neck pain enables healthcare providers to recommend ergonomic adjustments, postural exercises, and physical therapy to alleviate discomfort and promote better posture.

Degenerative conditions, such as cervical spondylosis or degenerative disc disease, can also cause neck pain. These conditions involve the gradual deterioration of the intervertebral discs, facet joints, and other structures in the cervical spine, leading to stiffness, inflammation, and potentially nerve compression. When healthcare providers identify a degenerative condition as the root cause of neck pain, treatment options may include medication, physical therapy, and in more severe cases, surgical intervention.

Nerve compression is another common cause of neck pain, often presenting as radicular pain that radiates down the arm. This can result from a herniated disc, spinal stenosis, or foraminal stenosis, which can compress or irritate the cervical nerve roots. Identifying nerve compression as the cause of neck pain allows healthcare providers to recommend targeted treatments, such as epidural steroid injections, nerve blocks, or surgical decompression, depending on the severity and duration of the condition.

Trauma, such as whiplash or a direct impact to the cervical spine, can also result in neck pain. Injuries may involve damage to the muscles, ligaments, facet joints, or intervertebral discs, leading to inflammation, instability, and potentially neurological symptoms. When healthcare providers identify trauma as the root cause of neck pain, treatment options may involve a combination of conservative measures, such as rest, immobilization, and medication, as well as more aggressive interventions like surgery or rehabilitation, depending on the severity of the injury and the patient's individual needs.

Accurately identifying the root cause of neck pain is essential for providing targeted and effective treatment. By carefully considering the patient's history, symptoms, and diagnostic findings, healthcare providers can tailor treatment plans that address the underlying issue, minimize the risk of recurrence, and promote long-term relief for patients suffering from neck pain.

A comprehensive understanding of the neck's anatomy is crucial for accurate diagnosis and treatment of neck pain. The cervical spine, or neck, is a complex structure consisting of bones, joints, muscles, ligaments, tendons, and nerves that work together to support the head and enable a wide range of motion.

The cervical spine is comprised of seven vertebrae, labeled C1 through C7. The first two vertebrae, C1 (atlas) and C2 (axis), are unique in their structure and function, allowing for the pivotal movements of the head, such as nodding and rotation. The remaining cervical vertebrae, C3 to C7, are more similar in structure and facilitate the neck's flexion, extension, and lateral bending.

Between each pair of vertebrae, intervertebral discs provide cushioning and support, absorbing shock and allowing for flexibility. Each disc is composed of a soft, gel-like center called the nucleus pulposus, surrounded by a tougher, fibrous outer layer called the annulus fibrosus. Over time, these discs may experience degenerative changes or damage, potentially leading to conditions such as herniated or bulging discs.

The spinal canal runs through the center of the cervical vertebrae, housing and protecting the spinal cord. The spinal cord is a vital part of the central nervous system, transmitting information between the brain and the rest of the body. At each level of the cervical spine, pairs of spinal nerves branch off from the spinal cord and exit through small openings called intervertebral foramina. These cervical nerves are responsible for controlling sensation and movement in the neck, shoulders, arms, and hands. Compression or irritation of these nerves can result in neck pain, as well as radiating pain or neurological symptoms in the upper extremities.

Various muscles, ligaments, and tendons in the neck region provide stability, support, and facilitate movement. The muscles of the neck are generally classified into three groups: superficial, intermediate, and deep. The superficial muscles, including the sternocleidomastoid and trapezius, are primarily responsible for larger movements such as head rotation and neck extension. The intermediate and deep muscles, such as the scalenes and the suboccipital muscles, provide more precise movements and help maintain proper alignment of the cervical vertebrae.

Ligaments, which are strong bands of connective tissue, connect the cervical vertebrae and help stabilize the spine. Key ligaments in the neck include the anterior and posterior longitudinal ligaments, which run along the front and back of the vertebral bodies, and the ligamentum flavum, which connects the laminae of adjacent vertebrae. Tendons, another type of connective tissue, attach muscles to bones, allowing for the transfer of force and movement.

The anatomy of the neck is a complex and interconnected system of bones, joints, muscles, ligaments, tendons, and nerves that work together to support the head and enable a wide range of motion. A thorough understanding of these structures and their functions is essential for accurate diagnosis and treatment of neck pain.

An accurate diagnosis of neck pain begins with a comprehensive patient history and physical examination. Obtaining a detailed patient history is essential to understand the context in which neck pain occurs and identify possible contributing factors. During the history-taking process, healthcare providers gather information on the onset, duration, severity, and location of pain. They also inquire about any associated symptoms, such as numbness or tingling in the upper extremities, headaches, or difficulty sleeping.

The patient's medical history plays a significant role in the diagnostic process. Healthcare providers consider previous injuries, surgeries, and comorbidities that might contribute to neck pain or predispose the patient to specific conditions. For example, a history of rheumatoid arthritis may suggest an inflammatory cause for neck pain, while a prior motor vehicle accident may raise suspicion of whiplash-associated disorders. Furthermore, a review of medications, allergies, and lifestyle factors, such as occupation and physical activity levels, can provide additional insights into potential causes and risk factors for neck pain.

During the physical examination, the healthcare provider assesses the patient's posture, paying close attention to any signs of forward head posture, rounded shoulders, or other misalignments that may contribute to neck strain. The patient's range of motion is evaluated, with the healthcare provider guiding the patient through various neck movements, such as flexion, extension, lateral flexion, and rotation, to identify any limitations or pain provocation.

Muscle strength and reflexes are assessed to evaluate the potential involvement of the cervical nerves. The healthcare provider may test the strength of the patient's neck, shoulder, and arm muscles and assess reflexes at specific points, such as the biceps, triceps, and brachioradialis. Any asymmetry or deficits in strength or reflexes can provide clues about potential nerve involvement.

Special tests, such as the Spurling test, may be performed to identify nerve root compression. In the Spurling test, the patient's head is gently extended and rotated toward the symptomatic side, and a downward force is applied to the top of the head. The test is considered positive if it reproduces the patient's arm pain or neurological symptoms, suggesting nerve root compression.

Palpation of the neck and shoulder muscles can help identify muscle strain, trigger points, or localized inflammation. The healthcare provider gently presses on various muscle groups, such as the trapezius, levator scapulae, and sternocleidomastoid, to assess for tenderness or tightness. Palpation can also reveal joint tenderness, which might suggest arthritis or other joint-related issues.

In some cases, additional assessments may be necessary to rule out other potential causes of neck pain. For instance, a thorough examination of the temporomandibular joint (TMJ) can help identify TMJ dysfunction as a contributing factor. Similarly, an evaluation of the shoulder joint and surrounding structures can help determine if the neck pain is referred from the shoulder or if both regions are independently affected.

Overall, a comprehensive patient history and physical examination are crucial components of the diagnostic process for neck pain. By carefully considering the patient's symptoms, medical history, and physical findings, healthcare providers can develop a working hypothesis of the underlying cause and direct further diagnostic tests and treatment accordingly.

Imaging studies play a crucial role in the diagnostic process for neck pain, as they allow healthcare providers to visualize the internal structures of the cervical spine and surrounding tissues. These imaging techniques can reveal the presence of fractures, dislocations, degenerative changes, and other abnormalities that may be contributing to neck pain.

One of the most common imaging techniques used in the evaluation of neck pain is the X-ray. This form of imaging uses a small amount of ionizing radiation to create images of the bony structures in the cervical spine. X-rays can help healthcare providers identify fractures or dislocations, which may occur due to trauma or injury. Additionally, X-rays can reveal degenerative changes in the cervical spine, such as the presence of arthritis or osteophyte (bone spur) formation. These degenerative changes can cause joint inflammation, reduced range of motion, and nerve compression, leading to neck pain and other symptoms. While X-rays are a valuable tool in the evaluation of neck pain, they do not provide detailed images of soft tissues, such as muscles, ligaments, and intervertebral discs.

It is important to note that although X-rays are a widely used diagnostic tool, they also have limitations. X-ray images can sometimes be challenging to interpret due to overlapping structures, and they may not capture subtle abnormalities or early-stage degenerative changes. As a result, additional imaging studies may be necessary to obtain a more comprehensive understanding of the underlying cause of neck pain.

Magnetic Resonance Imaging (MRI) is a powerful diagnostic tool that provides detailed images of the cervical spine, including the soft tissues such as muscles, ligaments, and intervertebral discs. It has become an invaluable tool for healthcare professionals in the accurate diagnosis of neck pain, as it allows for the visualization of structures that cannot be seen with traditional X-rays or CT scans.

MRI works by using a combination of a strong magnetic field, radio waves, and a computer to generate high-resolution images of the internal structures of the body. During the MRI scan, the patient lies down on a movable table that slides into the MRI machine, which is essentially a large, cylindrical magnet. The magnetic field aligns the hydrogen atoms in the body, and when radio waves are applied, the hydrogen atoms absorb and then release energy, producing signals that the MRI machine detects and uses to create images.

One of the primary benefits of MRI in the diagnosis of neck pain is its ability to visualize soft tissues, which is particularly useful for identifying disc herniation. A herniated disc, sometimes referred to as a slipped or ruptured disc, occurs when the soft inner core of an intervertebral disc protrudes through the outer fibrous layer. This can cause pressure on nearby nerves or the spinal cord, leading to pain, numbness, and weakness in the neck, shoulder, or arm. MRI can reveal the size, location, and extent of disc herniation, providing valuable information for planning appropriate treatment strategies.

MRI is also highly effective in diagnosing spinal stenosis, a condition where the spinal canal narrows, potentially compressing the spinal cord or nerve roots. Spinal stenosis can result from a variety of factors, including degenerative changes, bone spurs, or disc herniation. MRI can visualize the narrowing of the spinal canal, as well as any associated soft tissue abnormalities, such as thickened ligaments or bulging discs, that may be contributing to the compression.

Spinal cord compression, or myelopathy, is another critical condition that MRI can help identify. Myelopathy can have various causes, including spinal stenosis, disc herniation, or tumors, and can lead to significant neurological symptoms if left untreated. MRI provides an unparalleled view of the spinal cord, allowing healthcare professionals to assess the extent of compression, identify the cause, and plan for appropriate interventions, such as surgery or conservative management.

In addition to these specific conditions, MRI can also be used to diagnose other causes of neck pain, such as ligament injuries, muscle strains, and infections, or to rule out more serious conditions like tumors. Overall, the ability of MRI to provide detailed images of the cervical spine and its surrounding structures makes it an essential tool in the accurate diagnosis and management of neck pain.

A computed tomography (CT) scan is an advanced imaging technique that uses X-rays and computer technology to create detailed cross-sectional images, or "slices," of the cervical spine. By compiling these slices, a CT scan provides a comprehensive view of the bony structures in the neck, allowing healthcare providers to assess the cervical spine's overall condition.

One of the main advantages of a CT scan over standard X-rays is its ability to produce more detailed images of the bony structures in the cervical spine. This higher resolution enables healthcare providers to identify subtle fractures, degenerative changes, and bone spurs more accurately. Furthermore, a CT scan can provide additional information on the alignment and stability of the cervical spine, which may be crucial in cases of trauma or suspected instability.

In addition to fractures, CT scans can help identify other abnormalities in the cervical spine, such as degenerative changes. For example, a CT scan can reveal the presence of facet joint arthritis, spondylosis (spinal osteoarthritis), or the narrowing of the spinal canal (spinal stenosis). By visualizing these changes, healthcare providers can gain a better understanding of the underlying cause of neck pain and develop a targeted treatment plan.

CT scans can also be used to identify bone spurs, known as osteophytes, which can form due to degenerative processes or trauma. These bony growths can contribute to neck pain by compressing nerves, narrowing the spinal canal, or causing inflammation in the surrounding tissues. Identifying the presence of bone spurs through a CT scan allows healthcare providers to tailor treatment options to address these specific issues.

Although CT scans provide valuable information for the diagnosis of neck pain, it is important to note that they do have limitations. While CT scans excel at visualizing bony structures, they are not as effective at capturing images of soft tissues, such as muscles, ligaments, and intervertebral discs. In cases where soft tissue pathology is suspected, magnetic resonance imaging (MRI) may be a more appropriate imaging modality.

Additionally, CT scans expose patients to ionizing radiation, which can pose potential health risks, particularly with repeated exposure. As a result, healthcare providers must weigh the benefits of obtaining a CT scan against the potential risks, considering alternative imaging options when appropriate.

CT scans are a valuable diagnostic tool for assessing the bony structures of the cervical spine and identifying fractures, degenerative changes, and bone spurs. By providing detailed images of the neck's anatomy, CT scans can help healthcare providers pinpoint the underlying cause of neck pain and develop targeted treatment plans to address these issues. However, the limitations of CT scans and the potential risks associated with ionizing radiation must be considered when selecting the most appropriate imaging modality for each individual patient.

Myelography is an imaging technique that has been utilized for decades to visualize the spinal canal and its contents, including the spinal cord and nerve roots. This procedure is particularly helpful when other imaging methods, such as X-rays, CT scans, or MRI, are insufficient or contraindicated for a patient. Myelography can provide valuable information to healthcare providers, allowing for the detection of spinal cord compression, nerve root impingement, and spinal stenosis.

The myelography procedure begins with the patient lying on their side or stomach on the examination table. A healthcare provider administers local anesthesia to numb the skin and deeper tissues in the lower back. A thin, hollow needle is then carefully inserted into the spinal canal, and a small amount of cerebrospinal fluid (CSF) is removed to create space for the contrast dye.

Next, a radiopaque contrast dye is injected into the spinal canal through the needle. The contrast dye is designed to block X-rays, allowing for the clear visualization of the spinal canal, spinal cord, and nerve roots on X-ray or CT images. The patient may be asked to change positions during the injection to help the contrast dye flow through the spinal canal.

Once the contrast dye has been administered, X-rays or CT scans are performed. The X-ray images, known as myelograms, provide a detailed view of the spinal canal and its contents. The CT scans, which can be performed as part of a CT myelogram, offer additional detail and cross-sectional images of the spinal structures.

Myelography is particularly useful for identifying conditions that may not be easily visible on standard X-rays or MRI, such as spinal stenosis, nerve root impingement, or spinal cord compression caused by a herniated disc, tumor, or bone spur. This imaging technique can also be valuable in evaluating patients with metallic implants, which may cause artifacts on MRI images, or patients who cannot undergo MRI due to medical contraindications, such as having a pacemaker.

While myelography is a valuable diagnostic tool, it is an invasive procedure and carries some risks. These include infection, bleeding, headache, allergic reaction to the contrast dye, or damage to the spinal cord or nerve roots. However, advances in imaging techniques and improvements in the contrast dye have significantly reduced the risks associated with myelography. In many cases, MRI or CT scans without contrast may be used as alternatives to myelography, depending on the patient's specific needs and clinical presentation.

Myelography is a valuable imaging technique that can help visualize spinal cord compression, nerve root impingement, and spinal stenosis when other imaging methods are insufficient or contraindicated. By providing detailed information about the spinal canal and its contents, myelography can aid healthcare providers in making accurate diagnoses and developing targeted treatment plans for patients with neck pain.

Electrodiagnostic studies are essential tools for assessing the function of the nervous system, particularly in the context of neck pain. These tests help healthcare providers identify nerve-related causes of neck pain, such as cervical radiculopathy, brachial plexopathy, or peripheral nerve entrapment. Two primary electrodiagnostic studies are employed for this purpose: electromyography (EMG) and nerve conduction studies (NCS).

Electromyography (EMG) is a diagnostic procedure that evaluates the electrical activity produced by skeletal muscles. This test involves the insertion of a fine needle electrode into the muscle of interest, which records the muscle's electrical activity at rest and during contraction. In the context of neck pain, EMG can help identify abnormal muscle activity, denervation, or reinnervation, which may indicate nerve compression or damage. For example, EMG can demonstrate decreased recruitment or spontaneous activity in muscles innervated by a compressed nerve root, suggesting cervical radiculopathy.

Nerve conduction studies (NCS) assess the speed and amplitude of electrical signals traveling along peripheral nerves. This test involves stimulating a nerve at one point and recording the electrical response at another point along the nerve pathway, usually using surface electrodes. NCS can detect abnormalities in nerve conduction, such as slowed conduction velocities or reduced amplitude of the electrical response, which may indicate nerve compression or damage. In cases of neck pain, NCS can help differentiate between cervical radiculopathy and other nerve-related conditions, such as peripheral neuropathy or brachial plexopathy.

In some cases, healthcare providers may perform both EMG and NCS during the same diagnostic session, as the combination of these tests can provide a more comprehensive assessment of the patient's nerve function. The results of these studies, along with the patient's history and physical examination findings, can help healthcare providers develop a more accurate diagnosis and guide appropriate treatment strategies.

It is important to note that electrodiagnostic studies, while valuable, are not without limitations. These tests can be uncomfortable for patients, as they involve needle insertion and electrical stimulation. Furthermore, the sensitivity and specificity of EMG and NCS can vary depending on the specific clinical scenario, and false-negative or false-positive results are possible. Therefore, healthcare providers must interpret the results of electrodiagnostic studies within the context of the patient's overall clinical presentation.

Electrodiagnostic studies, such as EMG and NCS, play a crucial role in the evaluation of nerve-related causes of neck pain. By providing information about nerve function and identifying nerve compression or damage, these tests can help healthcare providers develop accurate diagnoses and implement targeted treatment plans to address the underlying cause of neck pain.

Understanding the different classifications of neck pain is essential for accurately diagnosing and effectively treating the condition. Based on diagnostic findings, neck pain can be classified into several categories.

Mechanical neck pain is one of the most common types of neck pain and encompasses a wide range of issues related to the cervical spine's structures and surrounding soft tissues. Mechanical neck pain can arise from muscle strains, which are often the result of overexertion, awkward movements, or prolonged static postures. Ligament sprains can also contribute to mechanical neck pain; these occur when the neck's supportive ligaments are overstretched or torn, often due to sudden movements or trauma.

Degenerative changes in the cervical spine, such as disc degeneration or facet joint arthritis, can cause mechanical neck pain as well. Disc degeneration occurs when the intervertebral discs lose their hydration and elasticity over time, reducing their ability to provide cushioning and support. This can lead to increased stress on the facet joints, which may result in the development of osteoarthritis.

Poor posture plays a significant role in mechanical neck pain, as it places additional strain on the muscles, ligaments, and joints of the cervical spine. Slouched or forward head posture, often seen in individuals who spend long hours at a computer or looking down at their phones, can contribute to chronic mechanical neck pain. Muscle imbalances, in which some muscles become tight and overactive while others are weak and underactive, can further exacerbate the problem.

Repetitive strain injuries, common in individuals who engage in activities requiring repetitive neck movements or sustained postures, can also lead to mechanical neck pain. These injuries may involve muscle fatigue, micro-tears in muscle fibers, or inflammation in tendons and ligaments, which can result in persistent pain and stiffness.

Mechanical neck pain encompasses a diverse range of issues related to the structures and function of the cervical spine. Accurate diagnosis of the specific cause of mechanical neck pain is essential for tailoring treatment approaches and providing long-term relief for patients.

Radicular pain, also known as radiculopathy, is a type of neck pain that arises from the compression or irritation of a cervical nerve root. This type of pain is commonly referred to as a "pinched nerve" and is often the result of conditions affecting the spinal structures, such as herniated discs or spinal stenosis. The cervical spine consists of seven vertebrae (C1-C7), and each level has a pair of nerve roots that branch off the spinal cord. When one of these nerve roots is affected, the pain and other symptoms often radiate down the arm, following the distribution of the affected nerve.

The pathophysiology of radicular pain involves mechanical compression or inflammation of the nerve root, leading to altered nerve function. Mechanical compression can result from a herniated disc, in which the gel-like nucleus of an intervertebral disc protrudes through its fibrous outer ring, putting pressure on the adjacent nerve root. Spinal stenosis, on the other hand, is a narrowing of the spinal canal or intervertebral foramina, which can also compress nerve roots. Inflammation and chemical irritation can further exacerbate the pain and dysfunction caused by mechanical compression.

The clinical presentation of radicular pain can vary depending on the affected nerve root level. Common symptoms include sharp, shooting pain that radiates from the neck down the arm, often accompanied by numbness, tingling, or weakness in the arm, hand, or fingers. The pain may be exacerbated by certain neck movements or positions, such as extending or rotating the neck.

To diagnose radicular pain, healthcare providers rely on a combination of patient history, physical examination, and imaging studies. During the history-taking process, the provider will gather information on the onset, nature, and distribution of pain, as well as any associated symptoms. The physical examination may involve assessing the patient's posture, neck range of motion, muscle strength, and reflexes. Special tests, such as the Spurling test, can help identify nerve root compression. Imaging studies, such as magnetic resonance imaging (MRI) or computed tomography (CT) scans, can provide detailed information about the spinal structures, allowing for the identification of herniated discs, spinal stenosis, or other potential causes of nerve root compression.

The treatment of radicular pain focuses on addressing the underlying cause of nerve root compression or irritation. Conservative treatment options include pain medication, such as nonsteroidal anti-inflammatory drugs (NSAIDs) or neuropathic pain medications, physical therapy, cervical traction, and activity modification. Epidural steroid injections can help reduce inflammation around the affected nerve root and provide temporary relief. In some cases, particularly when conservative treatments have been ineffective, or there is significant neurological dysfunction, surgical intervention may be necessary. Surgical options for radicular pain include microdiscectomy, in which the herniated disc material is removed, and decompression surgeries, such as laminectomy or foraminotomy, which aim to relieve pressure on the nerve root by enlarging the spinal canal or intervertebral foramina.

Radicular pain is a type of neck pain that occurs due to compression or irritation of cervical nerve roots. Accurate diagnosis and targeted treatment are essential for effectively managing radicular pain and preventing long-term complications. By addressing the underlying cause, healthcare providers can help patients achieve pain relief and restore function.

Myelopathy refers to spinal cord compression, which can result from severe spinal stenosis, trauma, or other conditions affecting the spinal canal. This condition can lead to neck pain and neurological symptoms such as muscle weakness, numbness, and coordination issues. It is essential to accurately diagnose and treat myelopathy to prevent further neurological deterioration and potential long-term complications.

Myelopathy can be categorized into different types based on the location of spinal cord compression. In the context of neck pain, the most relevant type is cervical myelopathy, which occurs when the spinal cord is compressed in the cervical spine. The causes of cervical myelopathy may include degenerative changes such as osteophyte formation or disc herniation, congenital spinal stenosis, spinal tumors, or conditions that affect the integrity of the spinal canal, such as spondylosis or ankylosing spondylitis.

The clinical presentation of myelopathy may vary depending on the severity and location of spinal cord compression. Patients with cervical myelopathy may experience neck pain, stiffness, or discomfort, along with neurological symptoms that can affect the upper and lower extremities. Common symptoms include muscle weakness, numbness or tingling, difficulty with fine motor tasks (such as buttoning a shirt), impaired balance, and gait disturbances. In advanced cases, patients may develop bowel or bladder dysfunction, indicating a more severe neurological impairment.

Diagnosing myelopathy requires a comprehensive patient history and physical examination, along with appropriate imaging studies. During the physical examination, the healthcare provider may assess the patient's reflexes, muscle strength, sensation, and coordination. Special tests, such as the Hoffmann's reflex or the Lhermitte's sign, may be performed to identify signs of spinal cord involvement. Magnetic resonance imaging (MRI) is the gold standard for diagnosing myelopathy, as it provides detailed images of the spinal cord, intervertebral discs, and surrounding structures. In some cases, additional imaging studies, such as computed tomography (CT) or myelography, may be necessary to further evaluate the spinal canal and identify the specific cause of compression.

Treatment for myelopathy depends on the severity of the condition and the underlying cause of spinal cord compression. In mild cases or when the compression is not progressing, conservative treatments such as physical therapy, medication, and activity modification may be recommended to manage symptoms and prevent further neurological decline. However, in cases of significant or progressive neurological impairment, surgical intervention may be necessary to decompress the spinal cord and prevent further damage. Surgical options for treating cervical myelopathy include anterior cervical discectomy and fusion (ACDF), posterior cervical laminectomy, or cervical laminoplasty, depending on the location and extent of the compression.

Postoperative care and rehabilitation play a crucial role in the recovery process following surgery for myelopathy. Patients may require physical therapy to regain strength, improve range of motion, and restore function in the affected areas. In some cases, occupational therapy may be necessary

51

to help patients adapt to any lingering neurological deficits and regain independence in daily activities.

Myelopathy is a serious condition that can result in neck pain and a wide range of neurological symptoms. Accurate diagnosis and timely intervention are essential to prevent further neurological deterioration and improve patients' quality of life. Treatment may involve conservative measures or surgical intervention, depending on the severity and progression of the condition.

Whiplash is a neck injury that occurs when the head and neck are rapidly and forcefully moved back and forth, typically during a motor vehicle accident, but also in sports, falls, and other trauma incidents. The sudden acceleration and deceleration forces can cause damage to the cervical spine's muscles, ligaments, tendons, intervertebral discs, and facet joints, resulting in a variety of symptoms collectively referred to as whiplash-associated disorders (WAD).

Whiplash-associated disorders encompass a range of symptoms and severity levels, which are commonly classified into four grades. This classification system helps healthcare providers assess the extent of the injury, tailor treatment plans, and monitor progress throughout the recovery process.

Grade 1 whiplash associated disorders are characterized by mild neck pain or stiffness without any observable physical signs. Patients in this category may experience discomfort during neck movement but typically have no significant limitations in their range of motion. Treatment for Grade 1 whiplash-associated disorders often includes self-care measures, such as over-the-counter pain medication, gentle stretching, and the application of heat or cold packs to the affected area.

Grade 2 whiplash associated disorders involve moderate neck pain accompanied by musculoskeletal signs, including reduced range of motion and tenderness in the neck muscles or surrounding structures. Patients may experience difficulty turning their head or maintaining proper posture due to pain and stiffness. In addition to self-care measures, treatment for Grade 2 whiplash-associated disorders may involve physical therapy, manual therapy, and prescription pain medication, as needed.

Grade 3 whiplash associated disorders are marked by severe neck pain with accompanying neurological signs, such as sensory deficits, muscle weakness, or reflex abnormalities. These symptoms indicate nerve involvement and may manifest as numbness, tingling, or burning sensations in the upper extremities, as well as muscle weakness or diminished reflexes. The treatment approach for Grade 3 whiplash-associated disorders is typically more comprehensive and may involve a combination of pain management, physical therapy, and manual therapy techniques. In some cases, further diagnostic tests or specialist consultations may be necessary to assess nerve involvement and determine the appropriate course of treatment.

Grade 4 whiplash associated disorders are the most severe, characterized by neck pain with a fracture or dislocation of one or more cervical vertebrae. This grade represents a significant injury to the cervical spine and may result in spinal instability, severe neurological symptoms, or the potential for spinal cord injury. The diagnosis of Grade 4 whiplash-associated disorders typically involves imaging studies, such as X-rays or CT scans, to confirm the presence of a fracture or dislocation. Treatment for this grade often requires surgical intervention to stabilize the spine, followed by a comprehensive rehabilitation program to restore function and manage pain.

The classification of whiplash-associated disorders into four grades is essential for understanding the severity of the injury, guiding treatment decisions, and monitoring progress throughout the recovery process. Each grade requires a tailored approach to treatment, ranging from self-care measures and physical therapy for milder cases to surgical intervention and extensive rehabilitation for the most severe injuries.

The symptoms of whiplash-associated disorders can be variable and may develop immediately after the injury or within a few days. Common symptoms include neck pain, stiffness, reduced range of motion, and headaches. Some individuals may also experience shoulder and upper back pain, dizziness, blurred vision, tinnitus (ringing in the ears), fatigue, and difficulty concentrating.

Diagnosing whiplash-associated disorders can be challenging, as there is no definitive diagnostic test for the condition. The diagnosis is typically based on the patient's history, the mechanism of injury, and a thorough physical examination. Imaging studies, such as X-rays, CT scans, or MRIs, may be used to rule out other potential causes of neck pain, such as fractures or dislocations, and to identify any structural abnormalities.

The management of whiplash-associated disorders aims to reduce pain and restore function while facilitating the patient's recovery. Conservative treatment approaches are often effective in achieving these goals and may involve a combination of pain management strategies, physical therapy, manual therapy, heat or cold applications, and education on self-management.

Pain management is an essential aspect of treating whiplash-associated disorders. Over-the-counter analgesics, such as acetaminophen or nonsteroidal anti-inflammatory drugs (NSAIDs), can help alleviate pain and reduce inflammation. In more severe cases, healthcare providers may prescribe medications like muscle relaxants to address muscle spasms or opioids for short-term pain relief. It is crucial to use these medications judiciously and under the guidance of a healthcare professional to minimize the risk of side effects and dependence.

Physical therapy plays a significant role in the conservative management of whiplash-associated disorders. A physical therapist can develop an individualized program tailored to the patient's needs and goals, with a focus on improving neck mobility, reducing pain, and strengthening the muscles that support the cervical spine. This program may involve gentle stretching exercises to improve flexibility, strengthening exercises to enhance muscular support, and range-of-motion exercises to restore normal neck movement. Additionally, the physical therapist can provide guidance on postural training and ergonomic advice to help patients adopt healthy habits and prevent further injury.

Manual therapy, including joint mobilization, soft tissue mobilization, and massage, can also be beneficial in managing whiplash-associated disorders. These techniques aim to relieve pain, improve neck mobility, and promote tissue healing by addressing restrictions in joint movement and soft tissue tightness. Manual therapy should be performed by a qualified healthcare professional, such as a physical therapist or chiropractor, to ensure safety and effectiveness.

The application of heat or cold can be a helpful adjunct to other treatment modalities for whiplash-associated disorders. Heat therapy, such as warm compresses or heating pads, can help relax muscles, increase blood flow to the affected area, and alleviate pain. Cold therapy, such as ice packs, can reduce inflammation and numb the area to provide pain relief. Patients should be advised on proper techniques for applying heat or cold to avoid burns, frostbite, or other complications.

Education and self-management are vital components of whiplash-associated disorder treatment. Healthcare providers should educate patients on proper posture, ergonomics, and self-care strategies to prevent symptom exacerbation and promote recovery. This may include guidance on maintaining a neutral spine while sitting or standing, adjusting workstations to reduce strain on the neck, and performing regular exercises to maintain flexibility and strength. Empowering patients with the knowledge and tools necessary to manage their condition can significantly contribute to a successful recovery and improved quality of life.

In most cases, individuals with whiplash-associated disorders will experience a gradual improvement in their symptoms over time. However, a small percentage of patients may continue to experience persistent symptoms, known as chronic whiplash syndrome. In these cases, a multidisciplinary approach involving pain management specialists, physical therapists, and mental health professionals may be necessary to address the complex nature of chronic pain and its associated psychological factors.

Inflammatory or infectious conditions can lead to neck pain by affecting the structures of the cervical spine, surrounding tissues, or the nervous system. Accurate diagnosis of these conditions is essential to ensure appropriate treatment and prevent complications. In this section, we will discuss some common inflammatory and infectious conditions that can cause neck pain, their symptoms, and the importance of accurate diagnosis.

Rheumatoid arthritis (RA) is an autoimmune disorder that primarily affects the joints, causing pain, stiffness, and inflammation. In the cervical spine, RA can lead to instability, joint degeneration, and compression of nerves or the spinal cord. Patients with rheumatoid arthritis may experience neck pain along with other symptoms such as fatigue, morning stiffness, and joint swelling. Accurate diagnosis of RA typically involves a combination of patient history, physical examination, blood tests for specific antibodies, and imaging studies such as X-rays, MRI, or ultrasound. Early diagnosis and appropriate treatment of RA, which may include medications, physical therapy, and in some cases, surgery, can help slow disease progression, alleviate pain, and maintain function.

Meningitis is an infection of the meninges, the protective membranes that cover the brain and spinal cord. Meningitis can be caused by various pathogens, including bacteria, viruses, fungi, or parasites. Neck pain and stiffness are common symptoms of meningitis, often accompanied by fever, headache, and sensitivity to light. Early diagnosis of meningitis is crucial, as bacterial meningitis, in particular, can be life-threatening if left untreated. Diagnostic tests for meningitis may include blood tests, imaging studies, and a lumbar puncture to obtain cerebrospinal fluid for analysis. Treatment for meningitis depends on the underlying cause and may involve antibiotics, antiviral medications, or antifungal agents, along with supportive care to manage symptoms.

Ankylosing spondylitis (AS) is a type of inflammatory arthritis that primarily affects the spine, causing pain and stiffness in the neck and lower back. Over time, AS can lead to the fusion of vertebrae, resulting in reduced spinal flexibility and, in some cases, impaired lung function due to reduced chest expansion. Diagnosis of AS typically involves patient history, physical examination, blood tests for inflammatory markers, and imaging studies such as X-rays or MRI. Early diagnosis and treatment of AS, which may include medications, physical therapy, and in some cases, surgery, can help manage symptoms, slow disease progression, and maintain function.

Infections of the cervical spine, such as vertebral osteomyelitis or discitis, can also cause neck pain. These conditions are often caused by bacterial infections that reach the spine through the bloodstream or as a result of a direct inoculation, such as during surgery. Symptoms of spinal infections may include neck pain, fever, and tenderness over the affected area. Accurate diagnosis of spinal infections typically involves a combination of patient history, physical examination, blood tests, and imaging studies, such as X-rays, MRI, or CT scans. Treatment for spinal infections usually involves antibiotics, and in some cases, surgical intervention to remove infected tissue or stabilize the spine.

Inflammatory and infectious conditions can cause neck pain by affecting the cervical spine, surrounding tissues, or the nervous system. Accurate diagnosis of these conditions is essential to ensure appropriate treatment and prevent complications. Early diagnosis and targeted treatment can help manage symptoms, slow disease progression, and maintain function, ultimately improving the quality of life for patients.

The differential diagnosis for neck pain involves considering a wide range of potential causes, as several conditions can mimic neck pain or present with similar symptoms. One such condition is thoracic outlet syndrome, a complex disorder resulting from the compression of nerves or blood vessels in the thoracic outlet, the anatomical space between the collarbone and first rib. Various factors can contribute to this compression, including congenital abnormalities, such as an extra cervical rib, muscle or tendon anomalies, and postural issues or muscle imbalances that lead to the narrowing of the thoracic outlet.

Thoracic outlet syndrome can be further divided into three subtypes based on the structures being compressed: neurogenic thoracic outlet syndrome, which involves compression of the brachial plexus nerves; vascular thoracic outlet syndrome, which affects the subclavian artery or vein; and non-specific or disputed thoracic outlet syndrome, which presents with similar symptoms but lacks clear diagnostic evidence of nerve or vascular compression.

Patients with thoracic outlet syndrome may experience a variety of symptoms, such as pain, numbness, and weakness in the neck, shoulder, and arm. Other symptoms may include swelling or discoloration of the affected arm, cold and pale fingers, and reduced range of motion in the shoulder. These symptoms may be exacerbated by certain activities, such as overhead movements, prolonged postures, or heavy lifting.

Diagnosing thoracic outlet syndrome can be challenging due to the overlap of symptoms with other conditions, such as cervical radiculopathy, rotator cuff injuries, or carpal tunnel syndrome. A thorough clinical examination is essential to evaluate the patient's posture, muscle strength, and the presence of tenderness or swelling in the thoracic outlet region. Special tests, such as the Adson's test, Roos test, or Wright's test, may be performed to assess for the presence of vascular or neurological compromise.

In addition to the clinical examination, imaging studies, such as X-rays, MRI, or ultrasound, may be used to visualize the thoracic outlet and identify potential causes of compression. In some cases, additional diagnostic tests, such as nerve conduction studies, electromyography, or angiography, may be necessary to confirm the diagnosis and assess the severity of nerve or vascular involvement.

Once thoracic outlet syndrome has been accurately diagnosed, a targeted treatment plan can be developed to address the underlying cause of compression and alleviate symptoms. Treatment options may include physical therapy, postural correction, exercises to improve muscle strength and flexibility, pain-relieving medication, or the use of assistive devices, such as cervical collars or ergonomic equipment. In more severe cases, or when conservative treatments fail to provide relief, surgical intervention may be necessary to decompress the affected structures and restore function.

Thoracic outlet syndrome is an important differential diagnosis to consider in patients presenting with neck pain and upper extremity symptoms. Accurate diagnosis requires a thorough clinical examination, appropriate imaging studies, and, in some cases, specialized diagnostic tests. With a targeted treatment approach, patients with thoracic outlet syndrome can experience significant relief from their symptoms and improved quality of life.

Cervicogenic headache is a secondary headache disorder, meaning it results from an underlying condition or structural problem. In the case of cervicogenic headaches, the pain originates from the cervical spine or surrounding muscles, specifically the upper cervical region (C1-C3). This type of headache is characterized by unilateral pain that typically starts at the base of the skull and radiates to the front of the head, temples, and sometimes the shoulder. The pain may be described as dull, aching, or throbbing, and it can vary in intensity.

The exact mechanism of cervicogenic headaches is not completely understood, but it is believed to involve a complex interaction between the nervous system and cervical structures. One possible explanation is the convergence of sensory input from the upper cervical nerves with sensory input from the trigeminal nerve, which is responsible for transmitting pain signals from the head and face. When dysfunction or irritation occurs in the cervical spine, it may result in the activation of pain pathways, leading to the sensation of headache.

There are several potential causes of cervicogenic headaches, including cervical disc degeneration, facet joint arthritis, muscle strain or spasm, and ligament injuries. Conditions such as whiplash, poor posture, and repetitive stress from occupational or sports activities can also contribute to the development of cervicogenic headaches. In some cases, the cause may not be identifiable, making diagnosis and treatment more challenging.

Diagnosis of cervicogenic headaches involves a thorough patient history, physical examination, and potentially diagnostic imaging or other tests. During the physical examination, the healthcare provider will assess the patient's range of motion, posture, and palpate the neck and surrounding muscles to identify tenderness or trigger points. Special tests, such as the flexion-rotation test, may be performed to help identify dysfunction in the upper cervical spine. Imaging studies, such as X-rays, MRI, or CT scans, may be necessary to evaluate the cervical spine for degenerative changes, disc herniation, or other structural abnormalities.

Treatment for cervicogenic headaches typically involves a combination of conservative therapies aimed at addressing the underlying cause and managing pain. Physical therapy plays a crucial role in the treatment process, focusing on improving posture, cervical mobility, and strengthening neck and upper back muscles to provide better support for the cervical spine. Manual therapies, such as massage, joint mobilizations, or spinal manipulations, may also be beneficial in addressing muscle tension, joint restrictions, and improving overall cervical function.

Pharmacological treatment options may include nonsteroidal anti-inflammatory drugs (NSAIDs), muscle relaxants, or analgesics to manage pain and inflammation. In some cases, nerve blocks or other interventional pain management techniques may be considered for more persistent or severe cervicogenic headaches. Cervicogenic headaches that haven't responded to other treatment options have a very high success rate with cervical spinal cord stimulation and the ability to reduce the frequency and intensity of headaches to near zero in many cases.

Lifestyle modifications, such as ergonomic adjustments to the workplace, stress management techniques, and regular exercise, can also play a significant role in the prevention and management of cervicogenic headaches. By addressing the underlying cause of cervicogenic headaches and implementing a targeted treatment plan, patients can experience a reduction in headache frequency and intensity, leading to improved quality of life.

Temporomandibular joint dysfunction, often abbreviated as TMJ or TMD, is a condition that affects the temporomandibular joint, which connects the jawbone to the skull. The temporomandibular joint is a complex, hinge-like structure that allows for a wide range of movements, including opening and closing the mouth, as well as side-to-side and forward-backward motions. TMJ dysfunction can cause pain in the jaw, face, and neck due to issues with the joint itself or the surrounding muscles, ligaments, and other supporting structures.

The precise cause of TMJ dysfunction can vary, and may include factors such as trauma or injury to the joint, excessive clenching or grinding of teeth (bruxism), misalignment of the jaw, arthritis, or muscle imbalances. TMJ dysfunction can present with various symptoms, including pain in the jaw, face, and neck, difficulty opening or closing the mouth, clicking or popping sounds when moving the jaw, ear pain, headaches, and even dizziness.

Accurate diagnosis of TMJ dysfunction is essential for providing targeted treatment and alleviating symptoms. The diagnostic process typically begins with a thorough patient history and physical examination, focusing on the jaw, face, and neck. Healthcare providers may ask about the onset, duration, and severity of symptoms, as well as any potential contributing factors or aggravating activities. During the physical examination, the healthcare provider will assess the range of motion of the jaw, palpate the joint and surrounding muscles for tenderness or abnormalities, and listen for clicking or popping sounds while the patient opens and closes their mouth.

In some cases, imaging studies may be necessary to further evaluate the temporomandibular joint and rule out other potential causes of symptoms. X-rays, magnetic resonance imaging (MRI), or computed tomography (CT) scans can provide detailed information about the joint's structure, as well as the surrounding bones and soft tissues.

Once a diagnosis of TMJ dysfunction is established, targeted treatment can be initiated to help alleviate symptoms and improve function. Treatment options for TMJ dysfunction are typically conservative, often involving a combination of strategies to address the specific needs of the patient.

One treatment option is the use of custom-made oral appliances, such as splints or bite guards. These devices are designed to stabilize the joint, reduce excessive clenching or grinding of teeth, and alleviate pressure on the jaw muscles. They work by providing a barrier between the upper and lower teeth, promoting a more neutral jaw position and reducing strain on the temporomandibular joint.

Physical therapy interventions can also play a vital role in the treatment of TMJ dysfunction. A physical therapist may prescribe stretching and strengthening exercises to improve muscle balance, joint mobility, and overall function. Additionally, manual therapy techniques, such as joint mobilization or soft tissue manipulation, may be utilized to address restrictions and promote optimal movement patterns. Posture training is another crucial aspect of physical therapy, as poor posture can contribute to TMJ dysfunction by placing undue stress on the joint and surrounding structures.

Medication management is another important component of TMJ dysfunction treatment. Over-the-counter or prescription medications, such as nonsteroidal anti-inflammatory drugs (NSAIDs), muscle relaxants, or analgesics, may be recommended to manage pain and inflammation associated with the condition. These medications can help alleviate discomfort and improve the patient's ability to participate in other therapeutic interventions, such as physical therapy.

Behavioral modification is an essential aspect of TMJ dysfunction treatment, as certain habits or behaviors can contribute to the condition. Healthcare providers may work with patients to identify and address factors, such as excessive gum chewing, nail-biting, or poor posture, that may exacerbate symptoms or impede recovery. By addressing these behaviors, patients can help to alleviate their symptoms and prevent the recurrence of TMJ dysfunction.

Finally, relaxation techniques and stress management play a crucial role in the treatment of TMJ dysfunction, as stress can exacerbate the condition by increasing muscle tension and promoting maladaptive behaviors, such as teeth clenching. Incorporating relaxation techniques, such as deep breathing exercises, progressive muscle relaxation, or meditation, can help to reduce muscle tension and alleviate symptoms. In some cases, healthcare providers may also recommend counseling or other psychological interventions to address underlying stressors and promote overall well-being.

A comprehensive approach to TMJ dysfunction treatment, including oral appliances, physical therapy, medication management, behavioral modification, and relaxation techniques, can help to alleviate symptoms and improve function. By addressing the specific underlying causes and contributing factors, patients can experience long-term relief and a better quality of life.

In cases where conservative treatments are unsuccessful or the underlying cause of TMJ dysfunction is severe, more invasive interventions, such as corticosteroid injections or surgery, may be considered. However, these options are typically reserved for patients who have not responded to conservative treatments and continue to experience significant pain and functional limitations.

Accurate diagnosis and targeted treatment of TMJ dysfunction are essential for alleviating pain in the jaw, face, and neck, and improving overall function. By addressing the specific underlying cause and implementing a comprehensive treatment plan, patients can experience significant relief from their symptoms and improved quality of life. It is important for healthcare providers to be aware of the potential connection between TMJ dysfunction and neck pain, as well as the various diagnostic and treatment options available, to ensure effective management of this complex condition. Ongoing collaboration between patients, healthcare providers, and other specialists, such as dentists or orthodontists, may be necessary to achieve the best possible outcomes for individuals suffering from TMJ dysfunction.

Referred pain is a phenomenon in which pain is perceived in a region of the body that is distinct from the source of the pain. This occurs due to the complex nature of the nervous system and the way pain signals are processed by the brain. In the context of neck pain, referred pain can sometimes complicate the diagnostic process, as it may lead healthcare providers to initially focus on the neck rather than the true source of the pain. Identifying the true source of pain is essential to provide appropriate treatment and relief.

Referred pain in the neck can arise from various sources, with the shoulder being one of the most common. Shoulder issues such as rotator cuff injuries, adhesive capsulitis (frozen shoulder), or tendonitis can lead to pain that is felt in the neck. This can occur due to the close proximity of the shoulder and neck, as well as the shared innervation by cervical nerves. For example, the suprascapular nerve, which originates from the C5 and C6 nerve roots, innervates key shoulder muscles and can contribute to referred neck pain if irritated or compressed.

Another possible source of referred neck pain is the thoracic spine. Issues in the upper and middle back, such as muscle strains or joint dysfunction, can sometimes manifest as pain in the neck. Furthermore, the facet joints in the cervical spine can refer pain to other areas, including the head, shoulders, and upper back.

Visceral organs, such as the lungs, heart, and gastrointestinal tract, can also cause referred pain in the neck. Cardiac-related pain, such as angina or myocardial infarction (heart attack), can sometimes present with neck pain, as well as pain in the chest, arms, or jaw. Similarly, conditions like gastroesophageal reflux disease (GERD) or lung issues may cause pain that is perceived in the neck region.

To accurately diagnose referred pain, healthcare providers must perform a thorough patient history and physical examination, taking into account any additional symptoms or factors that may point to a non-cervical source of pain. Imaging studies and other diagnostic tests may be necessary to rule out or confirm specific conditions. For example, shoulder X-rays, MRI, or ultrasound might be utilized to assess for rotator cuff injuries, while an electrocardiogram (ECG) could help identify cardiac issues.

Referred pain is an important consideration in the evaluation of neck pain. Identifying the true source of pain is crucial for providing appropriate treatment and relief. A comprehensive diagnostic approach, including a thorough patient history, physical examination, and appropriate diagnostic tests, can help healthcare providers accurately identify the cause of referred pain and develop an effective treatment plan.

In the management of neck pain, a multidisciplinary assessment can be crucial for accurately diagnosing and treating the condition. This approach involves the collaboration of various healthcare providers, including primary care physicians, physical therapists, chiropractors, and pain management specialists, to ensure a comprehensive evaluation and the development of an effective, individualized treatment plan.

Multidisciplinary assessment is particularly beneficial when the underlying cause of neck pain is complex or when conservative treatments have been unsuccessful. The collaboration between healthcare providers allows for a more holistic view of the patient's condition, taking into account different perspectives and expertise to identify the root cause of pain and develop an appropriate treatment plan.

Primary care physicians often serve as the initial point of contact for patients with neck pain, providing an overall assessment and initiating conservative treatments. They may refer patients to other specialists for further evaluation and management if the patient's condition does not improve or worsens.

Physical therapists play a vital role in the assessment and treatment of neck pain, focusing on the biomechanics, posture, muscle imbalances, and functional limitations associated with the condition. They may provide manual therapy, exercises, and other interventions to improve the patient's mobility, strength, and overall function. In addition, physical therapists can educate patients on proper body mechanics, ergonomics, and self-care techniques to prevent the recurrence of neck pain.

Chiropractors specialize in the diagnosis and treatment of musculoskeletal conditions, particularly those involving the spine. They may perform spinal manipulations, soft tissue techniques, and other therapies to address joint restrictions and muscle imbalances that contribute to neck pain. Chiropractors can also offer guidance on posture, ergonomics, and lifestyle modifications to promote spinal health and reduce the risk of future neck pain episodes.

Pain management specialists, such as anesthesiologists or physiatrists, may be involved in the diagnosis and treatment of neck pain when conservative treatments have been unsuccessful or when interventional pain management techniques are indicated. These specialists can provide targeted treatments, such as epidural steroid injections, nerve blocks, or radiofrequency ablation, to alleviate pain and improve function.

Other healthcare providers, such as rheumatologists, neurologists, or orthopedic surgeons, may also be involved in the multidisciplinary assessment and treatment of neck pain, particularly when there is an underlying medical condition, such as rheumatoid arthritis, that requires specialized care.

The role of multidisciplinary assessment in the management of neck pain is to provide a comprehensive and integrated approach to care, incorporating the expertise and perspectives of various healthcare providers to accurately diagnose and treat the condition. This collaborative approach helps to ensure that patients receive the most appropriate and effective care for their individual needs, promoting long-term relief and improved quality of life.

Accurate diagnosis of neck pain is vital for guiding appropriate treatment, as different underlying causes necessitate distinct approaches. Misdiagnosis can result in not only ineffective treatments but also potentially harmful interventions. By recognizing the root cause of neck pain, healthcare providers can tailor treatment plans to address the specific needs of each patient, promoting long-term relief and improved quality of life.

For mechanical neck pain, conservative treatments often form the first line of intervention. Physical therapy plays a crucial role in addressing issues such as muscle imbalances, poor posture, and limited range of motion. A skilled physical therapist can design a personalized exercise program to strengthen the neck muscles, improve flexibility, and promote optimal posture. In addition, manual therapy techniques, such as soft tissue mobilization and joint mobilizations, can help alleviate pain and improve function.

Medication management is another essential component of conservative treatment for mechanical neck pain. Nonsteroidal anti-inflammatory drugs (NSAIDs), analgesics, and muscle relaxants can provide temporary pain relief, allowing patients to engage in physical therapy and other rehabilitative interventions. It is important to note that long-term use of these medications should be approached cautiously, as they can lead to side effects and potential complications.

Lifestyle modifications can also significantly impact the management of mechanical neck pain. Ergonomic adjustments to the home and work environment, including the proper positioning of computer monitors, chairs, and other equipment, can help minimize strain on the cervical spine. Additionally, incorporating regular breaks and stretching exercises throughout the day can help maintain neck mobility and reduce discomfort.

In cases of radiculopathy or myelopathy, where conservative treatments fail to provide relief, surgical intervention may be necessary. Various surgical options exist, including cervical discectomy and fusion, cervical disc replacement, and laminoplasty. The choice of surgery depends on factors such as the severity of the condition, the patient's overall health, and the presence of other comorbidities. Accurate diagnosis is essential for determining the most appropriate surgical intervention and optimizing patient outcomes.

Targeted treatments for specific conditions, such as rheumatoid arthritis or TMJ dysfunction, can also play a crucial role in managing neck pain. In the case of rheumatoid arthritis, disease-modifying antirheumatic drugs

(DMARDs) and biologic agents can help slow disease progression and alleviate pain. Physical therapy and assistive devices may also be beneficial in maintaining joint function and mobility. For TMJ dysfunction, treatment may include oral appliances, medication management, and physical therapy exercises to address jaw muscle imbalances and improve joint function.

Accurate diagnosis of neck pain is essential for guiding appropriate treatment and ensuring optimal patient outcomes. By identifying the root cause of neck pain, healthcare providers can tailor treatment plans to each patient's specific needs, addressing the underlying issue and promoting long-term relief.

In conclusion, the accurate diagnosis of neck pain is an essential aspect of patient care, as it directly influences the choice of treatment and the potential for long-lasting relief. By conducting a thorough patient history, physical examination, and employing appropriate imaging or electrodiagnostic studies, healthcare providers can more effectively identify the root cause of neck pain and make informed treatment decisions. This comprehensive approach helps to avoid misdiagnosis, which could lead to inappropriate or even harmful treatment choices.

Given the wide range of potential causes for neck pain, healthcare providers must exercise diligence and expertise in their diagnostic process. This might involve considering less common causes of neck pain, such as referred pain from other areas of the body, or systemic inflammatory conditions that may present with neck pain as a secondary symptom. By remaining vigilant and open to the possibility of multiple contributing factors, healthcare providers can increase the likelihood of an accurate diagnosis and, subsequently, more effective treatment.

In some cases, a multidisciplinary approach may be necessary to ensure a comprehensive evaluation of a patient's neck pain. Collaboration between various healthcare providers, such as primary care physicians, physical therapists, chiropractors, and pain management specialists, can lead to a more complete understanding of the patient's condition and facilitate the development of an individualized treatment plan. This integrated approach often results in better patient outcomes and promotes a more efficient use of healthcare resources.

Ultimately, accurate diagnosis serves as the foundation for effective neck pain management. By identifying the root cause of a patient's neck pain, healthcare providers can offer targeted and evidence-based treatment options that address the underlying issue, minimize the risk of recurrence, and promote long-term relief. This not only improves the patient's physical well-being but also contributes to their overall quality of life.

In summary, accurate diagnosis plays a crucial role in neck pain management, guiding healthcare providers toward the most appropriate treatment options and promoting optimal patient outcomes. Through diligent diagnostic efforts and, when necessary, multidisciplinary collaboration, healthcare providers can make a meaningful difference in the lives of patients suffering from neck pain, offering them the best chance at long-term relief and improved quality of life.

Chapter 3

Conservative Treatment Approaches

Non-Invasive Methods to Alleviate Neck Pain

Conservative treatment approaches for neck pain primarily focus on non-invasive methods to alleviate discomfort, improve function, and promote healing. These approaches are designed to manage pain and restore the neck's normal range of motion without resorting to surgical intervention. Neck pain can result from various causes, including muscle strain, ligament sprains, joint dysfunction, nerve compression, and degenerative changes in the cervical spine. Identifying the underlying cause of neck pain is essential for selecting the most appropriate conservative treatment method and optimizing outcomes.

One of the most common conservative treatment methods for neck pain is pain medication. Both over-the-counter and prescription

69

medications can help manage pain and inflammation, providing temporary relief and allowing the individual to engage in other rehabilitative therapies. Pain medication is often used in conjunction with other conservative treatments, such as physical therapy, to address the root cause of neck pain and promote long-term recovery.

Physical therapy is another cornerstone of conservative neck pain treatment. A comprehensive physical therapy program can help to improve neck mobility, muscle strength, and endurance, addressing muscle imbalances and joint dysfunction contributing to neck pain. Physical therapy for neck pain often involves a combination of manual therapy techniques, therapeutic exercises, and modalities, such as heat and cold therapy or electrical stimulation. By targeting the specific impairments and limitations of the individual, physical therapy can help to alleviate neck pain and prevent its recurrence.

Heat and cold therapy are widely used conservative treatment methods for managing neck pain, as they provide readily accessible and low-cost options for pain relief. By alternating the application of heat and cold to the affected area, individuals can reduce inflammation, muscle tension, and pain. Understanding the appropriate indications and contraindications for heat and cold therapy, as well as the proper application techniques, is essential for maximizing their therapeutic benefits.

Ergonomic adjustments, including posture correction and modifications to the individual's work and sleep environments, can play a critical role in the conservative management of neck pain. Poor posture and improper ergonomics can place excessive strain on the cervical spine and surrounding muscles, contributing to neck pain and dysfunction. By making targeted adjustments to the individual's daily habits and surroundings, ergonomic interventions can help to reduce neck pain and promote long-term musculoskeletal health.

In addition to these primary conservative treatment methods, other non-invasive approaches, such as transcutaneous electrical nerve stimulation (TENS), acupuncture, and massage therapy, can also be beneficial for managing neck pain. These complementary therapies can help to alleviate pain, promote relaxation, and support the body's natural healing processes. Integrating these therapies into a comprehensive conservative treatment plan can help to optimize outcomes and enhance the individual's overall well-being.

This chapter aims to provide a comprehensive overview of these conservative treatment options, their underlying mechanisms, and the best practices for utilizing each method. By understanding the various conservative treatment approaches for neck pain, individuals and healthcare providers can work together to develop a personalized treatment plan that addresses the specific needs and goals of the individual, leading to improved function, reduced pain, and a better quality of life.

Over-the-counter (OTC) medications are typically the first line of treatment for mild to moderate neck pain. These medications can help reduce pain, inflammation, and muscle tension by targeting different pathways involved in pain perception and inflammation. The most common OTC medications for neck pain management include nonsteroidal anti-inflammatory drugs (NSAIDs), acetaminophen, and topical analgesics.

NSAIDs, such as ibuprofen and naproxen, work by blocking the production of prostaglandins, which are substances that promote inflammation and increase pain sensitivity. These drugs inhibit the cyclooxygenase (COX) enzymes responsible for the synthesis of prostaglandins. NSAIDs are particularly effective in reducing inflammation, making them an ideal choice for neck pain caused by conditions like muscle strains or cervical osteoarthritis.

Acetaminophen, also known as paracetamol, is another common OTC pain reliever. While it is not as effective at reducing inflammation as NSAIDs, it can still provide relief from mild to moderate pain. Acetaminophen works by inhibiting the synthesis of prostaglandins in the central nervous system, which in turn reduces the perception of pain. It can be used alone or in combination with NSAIDs to provide more comprehensive pain relief.

Topical analgesics, such as creams, gels, or patches, can also be used to manage neck pain. These products often contain active ingredients like menthol, camphor, or capsaicin, which work by stimulating nerve endings in the skin, creating a sensation of warmth or coolness and temporarily

71

reducing pain perception. Some topical analgesics also contain NSAIDs, which can provide localized anti-inflammatory effects.

It is essential to follow the recommended dosages for these medications and to be aware of potential side effects. For NSAIDs, common side effects include gastrointestinal issues like heartburn, nausea, and stomach ulcers. In some cases, long-term use of NSAIDs can also lead to kidney damage or increased risk of cardiovascular events. Acetaminophen, when used within recommended dosages, typically has fewer side effects. However, excessive use or combining it with alcohol can lead to liver toxicity.

To minimize the risk of side effects, it is crucial to use OTC pain relievers only as directed and for the shortest duration necessary. Long-term use should be avoided unless prescribed by a healthcare professional, who can monitor the individual's response to the medication and ensure that it is being used safely and effectively. In some cases, a healthcare provider may recommend alternative or additional treatment options to better address the underlying cause of the neck pain.

In cases where over-the-counter (OTC) medications do not provide sufficient relief from neck pain, healthcare providers may consider prescribing stronger medications. Prescription medications for neck pain management can include prescription-strength nonsteroidal anti-inflammatory drugs (NSAIDs), muscle relaxants, and opioids, each with their unique mechanisms of action and potential side effects.

Prescription-strength NSAIDs are similar to their OTC counterparts but have a higher dosage, providing more powerful anti-inflammatory and pain-relieving effects. Examples of prescription-strength NSAIDs include diclofenac, ketorolac, and celecoxib. These medications work by inhibiting the enzymes cyclooxygenase-1 (COX-1) and cyclooxygenase-2 (COX-2), which are responsible for the production of prostaglandins that promote inflammation and increase pain sensitivity. While these medications can be more effective in managing neck pain, they also carry a higher risk of side effects, such as gastrointestinal bleeding, ulcers, and kidney damage. Therefore, prescription-strength NSAIDs should be used with caution and only under the supervision of a healthcare provider.

Muscle relaxants, such as cyclobenzaprine, tizanidine, and baclofen, are another class of prescription medications that can be used for neck pain management. These medications work by acting on the central nervous system to decrease muscle tone and reduce muscle spasms, thereby providing relief from neck pain caused by muscle tension. Muscle relaxants can also help improve the range of motion and overall function of the neck. However, they can cause side effects such as drowsiness, dizziness, and dry mouth. Patients taking muscle relaxants should be monitored for these side effects, and dosage adjustments may be necessary to minimize adverse reactions.

Opioids, such as oxycodone, hydrocodone, and morphine, are potent pain relievers that can be prescribed for severe or persistent neck pain that has not responded to other treatments. Opioids work by binding to specific opioid receptors in the brain and spinal cord, inhibiting the transmission of pain signals and providing pain relief. They can be highly effective in managing severe pain, but due to their potential for addiction, abuse, and side effects, opioids should be prescribed with caution and only for short-term use.

Some common side effects of opioids include drowsiness, dizziness, constipation, and respiratory depression. Opioid-induced respiratory depression can be life-threatening, particularly in patients with pre-existing respiratory conditions or those who take other medications that can suppress respiration. Due to these risks, healthcare providers must closely monitor patients on opioid therapy and make appropriate dosage adjustments to ensure patient safety.

In some cases, healthcare providers may prescribe other types of medications, such as antidepressants or anticonvulsants, to manage neck pain. These medications, particularly tricyclic antidepressants and certain anticonvulsants like gabapentin and pregabalin, have been found to be effective in managing neuropathic pain, which can be a component of neck pain, particularly in cases of cervical radiculopathy. These medications work by modulating pain signaling pathways in the nervous system, providing pain relief without the risks associated with opioids.

Prescription medications can play an essential role in managing neck pain when OTC medications are insufficient. These medications include prescription-strength NSAIDs, muscle relaxants, opioids, and, in some cases, antidepressants or anticonvulsants. Each class of medication has its unique mechanisms of action, potential side effects, and considerations for use. Healthcare providers must carefully evaluate the risks and benefits of each medication, taking into account the individual patient's needs and medical history, to ensure safe and effective neck It is essential for patients to follow their healthcare provider's recommendations regarding the prescribed medication's dosage, frequency, and duration of use. Open communication between the patient and the healthcare provider can help ensure that the chosen medication is effectively managing neck pain while minimizing side effects. Regular follow-up appointments are crucial to monitor the patient's progress, evaluate the medication's effectiveness, and make any necessary adjustments to the treatment plan.

In some cases, a combination of medications may be prescribed to achieve optimal pain relief and address the different mechanisms contributing to neck pain. For instance, a patient may be prescribed a muscle relaxant to reduce muscle spasms and an NSAID to address inflammation. It is essential for patients to inform their healthcare providers of any other medications they are taking, including OTC medications and supplements, to avoid potential drug interactions and adverse effects.

Prescription medications should be used as part of a comprehensive neck pain management plan that may include physical therapy, ergonomic adjustments, and lifestyle modifications. By combining these different approaches, patients can maximize their chances of achieving pain relief, restoring neck function, and preventing future episodes of neck pain.

Prescription medications play a crucial role in the management of neck pain when conservative treatments, such as OTC medications, are insufficient. Through careful evaluation and monitoring by healthcare providers, patients can use prescription medications safely and effectively to manage their neck pain. By incorporating these medications into a comprehensive treatment plan, patients can work towards improved neck function, reduced pain, and an enhanced quality of life.

Manual therapy is a cornerstone of physical therapy and plays a vital role in the management of neck pain. It is a hands-on approach that involves skilled hand movements to manipulate joints and soft tissues, such as muscles, ligaments, and fascia, to alleviate pain, improve mobility, and restore function. Manual therapy techniques are often combined with other physical therapy modalities, such as therapeutic exercise, to address the multifaceted nature of neck pain. This section will provide a detailed overview of some of the primary techniques used in manual therapy for neck pain, including joint mobilization, soft tissue mobilization, and muscle energy techniques.

Joint mobilization is a technique that targets the joints of the cervical spine to reduce pain and improve joint mobility. During joint mobilization, the physical therapist applies gentle, controlled force to move the affected joint through its available range of motion. This technique can help to decrease pain by reducing joint stiffness and increasing joint lubrication. Additionally, joint mobilization can stimulate mechanoreceptors, sensory receptors that respond to mechanical pressure or distortion, leading to a reduction in pain perception and muscle guarding.

Soft tissue mobilization is another manual therapy technique used to address neck pain. This technique focuses on manipulating the muscles, ligaments, and fascia surrounding the cervical spine to reduce tension, break up scar tissue, and promote relaxation. Physical therapists utilize various soft tissue mobilization methods, such as myofascial release, trigger point therapy, and active release techniques. Myofascial release involves applying sustained pressure to the fascia, the connective tissue surrounding muscles, to release restrictions and improve tissue extensibility. Trigger point therapy targets specific, localized areas of muscle tightness or knots, known as trigger points, by applying direct pressure or using specific massage techniques to release tension and alleviate pain. Active release techniques involve a combination of manual pressure and guided movement of the affected muscles to break up adhesions and restore normal tissue function.

Muscle energy techniques (MET) are a unique subset of manual therapy that employs the patient's muscle contractions to improve muscle length, joint mobility, and overall function. In MET, the physical therapist positions the patient in a specific posture and instructs the patient to contract a targeted muscle group against the therapist's resistance. This is followed by a period of relaxation and a gentle, passive stretch of the

75

involved muscles. The process is repeated several times, with each subsequent stretch taking the muscles to a new range of motion. MET can be particularly effective for addressing neck pain related to muscle imbalances, postural dysfunction, and joint restrictions.

Manual therapy is a crucial component of physical therapy for managing neck pain. Techniques such as joint mobilization, soft tissue mobilization, and muscle energy techniques can help reduce muscle tension, improve joint mobility, and promote relaxation. When combined with other physical therapy modalities, manual therapy can play a significant role in alleviating neck pain and restoring function.

Therapeutic exercise is a critical component of physical therapy for neck pain management, aiming to restore and maintain the neck's range of motion, strength, and endurance. A physical therapist may assess an individual's specific needs and limitations before prescribing a personalized combination of stretching, strengthening, and stabilization exercises. This tailored approach ensures that the exercises are both safe and effective for the patient.

Stretching exercises are an essential part of therapeutic exercise for neck pain, as they help to maintain or improve flexibility and alleviate muscle tightness. Some common stretching exercises for the neck include neck flexion, extension, rotation, and lateral flexion. Neck flexion stretches the muscles at the back of the neck, while extension stretches the muscles at the front. Rotation stretches the muscles on either side of the neck, and lateral flexion stretches the muscles running along the side of the neck. It is crucial to perform these stretches slowly and gently, holding each position for 15-30 seconds, to prevent injury and ensure optimal results.

Strengthening exercises are another critical aspect of therapeutic exercise for neck pain management. These exercises aim to improve muscle strength and endurance, which can help support the cervical spine and alleviate pain. Isometric cervical exercises are a form of strengthening exercise that involves applying resistance without moving the joint. For example, an individual may press their hand against their forehead while attempting to flex their neck, creating resistance without actually moving the neck. This type of exercise can help to strengthen the neck muscles without placing excessive strain on the cervical spine.

76

Resistance training is another form of strengthening exercise that can be beneficial for neck pain management. This type of exercise involves using resistance bands or weights to challenge the neck muscles, promoting strength and endurance. Examples of resistance training exercises for the neck include seated rows, lateral raises, and shoulder shrugs. It is crucial to perform these exercises with proper form and technique, as improper execution can lead to further injury or exacerbation of pain.

Stabilization exercises are a vital component of therapeutic exercise for neck pain management, as they help to improve posture and alignment, thereby reducing neck pain. Deep neck flexor training is one example of a stabilization exercise that targets the deep muscles at the front of the neck, which are responsible for maintaining proper cervical spine alignment. To perform this exercise, an individual may lie on their back with their head supported and attempt to tuck their chin in toward their chest without lifting their head off the ground. This exercise should be performed slowly and with control, holding the position for several seconds before relaxing.

Scapular stabilization exercises are another form of stabilization exercise that can be beneficial for neck pain management. These exercises target the muscles around the shoulder blades, which play a crucial role in maintaining proper upper body posture and alignment. Examples of scapular stabilization exercises include scapular squeezes, where the individual attempts to bring their shoulder blades together while keeping their arms relaxed, and scapular retraction, where the individual pulls their shoulder blades back and down. These exercises can help to strengthen the muscles responsible for maintaining proper posture, thereby reducing strain on the neck and alleviating pain.

Therapeutic exercise is a vital aspect of physical therapy for neck pain management, encompassing a range of stretching, strengthening, and stabilization exercises. By incorporating these exercises into a comprehensive treatment plan, individuals with neck pain can improve their range of motion, muscle strength, and posture, ultimately reducing pain and enhancing their overall quality of life.

Heat and cold therapy, also known as thermotherapy and cryotherapy, respectively, are widely used conservative treatment methods for managing neck pain. These modalities can help reduce pain, inflammation, and muscle tension by affecting blood flow, metabolism, and nerve conduction in the treated area. Both heat and cold therapy have distinct therapeutic effects, making them suitable for different types of neck pain and inflammation.

Heat therapy, or thermotherapy, involves the application of heat to the affected area, which can be achieved through various methods such as heating pads, hot water bottles, warm towels, or even warm showers. The application of heat to the painful area can help to increase blood flow, which delivers oxygen and nutrients to the muscles and joints, thereby promoting healing and reducing muscle stiffness. Moreover, heat therapy can stimulate the sensory receptors in the skin, helping to block pain signals from reaching the brain and promoting a sense of relaxation and pain relief.

Heat therapy is particularly beneficial for chronic neck pain, muscle stiffness, and tension, as it can help to relax the muscles, improve range of motion, and decrease joint stiffness. To maximize the benefits of heat therapy, it is generally recommended to apply heat for 15-20 minutes at a time, with a 2-hour break between applications. It is essential to use a barrier, such as a towel or cloth, between the heat source and the skin to prevent burns or skin irritation. Individuals with certain medical conditions, such as diabetes or peripheral vascular disease, should consult with their healthcare provider before using heat therapy, as they may have an increased risk of burns or skin damage.

Cold therapy, or cryotherapy, involves the application of cold to the affected area, typically using ice packs, gel packs, or frozen vegetables. Cold therapy works by causing vasoconstriction, or the narrowing of blood vessels, which helps to reduce inflammation and numb the area, providing pain relief. Additionally, the application of cold can slow down nerve conduction, which may further contribute to pain reduction.

Cold therapy is often more effective for acute neck pain, injuries, or inflammation, as it can help to minimize swelling and prevent further tissue damage. To use cold therapy effectively, it is generally recommended to apply cold for 10-15 minutes at a time, with a 2-hour break between applications. It is crucial to avoid applying ice directly to the skin, as this can cause frostbite or skin damage. Instead, use a barrier such as a towel or cloth between the ice pack and the skin.

In some cases, healthcare providers may recommend alternating between heat and cold therapy, known as contrast therapy. This approach involves the application of heat followed by cold, which can help to improve circulation and promote healing. Contrast therapy can be particularly beneficial in cases of neck pain caused by inflammation, as the alternating temperatures can help to flush out inflammatory by-products and reduce swelling. Typically, the heat is applied for 15-20 minutes, followed by cold for 10-15 minutes, with a 2-hour break between cycles. As with heat and cold therapy, it is essential to use a barrier between the heat or cold source and the skin to prevent burns or skin damage.

Heat and cold therapy are widely used conservative treatment methods for managing neck pain, with each modality providing distinct therapeutic benefits. Heat therapy is particularly effective for chronic neck pain, muscle stiffness, and tension, while cold therapy is more suitable for acute neck pain, injuries, or inflammation. By understanding the underlying mechanisms and appropriate application techniques for heat and cold therapy, individuals suffering from neck pain can work with their healthcare providers to develop an effective treatment plan that includes these modalities.

Heat and cold therapy are widely used conservative treatment methods for managing neck pain. These modalities can help reduce pain, inflammation, and muscle tension.

Heat therapy, or thermotherapy, is a well-established conservative treatment approach for managing neck pain, particularly when it comes to chronic pain or stiffness. By applying heat to the affected area through various methods, such as heating pads, hot water bottles, or warm towels, this therapy offers a range of benefits that can help reduce discomfort and improve the overall function of the neck muscles and joints.

The primary mechanism behind heat therapy is the increase in blood flow to the treated area. When heat is applied to the neck, it causes the blood vessels to dilate, allowing for a higher volume of blood to flow through the region. This enhanced blood flow delivers vital oxygen and nutrients to the muscles and joints, promoting healing and recovery in the affected tissues. The increased temperature also helps to improve the elasticity of the connective tissues, including muscles, tendons, and ligaments, which can further contribute to reduced stiffness and improved range of motion.

Another significant benefit of heat therapy is its ability to promote relaxation in the neck muscles. When the muscles are exposed to heat, they tend to relax, which can help alleviate pain caused by muscle tension or spasms. This relaxation effect can also help improve the overall function of the neck, making it easier to perform daily activities without discomfort.

Heat therapy can be administered in various forms, each with its own advantages and considerations. Electric heating pads are a popular choice due to their convenience and ease of use. These devices typically offer adjustable temperature settings, allowing the user to find a comfortable level of heat. Moist heat, such as that provided by a hot water bottle or warm towel, can penetrate deeper into the tissues, potentially offering more significant relief for some individuals. It is essential to ensure that the heat source is not too hot, as excessive heat can cause burns or skin damage.

When using heat therapy for neck pain, it is important to follow the recommended guidelines to ensure safety and effectiveness. Typically, heat should be applied for 15-20 minutes at a time, allowing for a 2-hour break between applications to prevent overheating the tissues. This duration and frequency can be adjusted based on individual needs and the severity of the neck pain.

Heat therapy should not be used for acute injuries or inflammation, as it may exacerbate the issue by increasing blood flow and swelling. Additionally, individuals with certain medical conditions, such as diabetes, peripheral vascular disease, or open wounds, should consult with a healthcare professional before using heat therapy to ensure that it is safe and appropriate for their specific situation.

Heat therapy is a valuable conservative treatment option for managing chronic neck pain or stiffness. By increasing blood flow, promoting tissue elasticity, and inducing muscle relaxation, this approach can help alleviate discomfort and improve neck function for many individuals. By understanding the underlying mechanisms, advantages, and limitations of heat therapy, patients and healthcare providers can work together to develop an effective and safe treatment plan for neck pain management.

Cold therapy, also known as cryotherapy, is a popular and effective conservative treatment method for alleviating acute neck pain or injuries. The application of cold temperatures to the affected area, typically through the use of ice packs, gel packs, or even frozen vegetables, can provide numerous benefits for those experiencing neck pain.

One of the primary benefits of cold therapy is its ability to constrict blood vessels in the affected area. This vasoconstriction reduces blood flow and, consequently, inflammation. By limiting the inflammatory response, cold therapy can help to minimize swelling and decrease the pressure on nerves, which can contribute to pain relief. In addition to reducing inflammation, the application of cold temperatures also numbs the area, providing a localized anesthetic effect. This numbing sensation can help to block pain signals from reaching the brain, providing further relief from discomfort.

Cold therapy is particularly effective for acute neck pain or injuries that result from sudden trauma, such as whiplash, muscle strains, or ligament sprains. In these cases, the rapid onset of inflammation and swelling can exacerbate pain, making the use of cold therapy a valuable tool for pain management. However, it is important to note that cold therapy may not be as effective for chronic neck pain, which often has a more complex underlying cause and may require a combination of treatment methods.

When applying cold therapy, it is crucial to follow proper guidelines to ensure its effectiveness and prevent potential harm. Cold therapy should be applied for 10-15 minutes at a time, with a 2-hour break between applications to prevent tissue damage from prolonged exposure to cold temperatures. It is essential to avoid applying ice directly to the skin, as this can cause frostbite or skin damage. Instead, use a towel or cloth as a barrier between the ice pack and the skin, ensuring that the cold is applied evenly and safely.

Furthermore, it is crucial to monitor the skin for any signs of adverse reactions, such as redness, blistering, or excessive numbness. If any of these symptoms occur, discontinue cold therapy immediately and consult a healthcare professional. Additionally, individuals with circulatory problems, such as Raynaud's disease, or those with a history of frostbite should exercise caution when using cold therapy and consult with their healthcare provider before beginning this treatment method.

Cold therapy is a valuable conservative treatment option for acute neck pain or injuries. By constricting blood vessels, reducing inflammation, and providing a numbing effect, cold therapy can help to alleviate pain and promote healing. Proper application and adherence to guidelines are essential to maximize the benefits of this treatment method and ensure its safe use.

Poor posture is a common cause of neck pain, as it places additional stress on the cervical spine and surrounding muscles. Correcting one's posture can significantly help alleviate neck pain and prevent its recurrence. Achieving and maintaining proper posture involves several key principles that focus on maintaining a neutral spine position, engaging the core muscles, and fostering body awareness. By following these principles, individuals can distribute the weight of the head evenly and reduce strain on the neck muscles.

The first principle of posture correction is to maintain a neutral spine position, with the ears aligned over the shoulders and the shoulders aligned over the hips. This alignment minimizes the stress placed on the cervical spine and surrounding structures. To achieve this alignment, one should avoid slouching, hunching, or jutting the head forward while standing or sitting. Instead, individuals should focus on elongating the spine, lifting the chest, and relaxing the shoulders.

The second principle involves engaging the core muscles to provide additional support for the spine. The core muscles include the abdominal, pelvic floor, and back muscles, which work together to stabilize the spine and maintain proper posture. To engage the core muscles, individuals should gently draw the navel toward the spine and contract the pelvic floor muscles while maintaining a neutral spine position. This engagement should be maintained throughout the day, particularly when performing tasks that require bending, lifting, or carrying heavy loads.

The third principle of posture correction is fostering body awareness. Developing an awareness of one's posture throughout the day is crucial for identifying and correcting poor postural habits. Regularly checking in with the body's alignment and making adjustments as needed can help individuals maintain proper posture and reduce the risk of neck pain. Simple strategies to improve body awareness include setting reminders to check posture, using mirrors or video feedback to assess alignment, and practicing mindfulness techniques, such as yoga or meditation, which promote body awareness and relaxation.

In addition to these principles, several tools and techniques can be employed to facilitate posture correction. These include the use of lumbar rolls or cushions to support the natural curve of the lower back while sitting, standing desks that promote upright posture, and wearable devices or mobile apps that provide real-time feedback on postural alignment. By incorporating these tools and techniques into their daily routine, individuals can make significant strides toward improving their posture, alleviating neck pain, and preventing future episodes of discomfort.

Creating an ergonomic workstation is essential in reducing neck pain, as it promotes proper posture and minimizes strain on the neck and upper body. There are several key components to consider when setting up an ergonomic workstation, each playing a vital role in maintaining comfort and reducing the risk of neck pain.

One of the critical aspects of an ergonomic workstation is an adjustable chair that supports the natural curve of the spine. A chair with lumbar support helps maintain the spine's natural S-shape, while adjustable armrests can further reduce strain on the shoulders and neck. The chair's height should also be adjusted so that the feet are flat on the ground, and the knees are bent at a 90-degree angle, ensuring that the hips and thighs are parallel to the floor.

A desk at an appropriate height is another crucial element of an ergonomic workstation. The desk should be positioned to minimize reaching or bending, allowing for a comfortable distance between the user and their work equipment. Ideally, the desk should have enough space to accommodate a keyboard and mouse, with the user's elbows bent at a 90-

degree angle when typing. This positioning helps maintain a neutral wrist posture and minimizes strain on the forearms, shoulders, and neck.

The computer monitor's position is equally important in preventing neck pain. It should be positioned at eye level, with the top third of the screen aligned with the user's line of sight. This positioning prevents excessive neck flexion or extension, as the user can look straight ahead without tilting their head up or down. The monitor should also be placed approximately an arm's length away from the user, with the screen tilted slightly upward to reduce glare and minimize eye strain.

Incorporating accessories such as a telephone headset or speakerphone can help further reduce neck strain. These devices allow the user to avoid cradling the phone between the ear and shoulder, which can lead to muscle tension and neck pain. Similarly, using a document holder that positions papers at the same height and angle as the computer screen can help maintain proper neck alignment when reading or referencing materials.

In addition to the aforementioned components, it is essential to take regular breaks and change positions throughout the day. Prolonged sitting can contribute to neck pain and discomfort, so standing up, stretching, and moving around every 30 minutes to an hour can significantly reduce the risk of developing pain. Incorporating a sit-stand workstation or using an adjustable height desk can also help promote movement and postural changes throughout the day.

By paying attention to these critical components of an ergonomic workstation, individuals can significantly reduce the risk of neck pain and discomfort while promoting overall musculoskeletal health. Investing in an ergonomic workstation not only helps alleviate neck pain but can also increase productivity, as users are more likely to remain comfortable and focused on their work.

Sleep ergonomics plays a crucial role in managing neck pain, as the position of the cervical spine and the choice of pillow can significantly impact comfort and support during sleep. Proper sleep ergonomics can help maintain the natural curve of the cervical spine, thereby reducing discomfort and the risk of developing neck pain.

A supportive pillow is essential for maintaining the cervical spine's natural curve and alleviating pressure on the neck muscles and joints. A cervical pillow or a contoured pillow designed for neck pain can provide the necessary support to maintain proper alignment. These pillows often feature a curved design that supports the neck's natural curvature while cradling the head comfortably. The choice of pillow material, such as memory foam or latex, can also impact the level of support and comfort. Memory foam pillows, for instance, mold to the shape of the head and neck, providing personalized support and helping to reduce pressure points. Latex pillows, on the other hand, offer a more consistent level of support and tend to be more durable.

In addition to using a supportive pillow, it is essential to maintain a consistent sleep position that minimizes strain on the neck. The two most recommended sleep positions for individuals with neck pain are back sleeping and side sleeping.

Back sleeping allows the cervical spine to maintain its natural alignment and reduces the risk of developing pressure points. When sleeping on the back, a pillow with a lower loft can help support the neck without causing excessive flexion. Placing a small pillow or rolled-up towel under the neck can further enhance support, helping to maintain the cervical spine's natural curve.

Side sleeping is another suitable sleep position for individuals with neck pain, as it helps maintain the spine's overall alignment from the neck to the lower back. When side sleeping, it is crucial to use a pillow with a higher loft to fill the gap between the head and the mattress, ensuring that the neck remains in a neutral position. A contoured or cervical pillow can provide additional support by conforming to the natural curvature of the neck and head.

It is generally advised to avoid stomach sleeping, as this position can cause excessive neck rotation and extension, leading to increased strain on the cervical spine and surrounding muscles. If transitioning away from stomach sleeping is difficult, using a thin or no pillow can help minimize neck strain while adjusting to a new sleep position.

Proper sleep ergonomics, including the use of a supportive pillow and maintaining a consistent sleep position, can significantly impact neck pain management. By adopting suitable sleep habits, individuals can reduce the risk of developing or exacerbating neck pain, leading to more restful and comfortable sleep.

Transcutaneous Electrical Nerve Stimulation (TENS) is a non-invasive, conservative treatment method that has gained popularity as an adjunctive therapy for various types of pain, including neck pain. TENS involves the application of mild electrical currents to the skin through adhesive electrodes placed on or around the painful area. The underlying principle of TENS is that the electrical stimulation of peripheral nerves can help to block pain signals from reaching the brain, thereby providing pain relief.

The pain-relieving effects of TENS are primarily attributed to two mechanisms: the gate control theory of pain and the release of endogenous opioids. According to the gate control theory, TENS works by stimulating non-painful sensory nerve fibers, which then "close the gate" on pain signals by inhibiting the transmission of these signals through the spinal cord to the brain. This theory suggests that the electrical stimulation provided by TENS can effectively compete with pain signals, reducing the perception of pain.

Another proposed mechanism of action involves the release of endogenous opioids, such as endorphins, by the electrical stimulation of nerves. Endorphins are the body's natural painkillers, binding to opioid receptors in the brain and spinal cord and reducing the perception of pain. This mechanism suggests that TENS may help to alleviate pain by triggering the release of endorphins, which then act to dampen pain signals.

TENS has been studied for its efficacy in reducing neck pain, with mixed results. Some studies have reported positive effects of TENS on neck pain, particularly when used in conjunction with other conservative treatment methods such as physical therapy, medication, and ergonomic adjustments. However, other studies have found no significant difference in pain reduction between TENS and placebo treatments.

Despite these conflicting results, TENS remains a popular adjunctive therapy for neck pain due to its non-invasive nature, low risk of side effects, and potential for pain relief. TENS may be particularly beneficial for individuals who have not responded adequately to other conservative treatments or who wish to avoid the use of medications.

The intensity, frequency, and duration of TENS therapy can be adjusted to suit the individual's needs and tolerance. Generally, the electrical current should be strong enough to produce a tingling or buzzing sensation but not strong enough to cause discomfort or muscle contractions. The frequency of the electrical pulses can range from low-frequency (2-10 Hz) to high-frequency (80-120 Hz), with different frequencies thought to target different pain mechanisms.

The duration of TENS therapy may vary depending on the severity of the neck pain and the individual's response to treatment. Typical treatment sessions last 20-60 minutes and may be administered multiple times per day or on an as-needed basis.

It is essential for individuals using TENS therapy to be educated on the proper placement of electrodes, as well as the appropriate settings and duration for their specific needs. A healthcare professional, such as a physical therapist or physician, can provide guidance on the optimal use of TENS therapy for neck pain.

While TENS therapy is generally considered safe and well-tolerated, there are some precautions and contraindications to be aware of. TENS should not be used in individuals with a pacemaker, as the electrical currents may interfere with the device's function. Additionally, TENS should not be used on broken or irritated skin or applied directly over the eyes, carotid sinus, or other sensitive areas. Pregnant women should consult their healthcare provider before using TENS, as its safety during pregnancy has not been well-established. Individuals with epilepsy, heart conditions, or nerve disorders should also discuss the potential risks and benefits of TENS therapy with their healthcare provider before beginning treatment.

Although TENS therapy is generally considered safe, some individuals may experience mild side effects. The most common side effect is skin irritation or redness at the site of electrode placement, which can often be mitigated by using hypoallergenic electrodes, ensuring the skin is clean and dry before application, and rotating the electrode placement sites. In rare cases, individuals may experience an allergic reaction to the electrode adhesive, which may require the use of alternative electrodes or discontinuation of TENS therapy.

Further research is needed to better understand the efficacy of TENS therapy in managing neck pain and to identify the optimal parameters for treatment. This may include examining the effects of different frequencies, intensities, and durations of TENS therapy, as well as investigating the potential synergistic effects of TENS when combined with other conservative treatment methods. Advances in TENS technology, such as wireless devices and improved electrode materials, may also contribute to enhancing the convenience, comfort, and effectiveness of TENS therapy for neck pain management.

TENS therapy represents a non-invasive, conservative treatment option that may help to alleviate neck pain for some individuals. Although the evidence supporting its efficacy is mixed, TENS therapy may be a valuable adjunctive treatment when used alongside other conservative methods such as physical therapy, medication, and ergonomic adjustments. By understanding the mechanisms of action, potential benefits, and appropriate use of TENS therapy, individuals with neck pain can work with their healthcare providers to develop a comprehensive and personalized treatment plan.

Conservative treatment approaches for neck pain offer numerous non-invasive options that aim to manage discomfort and restore function. These approaches play a critical role in the early stages of neck pain management and can significantly improve the quality of life for those suffering from this condition. As each individual's experience with neck pain is unique, the effectiveness of these treatments may vary. Therefore, it is vital for healthcare providers and patients to work together to develop a comprehensive and personalized treatment plan.

Pain medication, such as over-the-counter and prescription-strength NSAIDs and muscle relaxants, is often the first line of defense in managing neck pain. These medications address inflammation and muscle tension, providing relief from discomfort. However, it is crucial to recognize that long-term use of these medications may have potential side effects, and they should be used judiciously under the guidance of a healthcare professional.

Physical therapy, including manual therapy and therapeutic exercises, addresses the underlying biomechanical issues contributing to neck pain. By improving joint mobility, reducing muscle tension, and promoting relaxation, physical therapy can provide long-lasting relief and help prevent future neck pain episodes. Furthermore, physical therapists can offer valuable guidance on posture correction and ergonomic adjustments, which can significantly reduce the strain on the neck during daily activities, both at work and home.

Heat and cold therapy can be easily administered at home and provide immediate relief for neck pain. By increasing blood flow to the affected area or numbing the pain, these modalities can reduce inflammation and muscle tension. It is essential to understand when and how to use heat and cold therapy effectively to maximize their benefits while avoiding potential harm.

Ergonomic adjustments, such as proper workstation setup and sleep ergonomics, can have a lasting impact on neck pain management. By promoting proper posture and alignment, these adjustments help distribute the weight of the head evenly and reduce strain on the neck muscles. Incorporating ergonomic principles into daily life can significantly improve neck pain and prevent its recurrence.

Transcutaneous electrical nerve stimulation (TENS) therapy is a valuable adjunct to other conservative treatment methods. By stimulating the nerves with mild electrical currents, TENS can help block pain signals from reaching the brain, providing relief from neck pain for some individuals. However, TENS therapy may not be effective for everyone and should be considered as a complementary treatment alongside other conservative approaches.

In conclusion, conservative treatment approaches for neck pain are essential in providing non-invasive options to alleviate discomfort and restore function. By understanding the underlying mechanisms and best practices for each treatment method, individuals suffering from neck pain can work with their healthcare providers to develop a comprehensive and effective treatment plan tailored to their specific needs. In many cases, conservative treatment approaches can lead to significant improvements in neck pain, allowing individuals to return to their daily activities with minimal discomfort and reduced risk of recurrence. These approaches underscore the importance of collaboration between patients and healthcare providers in addressing neck pain and promoting overall well-being.

Chapter 4

Physical Therapy and Rehabilitation

Techniques to Strengthen and Restore Neck Function

Physical therapy plays a crucial role in managing neck pain and improving the quality of life for affected individuals. Neck pain can arise from various causes, including muscle strain, poor posture, disc herniation, whiplash, and degenerative conditions such as osteoarthritis or spinal stenosis. As a non-invasive and holistic approach, physical therapy aims to address the root cause of the pain and employs a range of techniques tailored to each patient's specific needs.

The primary goals of physical therapy for neck pain are to restore neck function, decrease pain, and prevent future episodes of discomfort. To achieve these objectives, physical therapists utilize a combination of passive and active techniques that target the affected structures in the cervical spine and surrounding soft tissues. Passive techniques are those applied by the therapist, such as manual therapy or the use of modalities, while active techniques require the patient's participation, such as therapeutic exercises.

Manual therapy techniques encompass a variety of hands-on approaches, including soft tissue mobilization, joint mobilization, and cervical traction. These techniques aim to alleviate muscle tightness, improve joint mobility, and reduce pressure on the cervical spine, ultimately leading to decreased pain and increased function. In conjunction with manual therapy, physical therapists employ therapeutic exercises designed to improve the patient's range of motion, strengthen supporting muscles, and correct postural imbalances that may be contributing to neck pain.

In addition to manual therapy and therapeutic exercises, physical therapists also utilize various modalities to manage neck pain. These may include heat therapy, cold therapy, electrical stimulation, and ultrasound therapy. Heat and cold therapy can help to relax muscles, increase blood flow, reduce inflammation, and alleviate pain, while electrical stimulation and ultrasound therapy can provide additional pain relief and promote tissue healing.

An essential aspect of physical therapy for neck pain is the development of individualized treatment plans based on a comprehensive assessment of the patient's symptoms, lifestyle, and medical history. This personalized approach ensures that each patient receives the most appropriate interventions for their specific needs and goals, maximizing the effectiveness of the treatment plan. Furthermore, physical therapists emphasize patient education and the development of home exercise programs to empower patients to take an active role in their recovery and prevent future episodes of neck pain.

Physical therapy is a vital component of the comprehensive treatment plan for individuals experiencing neck pain. By employing a combination of manual therapy, therapeutic exercises, and modalities, physical therapists can address the underlying causes of neck pain, restore function, and improve the overall quality of life for affected individuals. With a focus on personalized treatment plans and patient education, physical therapy offers a holistic and non-invasive approach to managing neck pain and preventing future episodes.

The initial evaluation in physical therapy is a crucial step in understanding the patient's neck pain, as it allows the therapist to identify potential contributing factors and create a customized treatment plan. This comprehensive evaluation process involves several components, including the collection of the patient's history, a physical examination, and, when necessary, the use of diagnostic imaging.

The collection of the patient's history is an essential aspect of the initial evaluation. During this stage, the physical therapist will gather information about the patient's symptoms, including the onset, duration, frequency, and intensity of the pain. This may involve the use of pain scales or questionnaires to quantify the patient's pain levels. The therapist will also inquire about any previous episodes of neck pain, past treatments, and their outcomes.

The patient's lifestyle and occupational factors are also relevant, as these can significantly impact neck pain. For instance, a sedentary lifestyle or a job that requires prolonged sitting or repetitive neck movements can contribute to the development or exacerbation of neck pain. The therapist will consider these factors when designing the treatment plan, as addressing these lifestyle and occupational factors may be necessary for long-term pain relief and prevention.

The medical history of the patient is another critical aspect of the initial evaluation. The therapist will ask about any pre-existing medical conditions, previous surgeries or injuries, and the patient's current medication regimen. This information allows the therapist to identify potential contraindications to specific treatment approaches and to consider any comorbidities that may influence the patient's neck pain or treatment outcomes.

The physical examination is the next component of the initial evaluation. During this examination, the physical therapist will assess the patient's range of motion in the cervical spine, including flexion, extension, lateral flexion, and rotation. The therapist will also evaluate the strength of the neck and upper back muscles, as weakness in these muscles can contribute to pain and dysfunction. Postural assessment is another critical aspect of the physical examination, as poor posture can place excessive strain on the cervical spine and surrounding soft tissues.

Palpation of the cervical spine and surrounding soft tissues is an important technique used by the physical therapist during the initial evaluation. By manually examining the patient's neck, the therapist can identify areas of tenderness, muscle spasm, or joint restrictions that may be contributing to the patient's neck pain.

In some cases, the physical therapist may request diagnostic imaging, such as X-rays, MRI, or CT scans, to obtain a clearer understanding of the underlying cause of the patient's neck pain. These imaging studies can help to identify specific structural issues, such as disc herniations, bone spurs, or spinal stenosis, that may be contributing to the patient's symptoms. The therapist will use this information to guide the treatment plan and ensure that the most appropriate interventions are employed.

Overall, the initial evaluation is a comprehensive process that allows the physical therapist to gain a thorough understanding of the patient's neck pain and its potential contributing factors. This information is invaluable in creating a customized treatment plan that addresses the patient's specific needs and optimizes their rehabilitation outcomes.

Establishing realistic and achievable goals for rehabilitation is a crucial aspect of the physical therapy process. By working together with the patient, the physical therapist can better understand the patient's priorities, expectations, and limitations, which will inform the development of an individualized treatment plan.

During the goal-setting process, the therapist and patient will discuss both short-term and long-term objectives. Short-term goals may focus on immediate pain relief, improving range of motion, and reducing muscle stiffness or spasms. Long-term goals, on the other hand, often involve restoring full neck function, enhancing strength and flexibility, improving posture, and preventing future episodes of neck pain.

The therapist will consider several factors when setting these goals, such as the patient's age, general health, occupation, and daily activities. For instance, an office worker who spends long hours in front of a computer may require specific ergonomic adjustments and posture correction exercises, while an athlete may need sport-specific rehabilitation to return to their pre-injury level of performance.

Once goals have been established, the therapist will design a customized treatment plan tailored to the patient's unique needs. This plan will include a combination of evidence-based techniques, such as manual therapy, therapeutic exercises, and adjunctive therapies, to optimize neck function, alleviate pain, and prevent recurrence.

The treatment plan will begin with a focus on pain relief and management, which may involve the use of modalities like heat, cold, or electrical stimulation, as well as gentle manual therapy techniques. As the patient's pain subsides and their tolerance for movement increases, the therapist will gradually introduce therapeutic exercises to improve range of motion, flexibility, and strength. The choice of exercises will be based on the patient's specific deficits and functional limitations, as identified during the initial evaluation.

In addition to addressing the physical aspects of neck pain, the therapist will also consider the patient's psychosocial factors, such as stress, anxiety, and depression, which may contribute to or exacerbate their symptoms. The treatment plan may incorporate strategies for stress management, relaxation techniques, and coping skills to help the patient manage these factors more effectively.

Throughout the course of treatment, the physical therapist will continuously monitor and reassess the patient's progress, making adjustments to the treatment plan as needed. This ongoing evaluation ensures that the patient's goals remain realistic and achievable, and that the treatment plan remains effective in addressing their specific needs. Regular communication between the patient and the therapist is essential to facilitate this process and ensure that the patient remains engaged and committed to their rehabilitation journey.

Soft tissue mobilization (STM) is a fundamental manual therapy technique used by physical therapists to address neck pain and dysfunction. STM focuses on manipulating the muscles, ligaments, and fascia in the cervical region, which can help alleviate discomfort, improve mobility, and enhance the overall function of the neck. This hands-on approach employs a variety of techniques, including gentle pressure, rhythmic stretching, and sustained holds, to target soft tissues that may be contributing to neck pain.

The primary goals of soft tissue mobilization are to release tightness, alleviate muscle spasms, and promote blood flow to the affected area. By applying targeted pressure to specific areas of tension, the therapist can encourage the relaxation of contracted muscles and increase the extensibility of the surrounding connective tissue. This can result in improved muscle balance and reduced strain on the cervical spine. Additionally, promoting blood flow to the area helps deliver essential nutrients and oxygen, which can support the healing process and reduce inflammation.

Soft tissue mobilization can also help to break up scar tissue and adhesions that may be contributing to neck pain. Scar tissue and adhesions are the body's natural response to injury and can form as a result of trauma, surgery, or chronic inflammation. While these formations help to stabilize and protect the injured area, they can also lead to restricted movement, decreased tissue flexibility, and increased pain. By using specialized STM techniques, such as cross-friction massage and myofascial release, the therapist can gently break down these restrictive structures and restore normal tissue mobility.

It is essential to note that the effectiveness of soft tissue mobilization depends on the skill and expertise of the therapist, as well as the patient's individual needs and tolerance. To achieve optimal results, the therapist must use appropriate techniques and pressure, tailored to the patient's comfort level and specific condition. Furthermore, ongoing communication between the therapist and the patient is crucial to ensure that the treatment remains effective and comfortable throughout the process.

Soft tissue mobilization is a valuable manual therapy technique that can help alleviate neck pain and improve mobility by addressing tight muscles, ligaments, and fascia in the cervical region. By using targeted pressure and stretching techniques, the therapist can release tension, promote blood flow, and break up scar tissue and adhesions, ultimately enhancing neck function and reducing discomfort.

Joint mobilization is a widely used manual therapy technique that focuses on restoring normal movement in the cervical spine by addressing joint restrictions and stiffness. This technique involves the physical therapist applying controlled, passive movements to the cervical vertebrae to increase joint mobility, decrease stiffness, and ultimately improve overall neck function.

Joint mobilization techniques are based on the principles of biomechanics and joint kinematics. The therapist uses their understanding of joint anatomy, the direction of joint movement, and the patient's specific condition to choose the most appropriate technique for each situation. These techniques are designed to target specific joint restrictions and improve the overall quality and range of motion in the cervical spine.

There are various grades of joint mobilization, ranging from gentle oscillations to more forceful, sustained stretches. The choice of technique depends on the patient's tolerance, the therapist's assessment, and the desired outcome. For instance, lower-grade techniques, such as Grade I and II oscillations, are typically used to alleviate pain and muscle guarding. These gentle oscillations can help to stimulate mechanoreceptors in the joint capsule, which in turn can reduce pain and promote relaxation.

Higher-grade techniques, such as Grade III and IV mobilizations, are used to improve joint mobility and range of motion. Grade III mobilizations involve more significant joint movement and are performed at the end of the available range, while Grade IV mobilizations involve small amplitude movements within the restricted range. These higher-grade techniques can help to break up adhesions, stretch tight joint capsules, and mobilize restricted joint surfaces, ultimately leading to improved joint mobility and decreased stiffness.

Joint mobilization should be performed by a skilled physical therapist who has undergone specialized training in manual therapy techniques. It is essential for the therapist to continuously monitor the patient's response to treatment, as well as to adjust the intensity and duration of the mobilization based on the patient's tolerance and feedback. In some cases, joint mobilization may be contraindicated, such as in instances of joint instability, acute inflammation, or severe osteoporosis. The therapist will carefully assess the appropriateness of joint mobilization based on the patient's specific condition and medical history.

Joint mobilization is an effective manual therapy technique used to address joint restrictions and stiffness in the cervical spine. By applying controlled, passive movements to the cervical vertebrae, physical therapists can help to increase joint mobility, decrease stiffness, and improve overall neck function. When performed correctly and tailored to the patient's specific needs, joint mobilization can be an essential component of a comprehensive treatment plan for individuals experiencing neck pain.

Cervical traction is a widely used technique in physical therapy that focuses on relieving pressure on the cervical spine by gently stretching the neck. This method has been proven effective in addressing various neck conditions, such as cervical radiculopathy, degenerative disc disease, and muscle spasms. It works by creating space between the cervical vertebrae, which can help to decompress the discs, alleviate pressure on nerve roots, and reduce muscle tension.

There are two main types of cervical traction: manual and mechanical. Manual cervical traction is performed by the physical therapist using their hands to apply a controlled force to the patient's head, gradually stretching the neck. The therapist will carefully monitor the patient's response to the traction and adjust the force accordingly to ensure comfort and safety. This type of traction can be performed in various positions, such as sitting or lying down, depending on the patient's specific needs and preferences.

Mechanical cervical traction utilizes specialized devices to apply a consistent, controlled force to the neck. These devices can range from over-the-door pulley systems to more sophisticated motorized units. Some mechanical traction devices are designed for use in a clinical setting under the supervision of a physical therapist, while others are intended for home use, allowing the patient to perform traction independently as part of their home exercise program. When using a mechanical traction device, the physical therapist will provide the patient with detailed instructions on proper setup, positioning, and the appropriate amount of force to be applied.

The effectiveness of cervical traction depends on various factors, including the patient's specific condition, the cause of their neck pain, and the duration and frequency of traction sessions. In general, traction is most effective when used in conjunction with other physical therapy techniques, such as manual therapy, therapeutic exercises, and patient education on proper body mechanics and posture.

It is crucial to note that cervical traction is not suitable for all patients. Certain conditions, such as spinal instability, acute neck injuries, or the presence of certain medical devices, may contraindicate the use of traction. The physical therapist will carefully assess the patient's specific condition and medical history to determine if cervical traction is an appropriate and safe intervention. In some cases, the therapist may need to consult with the patient's primary healthcare provider or a specialist before initiating traction therapy.

Cervical traction is a valuable technique for alleviating pressure on the cervical spine and addressing various neck conditions. By decompressing the cervical discs, reducing pressure on nerve roots, and relieving muscle spasms, traction can significantly contribute to improving a patient's neck function and reducing pain. As part of a comprehensive physical therapy program, cervical traction can enhance the overall quality of life for individuals experiencing neck pain. However, it is essential for the physical therapist to carefully assess each patient's specific condition and needs to ensure the safe and effective application of this technique.

The goal of range of motion exercises is to improve the neck's mobility and flexibility, which is essential for maintaining proper cervical spine function and preventing stiffness and pain. These exercises involve moving the head and neck through their full range of motion, including flexion, extension, lateral flexion, and rotation.

During flexion exercises, patients are guided to gently tilt their head forward, bringing their chin towards their chest. This movement stretches the muscles of the neck and upper back and helps to maintain flexibility in the cervical spine. Extension exercises involve moving the head backward, looking up towards the ceiling. This motion can help to stretch and strengthen the muscles in the front of the neck.

Lateral flexion exercises require patients to tilt their head to one side, attempting to touch their ear to their shoulder without raising the shoulder. This movement can help to improve the mobility of the cervical spine and stretch the muscles on the side of the neck. Rotation exercises involve turning the head from side to side, as if looking over each shoulder. This motion helps to maintain the cervical spine's ability to rotate and engages the muscles responsible for stabilizing the neck.

The therapist may guide the patient through these movements or instruct the patient to perform them independently, depending on the individual's comfort level and the therapist's assessment of the patient's needs. In some cases, the therapist may use manual resistance to facilitate improvements in range of motion. This technique involves the therapist gently applying pressure against the patient's head as they perform the range of motion exercises, which can help to increase the challenge of the exercise and promote greater improvements in flexibility and mobility.

To ensure safety and effectiveness, range of motion exercises should be performed in a controlled and slow manner, with the focus on maintaining proper form and alignment. Patients should avoid forcing their neck into uncomfortable or painful positions, as this can exacerbate symptoms and impede progress. It is also important to note that individual results may vary, and some patients may require more time and practice to achieve significant improvements in their neck's range of motion.

Incorporating range of motion exercises into a physical therapy program for neck pain can help to alleviate symptoms and improve overall neck function. By regularly practicing these exercises, patients can maintain their cervical spine's flexibility and mobility, reducing the risk of recurrent neck pain and stiffness.

Strengthening exercises play a vital role in the rehabilitation of neck pain, as they target the muscles responsible for supporting the cervical spine. These muscles include the deep neck flexors, extensors, and the muscles of the upper back and shoulders. By improving the strength and endurance of these muscles, patients can maintain proper posture, reduce strain on the cervical spine, and decrease the risk of recurring neck pain.

Isometric exercises are a type of strengthening exercise that involves contracting the muscles without moving the joints. These exercises can be particularly beneficial for individuals experiencing neck pain, as they help to stabilize the cervical spine and minimize excessive movement. An example of an isometric exercise for the neck is the chin tuck, where the patient gently presses their head backward while maintaining a neutral position, as if trying to create a double chin. This exercise targets the deep neck flexors and can be performed in various positions, such as sitting or lying down.

Dynamic strengthening exercises are essential in a comprehensive rehabilitation program for neck pain, as they challenge the muscles of the cervical spine and surrounding regions. These exercises aim to improve muscle coordination, balance, and functional strength, which contribute to maintaining proper neck posture and preventing neck pain.

One such exercise is scapular retraction, which targets the muscles of the upper back and shoulders. These muscles play a crucial role in maintaining proper neck posture by supporting the cervical spine. To perform scapular retraction, the patient pulls their shoulder blades back and down, as if trying to squeeze them together, while maintaining a neutral neck position. This movement can be performed in various positions, such as standing, sitting, or lying on one's back, allowing the patient to practice the exercise in different settings and postures. Regular practice of scapular retraction can help to reinforce proper posture, reducing the risk of neck pain and promoting overall spinal health.

Another dynamic strengthening exercise that focuses on the neck extensors, which support the back of the cervical spine, is cervical extension. The patient gently extends their neck backward, lifting the chin upward while maintaining proper alignment. This exercise can be performed in various positions, such as sitting, standing, or lying on one's back with a rolled towel or small pillow under the neck for support. By strengthening the neck extensors, the cervical extension exercise helps to improve neck stability and support the natural curvature of the cervical spine.

The prone cobra exercise is another example of a dynamic strengthening exercise that targets the neck extensors and the muscles of the upper back and shoulders. To perform this exercise, the patient lies face down with their arms by their sides and their forehead resting on a small towel or pillow. They then lift their head, neck, and shoulders off the floor, squeezing their shoulder blades together and extending the neck. This movement engages the neck extensors, as well as the muscles of the upper back and shoulders, improving overall neck strength and stability. The patient should maintain a neutral spine and avoid excessive extension in the lower back to ensure proper form and minimize the risk of injury.

Incorporating dynamic strengthening exercises into a rehabilitation program for neck pain can lead to significant improvements in muscle coordination, balance, and functional strength. These exercises help to create a strong foundation for maintaining proper neck posture, reducing the risk of future neck pain and promoting overall spinal health. Physical therapists will carefully select and adjust these exercises based on the patient's individual needs and progress, ensuring optimal outcomes and long-term benefits.

Poor posture is a common contributing factor to neck pain, often resulting from prolonged periods of sitting or standing in improper positions, such as working at a computer or looking down at a smartphone. Over time, these positions can lead to muscle imbalances, strain on the cervical spine, and neck pain. Postural correction exercises aim to retrain and strengthen the muscles responsible for maintaining proper alignment of the cervical spine, ultimately reducing strain and discomfort.

Postural correction exercises focus on various muscle groups to ensure proper neck alignment. These exercises often target the muscles of the upper back and shoulders, such as the trapezius, rhomboids, and serratus anterior, as well as the deep neck flexors, including the longus colli and longus capitis. By strengthening these muscles, patients can improve their posture and reduce the likelihood of neck pain caused by poor alignment.

One common postural correction exercise is the chin tuck, which targets the deep neck flexors. To perform a chin tuck, the patient sits or stands with their back against a wall, ensuring that their head is also touching the wall. The patient then gently tucks their chin in towards their chest, creating a double chin, while maintaining contact between the back of their head and the wall. This position should be held for a few seconds before relaxing and repeating the exercise. Chin tucks can help to strengthen the deep neck flexors and promote proper cervical alignment.

Another effective postural correction exercise is the scapular retraction, which focuses on the muscles of the upper back and shoulders. To perform scapular retractions, the patient sits or stands with their arms relaxed at their sides. They then draw their shoulder blades together, as if trying to pinch a pencil between them, and hold this position for a few seconds before relaxing. This exercise can be repeated several times to strengthen the muscles responsible for maintaining proper shoulder and upper back positioning.

Thoracic extension exercises can also help to improve posture and alleviate neck pain by addressing stiffness in the mid and upper back. One simple thoracic extension exercise involves sitting on a chair with a rolled-up towel or foam roller placed vertically along the spine. The patient then places their hands behind their head and gently extends their upper back over the towel or roller, focusing on moving through the thoracic spine rather than the lower back or neck. This exercise can be performed in a series of repetitions, gradually increasing the range of motion as the patient becomes more comfortable.

In addition to these specific exercises, patients should also be educated on proper ergonomics and body mechanics in their daily activities. This may include adjusting the height of their computer monitor, using a lumbar roll for support when sitting, and practicing good lifting techniques. These lifestyle modifications, combined with postural correction exercises, can help to alleviate neck pain and prevent future episodes caused by poor posture.

By incorporating postural correction exercises into a rehabilitation program, patients can reduce strain on the cervical spine, alleviate neck pain, and prevent future episodes. It is important for patients to perform these exercises consistently and with proper technique to achieve optimal results. Physical therapists can provide guidance and support, helping patients to develop good postural habits that will benefit them in the long term.

Neuromuscular retraining is an essential aspect of physical therapy for individuals with neck pain, as it aims to reestablish proper movement patterns and muscle activation to improve overall neck function. This approach can be particularly beneficial for patients who have developed compensatory patterns of movement due to pain or dysfunction. These compensatory patterns can lead to muscle imbalances and further strain on the cervical spine, exacerbating neck pain and potentially leading to chronic issues. Therefore, neuromuscular retraining plays a crucial role in addressing these imbalances and promoting long-term pain relief.

One key component of neuromuscular retraining is proprioceptive exercises. Proprioception is the body's ability to sense its position and movements in space, which is essential for maintaining balance, coordinating movements, and performing daily activities safely and efficiently. Proprioceptive exercises aim to improve the patient's awareness of their body's position in space, focusing on joint position sense and muscle activation patterns. Examples of proprioceptive exercises for neck pain may include maintaining proper head and neck alignment while performing various movements or tasks, such as reaching overhead or turning the head to look over the shoulder. The therapist may also use tactile cues or verbal feedback to guide the patient in refining their proprioceptive abilities.

Another vital aspect of neuromuscular retraining is motor control exercises. These exercises focus on coordinating muscle activation and movement patterns to improve overall neck function. Motor control exercises aim to target the deep cervical stabilizing muscles, which play a significant role in maintaining proper alignment of the cervical spine and controlling head and neck movements. These exercises may include performing isolated contractions of specific neck muscles, such as the deep neck flexors, while maintaining proper head and neck alignment. Additionally, motor control exercises may involve integrating neck muscle activation into more complex movements or functional tasks, such as lifting objects or turning the head while walking.

Neuromuscular retraining is a progressive process, and the therapist will carefully guide the patient through increasingly challenging exercises as their abilities and confidence improve. The goal is to help the patient develop the skills, strength, and endurance necessary to perform daily activities without experiencing pain or exacerbating their neck symptoms. By addressing compensatory movement patterns, muscle imbalances, and proprioceptive deficits, neuromuscular retraining can play a crucial role in the successful rehabilitation of individuals with neck pain and contribute to their long-term well-being.

Heat and cold therapy are commonly used in physical therapy to manage pain and inflammation, as both modalities can provide therapeutic benefits depending on the patient's specific condition and stage of recovery.

Heat therapy, which includes the use of hot packs, warm towels, and heating pads, is effective in relaxing tight muscles and reducing pain. When applied to the affected area, heat increases blood flow, delivering vital oxygen and nutrients to the tissues while promoting the removal of metabolic waste products. This increase in blood flow can help to facilitate the healing process and improve the overall flexibility of the soft tissues surrounding the cervical spine. In addition, heat therapy can aid in reducing muscle spasms and decreasing the sensitivity of nerve endings, resulting in decreased pain perception.

Cold therapy, which involves the use of ice packs, cold gel packs, or ice massage, is particularly beneficial for reducing inflammation and swelling in acute injuries or flare-ups of neck pain. The cooling effect of cold therapy constricts blood vessels, reducing blood flow to the affected area, which in turn helps to minimize inflammation and limit the extent of tissue damage. Cold therapy also has a numbing effect on the area, providing temporary pain relief by slowing down nerve conduction and reducing the perception of pain.

In many cases, physical therapists may recommend a combination of heat and cold therapy, known as contrast therapy, to optimize therapeutic benefits. Contrast therapy alternates between hot and cold applications, which helps to create a pumping action in the blood vessels that can enhance circulation, reduce edema, and promote tissue healing.

When employing heat or cold therapy, it is essential to consider proper application methods and precautions. For instance, heat and cold modalities should never be applied directly to the skin, as this can result in burns or frostbite. Instead, a barrier such as a towel or cloth should be placed between the skin and the heat or cold source. Additionally, the duration of each application should generally be limited to 15-20 minutes, with breaks in between to allow the skin to return to its normal temperature.

The physical therapist will determine the most appropriate use of heat and cold therapy based on the patient's specific condition, the stage of recovery, and individual preferences. It is crucial for patients to follow their therapist's recommendations and closely monitor their response to these modalities to ensure safe and effective treatment.

Electrical stimulation is a versatile modality that encompasses various techniques, such as transcutaneous electrical nerve stimulation (TENS), neuromuscular electrical stimulation (NMES), and interferential current (IFC). These non-invasive methods can be effectively used to manage neck pain, support muscle function, and promote healing.

Transcutaneous electrical nerve stimulation (TENS) is one of the most widely used forms of electrical stimulation for pain management. This technique involves the application of a low-voltage electrical current to the skin via electrodes placed on or around the painful area. The electrical current is thought to interfere with pain signals being sent to the brain, thereby reducing the perception of pain. This process, known as the gate control theory, suggests that TENS can effectively "close the gate" on pain signals, preventing them from reaching the central nervous system.

In addition to its pain-blocking effects, TENS can also stimulate the release of endorphins, the body's natural pain-relieving chemicals. Endorphins are neurotransmitters that interact with opioid receptors in the brain, producing analgesic effects similar to those of opioid medications. By enhancing the release of endorphins, TENS can provide an additional level of pain relief for patients experiencing neck pain.

Neuromuscular electrical stimulation (NMES) is another form of electrical stimulation that targets muscle function rather than pain modulation. NMES involves the application of an electrical current to the skin via electrodes placed on the target muscles, causing them to contract. This technique can be particularly beneficial for patients with muscle weakness or imbalances due to neck pain or associated conditions, such as cervical radiculopathy. By promoting muscle activation and strengthening, NMES can help to restore normal movement patterns and reduce the risk of further injury.

Interferential current (IFC) is a form of electrical stimulation that uses two separate currents to generate a deeper, more focused effect within the tissues. The intersecting currents create an interference pattern, which is thought to penetrate deeper into the muscles and provide more effective pain relief compared to TENS alone. IFC may be particularly useful for patients with chronic neck pain or those who have not responded adequately to TENS treatment.

It is important to note that electrical stimulation is not suitable for all patients. Contraindications for the use of electrical stimulation include the presence of a pacemaker or other implanted electronic devices, broken or irritated skin, and certain medical conditions, such as epilepsy or deep vein thrombosis. The physical therapist will carefully assess the appropriateness of electrical stimulation for each patient based on their specific condition and medical history.

Electrical stimulation is a valuable tool in the management of neck pain, offering multiple techniques for pain relief and muscle function improvement. By incorporating electrical stimulation into a comprehensive treatment plan, physical therapists can enhance the effectiveness of their interventions and help patients achieve optimal outcomes in their rehabilitation journey.

Ultrasound therapy is a non-invasive modality used in physical therapy to treat various musculoskeletal conditions, including neck pain. It works by utilizing high-frequency sound waves to generate heat within the body's tissues. When applied to the cervical region, ultrasound therapy can offer several therapeutic benefits, such as increasing blood flow, reducing muscle spasms, and promoting healing.

The therapist applies a handheld device called an ultrasound transducer to the skin over the affected area. A water-soluble gel is used to facilitate better contact between the transducer and the skin, ensuring that the sound waves can penetrate the tissues effectively. The sound waves emitted by the transducer are absorbed by the body's tissues, resulting in a warming effect at the cellular level. This process, called deep heating, can improve the extensibility of collagen fibers, relax tight muscles, and enhance blood flow to the treated area. The increased blood flow delivers oxygen and nutrients to the injured tissues while also promoting the removal of waste products, thus facilitating the healing process.

In addition to its thermal effects, ultrasound therapy can also produce non-thermal effects, which are primarily attributed to a phenomenon called cavitation. Cavitation occurs when the sound waves create microscopic gas bubbles in the body's tissues that expand and contract rapidly. This process can stimulate cell membranes, increase cellular activity, and promote tissue repair.

Ultrasound therapy can be administered in two primary modes: continuous and pulsed. Continuous ultrasound delivers a constant flow of sound waves, providing a more pronounced thermal effect. In contrast, pulsed ultrasound alternates between periods of sound wave emission and periods of rest, offering a more gentle treatment with reduced thermal effects. The choice between continuous and pulsed ultrasound depends on the patient's specific condition and the desired therapeutic outcome.

Although ultrasound therapy can be beneficial for many patients with neck pain, it is not suitable for everyone. Certain medical conditions and factors may contraindicate its use. For instance, patients with deep vein thrombosis, malignancy, or active infection should not receive ultrasound therapy. Additionally, ultrasound should not be applied over areas with impaired sensation, open wounds, or fractures. Furthermore, it is generally not recommended for patients with implanted devices, such as pacemakers, as the sound waves may interfere with the function of these devices.

Ultrasound therapy can be a valuable tool in the management of neck pain when used as part of a comprehensive physical therapy program. By generating heat within the body's tissues and stimulating cellular activity, it can help to alleviate muscle tightness, increase blood flow, and promote the healing process. However, it is essential to consider each patient's unique needs and medical history when determining the appropriateness of ultrasound therapy in their treatment plan.

An essential component of physical therapy for neck pain is patient education. This involves not only teaching patients the exercises they need to perform but also helping them understand the importance of proper body mechanics, posture, and ergonomic principles in preventing future episodes of neck pain.

One aspect of patient education involves instructing patients on proper body mechanics, which refers to the way individuals use their bodies to perform daily activities efficiently and safely. This can include lifting objects correctly, turning the head and neck with care, and maintaining a neutral spine position during various tasks. By learning and implementing proper body mechanics, patients can minimize the risk of aggravating their neck pain or causing new injuries.

Posture education is another vital component of patient education. The therapist will work with the patient to identify and correct any postural imbalances that may be contributing to neck pain. This may involve retraining the muscles responsible for maintaining proper alignment of the cervical spine, as well as addressing any muscular imbalances in the upper back and shoulders. Patients will learn techniques to maintain proper posture while sitting, standing, and sleeping. For example, they may be instructed to keep their computer screens at eye level, use lumbar rolls to support their lower back while sitting, or utilize a cervical pillow to maintain optimal neck alignment during sleep.

Ergonomic principles are also an essential part of patient education. The therapist will assess the patient's work environment and provide recommendations for modifications to reduce strain on the neck. These recommendations may include adjusting the height of the chair and desk, using a headset for phone calls, or taking regular breaks to stretch and move throughout the workday. By implementing these ergonomic strategies, patients can create a workspace that minimizes stress on the cervical spine and reduces the risk of neck pain.

In addition to providing education on body mechanics, posture, and ergonomics, the therapist will also develop a tailored home exercise program for the patient. This program will include a combination of stretching, strengthening, and postural correction exercises that the patient can perform independently at home. Stretching exercises will focus on improving the flexibility of the muscles and soft tissues surrounding the cervical spine, while strengthening exercises will target the muscles that support the neck and upper back. Postural correction exercises will help to retrain the muscles responsible for maintaining proper spinal alignment and reinforce the principles learned during therapy sessions.

Adherence to the home exercise program is crucial for maintaining the gains made during therapy sessions and ensuring long-term improvements in neck function and pain reduction. The therapist will provide the patient with clear instructions, demonstrations, and any necessary handouts or resources to support the successful completion of the home exercise program. The patient should maintain open communication with their therapist regarding any challenges or concerns they may have about their home exercise program. By being proactive and taking responsibility for their recovery, patients can maximize the benefits of physical therapy and achieve lasting improvements in their neck function and overall quality of life.

Monitoring the patient's progress throughout the course of treatment is essential in ensuring the effectiveness of the physical therapy plan for neck pain. The physical therapist will use various assessment tools and outcome measures to track changes in the patient's range of motion, strength, and pain levels during the rehabilitation process. This ongoing evaluation allows the therapist to make necessary adjustments to the treatment plan, ensuring that the patient's goals are met and that optimal outcomes are achieved.

One of the key components of progress monitoring is reassessing the patient's range of motion. The physical therapist will periodically measure the patient's neck flexibility in all directions, comparing these measurements to baseline values obtained during the initial evaluation. Improvements in range of motion can be indicative of reduced stiffness, increased mobility, and overall progress in the patient's recovery.

Strength assessment is another critical aspect of progress monitoring. The physical therapist will evaluate the strength of the muscles that support the cervical spine, including the deep neck flexors, extensors, and the muscles of the upper back and shoulders. By tracking changes in muscle strength over time, the therapist can determine the effectiveness of the prescribed strengthening exercises and make adjustments as needed.

Monitoring pain levels is also an important aspect of evaluating progress in physical therapy. The physical therapist will regularly ask the patient to rate their pain on a scale, such as the Visual Analog Scale (VAS) or the Numeric Pain Rating Scale (NPRS). These self-reported pain ratings can provide valuable insight into the patient's subjective experience of pain, allowing the therapist to determine the effectiveness of various treatment techniques and make modifications as necessary.

In addition to these assessments, various outcome measures can be used to quantify improvements in neck function and overall quality of life. The Neck Disability Index (NDI) is a widely used outcome measure that evaluates the patient's self-reported disability related to neck pain. The NDI consists of 10 items addressing various aspects of daily living, including pain intensity, personal care, lifting, reading, headaches, concentration, work, driving, sleeping, and recreation. The patient rates their level of disability for each item on a scale, with higher scores indicating greater disability. By comparing NDI scores over time, the physical therapist can assess the patient's progress and the effectiveness of the treatment plan.

Another valuable outcome measure is the Patient-Specific Functional Scale (PSFS). The PSFS is a self-report measure that allows patients to identify specific activities that are limited or restricted due to neck pain. The patient rates their ability to perform each activity on a scale, with higher scores indicating better function. The PSFS is a useful tool for monitoring functional improvements in the context of the patient's individual goals and priorities.

These outcome measures, combined with the ongoing assessments of range of motion, strength, and pain levels, can help both the therapist and the patient to track progress and determine the effectiveness of the treatment plan. By carefully monitoring the patient's progress and making necessary adjustments to the treatment plan, the physical therapist can ensure that the patient achieves the best possible outcomes in their recovery from neck pain.

Determining the appropriate duration and frequency of physical therapy sessions for neck pain is a critical aspect of designing an effective treatment plan. The individual needs of the patient, the severity of their neck pain, and the underlying cause of their symptoms will all play a significant role in shaping the course of therapy. In this section, we will discuss the factors

111

that influence the duration and frequency of physical therapy for neck pain and the typical progression of treatment.

One of the primary factors influencing the duration and frequency of physical therapy sessions is the patient's individual needs. Each patient will present with a unique set of symptoms, functional limitations, and treatment goals. The physical therapist will consider these factors when designing a treatment plan tailored to the patient's specific requirements. For instance, a patient with severe neck pain and limited range of motion may require more frequent sessions initially, while a patient with mild pain and fewer functional limitations may benefit from a less intensive therapy schedule.

The severity of the patient's neck pain is another important consideration in determining the duration and frequency of physical therapy sessions. Patients with severe or chronic neck pain may require more intensive and prolonged treatment to address the underlying causes of their symptoms and restore neck function. In such cases, the patient may attend therapy sessions two to three times per week for several months or even longer. Conversely, patients with mild or acute neck pain may experience rapid improvements in their symptoms and may only require a few weeks of therapy sessions.

The underlying cause of the patient's neck pain is also a crucial factor in determining the duration and frequency of physical therapy. Some causes of neck pain, such as muscle strains or poor posture, may respond more quickly to therapy than others, like herniated discs or degenerative disc disease. In cases where the cause of neck pain is more complex or persistent, the physical therapist may need to adjust the therapy plan accordingly, incorporating additional techniques or modalities to address the specific issue.

As the patient progresses through their physical therapy program and demonstrates improvements in neck function and pain levels, the frequency of therapy sessions may be reduced. This reduction in frequency allows the patient to transition from a therapist-guided program to a more independent approach, emphasizing the importance of a home exercise program and self-management strategies. By gradually reducing the frequency of therapy sessions, the physical therapist can empower the patient to take greater ownership of their recovery and equip them with the knowledge, skills, and confidence to manage their neck pain independently.

Ultimately, the goal of physical therapy for neck pain is to help the patient achieve their treatment goals, restore neck function, and prevent future episodes of discomfort. The duration and frequency of physical therapy sessions will vary for each individual but will be guided by the patient's needs, the severity of their pain, and the underlying cause of their symptoms. By carefully considering these factors and adapting the treatment plan as needed, physical therapists can optimize the patient's recovery and improve their overall quality of life.

In conclusion, physical therapy plays a critical role in the management and treatment of neck pain, offering a safe and effective approach to addressing a wide range of cervical issues. By leveraging a combination of manual therapy techniques, therapeutic exercises, and modalities, physical therapists can develop personalized treatment plans designed to restore neck function, alleviate pain, and prevent the recurrence of discomfort.

The comprehensive assessment conducted by physical therapists ensures that each patient receives a treatment plan tailored to their specific needs and goals. This individualized approach not only addresses the underlying cause of neck pain but also takes into account factors such as the patient's lifestyle, occupation, and overall health. As a result, physical therapy can lead to significant improvements in patients' overall quality of life, enabling them to return to their daily activities with less pain and discomfort.

Patient engagement and active participation in the rehabilitation process are crucial to achieving optimal outcomes. Adhering to a prescribed home exercise program, for instance, is essential in reinforcing the progress made during in-person therapy sessions and maintaining the gains achieved over the long term. Regularly performing these exercises can help patients build strength, improve flexibility, and ultimately minimize the risk of future neck pain episodes.

Open communication between patients and their physical therapists is also of paramount importance. By discussing their concerns, asking questions, and providing feedback, patients can help therapists fine-tune treatment plans and better address their individual needs. Moreover, maintaining a strong therapeutic alliance can lead to better adherence to treatment recommendations and improved patient satisfaction.

Furthermore, as research into the field of physical therapy continues to evolve, new techniques and approaches are being developed to enhance the effectiveness of neck pain treatment. Staying informed about these advancements and incorporating evidence-based practices into physical therapy sessions can further improve patient outcomes and overall satisfaction with the rehabilitation process.

In summary, physical therapy offers a multifaceted and patient-centered approach to treating neck pain, providing individuals with the tools and knowledge necessary to manage their symptoms and improve their overall quality of life. By engaging in the process, adhering to home exercise programs, and maintaining open communication with their therapist, patients can maximize their chances of achieving lasting pain relief and restored neck function.

Chapter 5

Alternative and Complementary Therapies

Acupuncture, Massage, and Chiropractic Care for Neck Pain Relief

Neck pain is a prevalent musculoskeletal disorder that affects a significant portion of the population. Various factors can contribute to neck pain, such as muscle strains, degenerative disc disease, herniated discs, and spinal stenosis. Conventional medical treatments like medication and physical therapy are often the first line of defense for managing neck pain. However, alternative and complementary therapies can also play a crucial role in addressing this condition. These therapies, which include acupuncture, massage, and chiropractic care, have increasingly gained attention due to their potential benefits in pain relief and overall well-being. This chapter aims to provide a comprehensive overview of these therapies and the current scientific evidence supporting their efficacy in treating neck pain.

Alternative and complementary therapies encompass a diverse range of treatment modalities that are not typically considered part of conventional medicine. They are often used in conjunction with standard medical treatments to enhance their effectiveness, address potential side effects, and improve the overall quality of life for patients. In the context of neck pain, alternative and complementary therapies can help reduce pain intensity, improve functional mobility, and promote a sense of relaxation and stress relief. These benefits can be especially valuable for individuals with chronic neck pain, who often experience a complex interplay of physical, psychological, and social factors that contribute to their condition.

The growing interest in alternative and complementary therapies for neck pain can be attributed to several factors. First, there is increasing public awareness and demand for non-pharmacological and non-invasive treatment options, particularly in light of the opioid crisis and concerns about the long-term safety and efficacy of certain medications. Second, a growing body of scientific research has begun to elucidate the mechanisms and clinical benefits of these therapies, lending credibility to their use in medical practice. Third, many healthcare providers and patients are embracing a more holistic and patient-centered approach to care, which recognizes the importance of addressing the whole person, including their physical, emotional, and social well-being.

Despite the potential benefits of alternative and complementary therapies for neck pain, their use in clinical practice is not without challenges. One significant challenge is the variability in the quality and rigor of research studies, which can make it difficult to draw definitive conclusions about the efficacy and safety of certain therapies. Additionally, there is often a lack of standardized treatment protocols and guidelines, making it challenging for healthcare providers to determine the most appropriate treatment course for their patients. Finally, access to alternative and complementary therapies can be limited by factors such as insurance coverage, provider availability, and patient knowledge and preferences.

In light of these challenges, it is crucial to critically appraise the available scientific evidence for alternative and complementary therapies for neck pain and to engage in a collaborative and informed decision-making process with patients. This chapter will delve deeper into three widely used therapies – acupuncture, massage, and chiropractic care – examining their theoretical foundations, clinical evidence, and practical considerations for neck pain treatment. By understanding the current state of knowledge and remaining open to new research and perspectives, healthcare providers can better support their patients in navigating the complex landscape of neck pain management and achieving optimal outcomes.

Acupuncture is a traditional Chinese medicine practice that has been used for thousands of years to treat various health conditions, including neck pain. It involves the insertion of thin needles into specific points on the body, known as acupuncture points or acupoints. The underlying theory of acupuncture is based on the concept of Qi (pronounced "chee"), which is considered vital energy or life force that flows through channels, or meridians, in the body. These meridians form a complex network that connects various organs and body parts. When Qi is blocked or disrupted, it can lead to pain, illness, or dysfunction. Acupuncture aims to restore the balance and flow of Qi by stimulating acupoints, thus promoting healing and pain relief.

Recent research has provided insights into the possible mechanisms through which acupuncture may provide pain relief. One of the primary mechanisms is the release of endogenous opioids, which are the body's natural painkillers. When acupuncture needles are inserted into acupoints, they stimulate the release of endorphins, enkephalins, and dynorphins, which are endogenous opioid peptides. These substances bind to opioid receptors in the nervous system and effectively reduce the perception of pain.

Another proposed mechanism of acupuncture's pain-relieving effect is the modulation of the pain signaling pathway. Pain signals are transmitted from the site of injury or inflammation to the brain through a series of nerve fibers and synapses. Acupuncture is thought to alter the pain transmission process by inhibiting the activation of certain pain pathways or by stimulating the release of neurotransmitters, such as serotonin and norepinephrine, which have analgesic effects.

Additionally, acupuncture has been shown to improve local blood circulation, which can help promote healing and reduce inflammation at the site of pain. By increasing blood flow, acupuncture can deliver oxygen and

117

nutrients to the affected area more effectively and facilitate the removal of waste products and inflammatory mediators, which may contribute to the reduction of pain and discomfort.

Furthermore, acupuncture has been found to have anti-inflammatory effects, which may play a role in its ability to alleviate neck pain. It is suggested that acupuncture can modulate the release of pro-inflammatory cytokines, such as tumor necrosis factor-alpha (TNF-α) and interleukin-6 (IL-6), which are involved in the inflammatory response. By reducing the levels of these pro-inflammatory cytokines, acupuncture may help to reduce inflammation and, consequently, alleviate pain.

It should be noted that the exact mechanisms through which acupuncture relieves neck pain are still not fully understood, and more research is needed to elucidate the precise pathways and processes involved. Nonetheless, the current evidence suggests that acupuncture can provide pain relief through a combination of neurochemical, neurophysiological, and circulatory mechanisms, making it a potentially valuable treatment option for those suffering from neck pain.

The effectiveness of acupuncture in treating neck pain has been a topic of interest in numerous clinical trials and systematic reviews. A notable systematic review and meta-analysis published in 2017 analyzed data from 22 randomized controlled trials (RCTs) to evaluate the efficacy of acupuncture for neck pain. This comprehensive review found that acupuncture outperformed sham acupuncture, inactive treatment, and waiting list control in reducing neck pain intensity and improving function. The researchers concluded that acupuncture could be considered a viable treatment option for neck pain relief.

Another systematic review, published in 2020, further investigated the effectiveness of acupuncture in treating neck pain. This review included 27 RCTs and similarly concluded that acupuncture was effective in alleviating neck pain and improving neck function, with a particular emphasis on its benefits for patients with chronic neck pain. This review also highlighted that acupuncture could potentially reduce the need for pain medications and improve the overall quality of life for patients suffering from neck pain.

Despite these encouraging findings, the quality of evidence supporting acupuncture's efficacy in neck pain treatment is not consistent across all studies. Some research has reported small effect sizes or conflicting results, leading to a degree of uncertainty in the evidence base. For instance, a 2016 Cochrane review evaluating the effects of acupuncture for neck pain found that while there was some evidence for short-term pain relief, the long-term benefits remained unclear.

Several factors may contribute to these inconsistencies, including differences in study design, sample sizes, acupuncture techniques, treatment duration, and the use of sham acupuncture controls. Furthermore, the lack of standardization in acupuncture protocols makes it challenging to compare the results of different studies directly.

As a result, more high-quality research is needed to establish the optimal acupuncture protocols for neck pain management. Future studies should focus on addressing the methodological limitations of previous research, such as improving study design, adequately blinding participants and assessors, and using standardized treatment protocols. Additionally, research should explore the potential mechanisms underlying acupuncture's pain-relieving effects to better understand how it can be most effectively applied in clinical practice.

While there is a growing body of evidence suggesting that acupuncture can be effective in alleviating neck pain and improving function, particularly for patients with chronic neck pain, more high-quality research is needed to confirm these findings and determine the most effective treatment protocols. Despite the current limitations in the evidence, acupuncture may still be a valuable addition to a comprehensive neck pain treatment plan, particularly for patients seeking alternative or complementary approaches to pain management.

Massage therapy is a widely practiced manual therapy that involves the manipulation of soft tissues, such as muscles, tendons, and ligaments, to promote relaxation, improve circulation, and alleviate pain. The application of pressure, friction, and various movements on the body's soft tissues helps in the reduction of muscle tension, the improvement of flexibility, and the promotion of overall well-being. Massage therapy is rooted in the understanding that muscular imbalances, poor posture, and emotional stress can contribute to neck pain. By addressing these factors, massage can help relieve pain, promote healing, and prevent future occurrences of neck pain.

Swedish massage is a common technique that employs long, gliding strokes, kneading, friction, tapping, and shaking motions to promote relaxation and improve circulation. This gentle form of massage can be beneficial for neck pain as it helps to release muscle tension, improve blood flow, and reduce stress. It is generally considered the foundation of most massage techniques and is often combined with other methods for a comprehensive treatment.

Deep tissue massage targets the deeper layers of muscles and connective tissue, using slow, deep strokes and sustained pressure to break up adhesions and scar tissue that can contribute to neck pain. This type of massage is particularly useful for chronic neck pain caused by muscular tension or strain, as it can help to release tight muscle fibers and improve range of motion.

Myofascial release is a technique that focuses on the fascia, the thin, connective tissue that surrounds and supports the muscles, organs, and bones in the body. In cases of neck pain, the fascia may become restricted, contributing to muscle stiffness and reduced mobility. Myofascial release involves the application of gentle, sustained pressure on the fascia to release restrictions, promote flexibility, and relieve pain. This technique can be especially helpful for individuals with chronic neck pain caused by poor posture or repetitive strain injuries.

Trigger point therapy, also known as neuromuscular therapy, targets specific areas of tightness or "knots" within the muscles, which can refer pain to other areas of the body. Trigger points in the neck and shoulder muscles can contribute to neck pain and may even cause headaches or radiating pain in the arms. In trigger point therapy, the therapist applies focused pressure on these tight spots to release muscle tension, alleviate pain, and improve function.

Each of these massage techniques has its own specific approach and goals, but all share the common aim of reducing muscle tension, improving flexibility, and promoting overall well-being. A skilled massage therapist can assess an individual's specific needs and tailor a treatment plan that combines these techniques to provide the most effective relief for neck pain.

The effectiveness of massage therapy in treating neck pain has been a subject of extensive research, with numerous clinical trials and systematic reviews conducted to evaluate its efficacy. A 2014 systematic review and meta-analysis of 15 randomized controlled trials assessed the impact of massage therapy on pain relief and functional improvement in patients with neck pain. The results demonstrated that massage therapy led to significant pain relief and improved function when compared to no treatment or inactive controls, such as relaxation or attention control.

In a more recent systematic review and meta-analysis conducted in 2019, researchers analyzed 27 randomized controlled trials to evaluate the effectiveness of massage therapy on neck pain. The findings of this review indicated that massage therapy was effective in reducing pain intensity, increasing range of motion, and improving the quality of life for patients with neck pain, particularly for those suffering from chronic neck pain. These results further support the use of massage therapy as a viable treatment option for neck pain relief.

Despite the generally supportive evidence for massage therapy in neck pain treatment, the optimal frequency, duration, and type of massage technique may differ among individuals. Some studies have suggested that multiple massage sessions per week, lasting between 30 to 60 minutes each, may be more effective in reducing neck pain than single sessions or sessions of shorter duration. Additionally, the type of massage technique employed, such as Swedish massage, deep tissue massage, myofascial release, or trigger point therapy, may also influence treatment outcomes.

For example, a randomized controlled trial published in 2012 compared the effectiveness of Swedish massage and deep tissue massage in patients with chronic neck pain. The results indicated that both techniques led to significant improvements in pain intensity and neck disability, but deep tissue massage was more effective in improving range of motion. Another study published in 2013 compared the effects of myofascial release and ischemic compression (a form of trigger point therapy) on neck pain and functional disability. The study found that both techniques significantly improved neck pain and disability, but myofascial release was more effective in improving cervical range of motion.

It is essential to consider individual patient factors, such as pain severity, duration, and underlying causes, when determining the most appropriate massage therapy approach. Moreover, patient preferences and treatment goals should also be taken into account to ensure optimal outcomes.

While the evidence generally supports the use of massage therapy for neck pain relief, further research is needed to determine the most effective massage protocols for different types of neck pain and patient populations. By considering individual patient factors and preferences, healthcare providers and massage therapists can work together to develop tailored treatment plans that maximize the potential benefits of massage therapy for neck pain relief.

Chiropractic care is a form of manual therapy that focuses on the diagnosis, treatment, and prevention of musculoskeletal disorders, particularly those involving the spine. The foundation of chiropractic care is the premise that proper alignment and functioning of the spine are essential for overall health and well-being. Chiropractors primarily utilize spinal manipulation, also known as chiropractic adjustments, to correct misalignments or subluxations in the spine, which are thought to interfere with nerve function and cause pain.

Spinal manipulation is a technique that involves the application of controlled force to specific joints in the spine, often accompanied by a popping or cracking sound. This sound is caused by the release of gas bubbles from the joint fluid, known as cavitation. The primary goal of spinal manipulation is to restore joint mobility, decrease inflammation, and alleviate pain by addressing biomechanical dysfunction in the spinal joints.

In addition to spinal manipulation, chiropractors employ a variety of manual techniques to address neck pain and related issues. One such technique is mobilization, which involves the gentle, passive movement of joints and soft tissues within their normal range of motion. By doing so, mobilization aims to improve joint flexibility, reduce muscle stiffness, and promote relaxation, ultimately contributing to neck pain relief.

Chiropractors also utilize various soft tissue techniques to address muscle and connective tissue tightness or dysfunction. Techniques such as myofascial release, trigger point therapy, and active release techniques are employed to help relieve muscle tension, break up scar tissue, and improve blood flow to the affected area. Myofascial release focuses on releasing restrictions in the fascia, a connective tissue that surrounds muscles, while trigger point therapy targets specific tight spots within muscles that cause pain and discomfort. Active release techniques involve the combination of manual pressure and specific patient movements to address muscle and soft tissue adhesions.

Another component of chiropractic care is the prescription of therapeutic exercises and stretches to be performed at home. These exercises are designed to help strengthen and stabilize the muscles supporting the spine, ultimately improving flexibility and range of motion. By doing so, they contribute to long-term neck pain relief and prevention, as well as overall spinal health.

Chiropractors also focus on postural correction as a part of their treatment approach. They often assess and address postural imbalances that may contribute to neck pain by providing guidance on ergonomic adjustments. For example, they may suggest optimizing workstation setup, such as adjusting the height of a computer monitor or the position of a keyboard, to promote proper spinal alignment and minimize strain on the neck. They may also recommend using supportive pillows while sleeping to maintain a neutral spine position and reduce nighttime discomfort.

Some chiropractors incorporate instrument-assisted techniques into their treatment plans. Specialized instruments, such as the Activator or Graston Technique, are used to apply controlled force to the spine or release soft tissue adhesions. The Activator is a small, handheld device that delivers a low-force impulse to the spine, while the Graston Technique involves the use of stainless steel tools to break up scar tissue and fascial restrictions. These instruments can provide a more targeted and precise treatment while minimizing discomfort, making them an appealing option for some patients and practitioners.

Overall, chiropractors employ a diverse range of manual techniques to address neck pain and its underlying causes. By combining these techniques and tailoring treatment plans to individual patient needs, chiropractors aim to provide comprehensive, effective care for those suffering from neck pain and related issues.

It is essential to note that chiropractic care is not a one-size-fits-all approach, and treatment plans are typically tailored to the individual patient's needs and preferences. Chiropractors typically perform a thorough physical examination, review the patient's medical history, and may utilize diagnostic imaging, such as X-rays or MRI, to inform their treatment approach and ensure the safety and effectiveness of the chosen techniques.

The growing body of research supporting the effectiveness of chiropractic care for neck pain comprises various study designs and patient populations. In the 2012 systematic review, the analysis of 12 randomized controlled trials demonstrated that spinal manipulation outperformed medication or home exercise with advice in terms of pain relief and functional improvement for patients with acute and subacute neck pain. One of the trials in this review, which involved 272 participants, revealed that spinal manipulation led to a more significant reduction in pain scores compared to both medication and home exercise at eight and 26 weeks follow-up.

The 2019 systematic review, which included 51 randomized controlled trials, provided further evidence supporting the use of chiropractic care in patients with chronic neck pain. This review highlighted that spinal manipulation led to moderate to strong evidence of pain relief and functional improvement in this patient population. In addition to spinal manipulation, the review also found moderate evidence supporting the use of other manual therapies, such as mobilization and soft tissue techniques, for neck pain relief.

Despite these promising findings, inconsistencies in study results and methodological limitations should be considered. Some studies have reported conflicting results, with small effect sizes or no significant differences between chiropractic care and other treatments for neck pain. For example, a 2015 randomized controlled trial involving 183 participants found no significant differences in pain relief or functional improvement between spinal manipulation and a home exercise program for patients with chronic neck pain. Additionally, the heterogeneity in chiropractic techniques and treatment protocols across studies makes it challenging to draw definitive conclusions about the most effective approaches for different types of neck pain.

Moreover, the existing literature has some limitations, such as small sample sizes, short follow-up periods, and potential biases, which may impact the generalizability and robustness of the findings. To better establish the role of chiropractic care in neck pain treatment and optimize its therapeutic potential, future research should focus on conducting high-quality, large-scale randomized controlled trials with longer follow-up periods. These studies should aim to compare different chiropractic techniques and treatment protocols, as well as their effectiveness in various patient populations, such as those with acute, subacute, or chronic neck pain, and those with different underlying causes of neck pain, such as disc herniation or cervical spondylosis.

The clinical evidence for chiropractic care in neck pain treatment is promising, with numerous studies demonstrating its effectiveness in providing pain relief and functional improvement, particularly for patients with chronic neck pain. However, more high-quality research is needed to identify the most effective chiropractic techniques and treatment protocols for different types of neck pain and patient populations, as well as to resolve inconsistencies in study results and address methodological limitations in the existing literature.

While acupuncture, massage therapy, and chiropractic care are generally considered safe for neck pain treatment, potential risks and adverse effects should be considered to ensure patient safety and appropriate care.

For acupuncture, the low risk of complications is attributed to the procedure being performed by a qualified practitioner using sterile needles. Some of the most common side effects of acupuncture include temporary pain, bleeding, or bruising at the needle insertion site. More severe complications, such as infection, pneumothorax, or nerve injury, are extremely rare but can occur if the practitioner fails to follow proper technique or hygiene practices. To minimize the risk of complications, patients should seek treatment from a licensed acupuncturist with appropriate training and credentials.

Massage therapy, in general, is considered safe; however, temporary soreness or discomfort may arise, particularly after deep tissue or more intense techniques. In some cases, massage therapy can exacerbate existing conditions, such as muscle strains or inflammation. It is crucial for patients to communicate with the massage therapist about their medical history, current symptoms, and comfort level during the session to minimize potential discomfort and ensure a safe and effective treatment. Additionally, the massage therapist should have proper training and certification to provide the most appropriate care for each patient's needs.

Chiropractic care, specifically spinal manipulation, has been associated with a low risk of mild to moderate adverse effects, such as temporary pain, stiffness, or headache. However, in rare cases, more severe complications can occur, such as vertebral artery dissection, which can lead to stroke. This risk is higher in patients with certain predisposing factors, such as a history of stroke or vascular disease, connective tissue disorders, or cervical spine instability. It is essential for patients to discuss their medical history and potential risk factors with their healthcare provider before receiving chiropractic care for neck pain. The chiropractor should also be informed of any concurrent medical conditions, medications, or previous surgical interventions that may affect the safety or appropriateness of spinal manipulation.

To ensure the safety and effectiveness of alternative and complementary therapies for neck pain, patients should consult with their healthcare provider to determine the most suitable treatment options based on their individual needs, medical history, and potential risk factors. Furthermore, it is crucial to select qualified practitioners with appropriate training, credentials, and experience to provide the highest quality care and minimize the risk of complications.

In conclusion, alternative and complementary therapies have emerged as significant contributors to the management of neck pain. Acupuncture, massage therapy, and chiropractic care have gained popularity due to the growing body of scientific evidence supporting their efficacy in providing pain relief and improving function, particularly in cases of chronic neck pain. These therapies have shown promising results, as they address not only the physical aspects of neck pain but also the holistic well-being of the individual. Furthermore, these therapies often have fewer side effects compared to conventional treatments such as medication, making them an appealing option for patients seeking non-pharmacological interventions.

Despite the positive findings in current research, there is still a need for additional high-quality studies to determine the optimal treatment protocols and techniques for different types of neck pain and patient populations. Factors such as the duration and frequency of treatment, specific techniques, and individual patient characteristics may play a crucial role in the effectiveness of these therapies. Further research will help refine our understanding of how to best integrate acupuncture, massage therapy, and chiropractic care into comprehensive neck pain management plans, which may also include conventional treatments such as medication and physical therapy.

As with any treatment approach, it is essential to discuss the potential benefits, risks, and suitability of alternative and complementary therapies with a qualified healthcare professional before incorporating them into a neck pain treatment plan. This ensures that the chosen therapies align with the patient's specific needs, medical history, and preferences. Additionally, the healthcare professional can monitor the patient's progress and make any necessary adjustments to the treatment plan to ensure the best possible outcomes.

Incorporating alternative and complementary therapies into a comprehensive neck pain treatment plan can offer patients a well-rounded approach to pain management, addressing the physical, emotional, and psychological components of their condition. By combining these therapies with conventional treatments, patients may experience improved pain relief, enhanced function, and a better overall quality of life. Ultimately, the integration of various therapeutic modalities tailored to the individual's needs is key to achieving optimal results in the management of neck pain.

Chapter 6

Cervical Traction and Orthotic Devices

The Role of Supportive Aids in Neck Pain Treatment

Cervical traction and orthotic devices have gained prominence in recent years due to their potential to alleviate neck pain and discomfort, promote healing, and restore the normal functioning of the cervical spine. These supportive aids are an integral part of a comprehensive treatment plan that typically includes other conservative interventions such as medication management, physical therapy, and lifestyle modifications.

Cervical traction is a therapeutic technique that aims to decompress the cervical spine by gently stretching the neck muscles and ligaments. This process helps reduce pressure on the nerves, alleviate pain, improve blood circulation, and facilitate the healing of injured tissues. Cervical traction can be performed using mechanical devices or manual techniques, depending on the patient's needs and the healthcare professional's recommendations.

Orthotic devices, commonly known as cervical collars or neck braces, are designed to provide support and stability to the neck by restricting movement and maintaining proper alignment. These devices can be employed for various purposes, such as immobilization following trauma or surgery, providing temporary relief from pain during daily activities, and maintaining alignment during the healing process.

Both cervical traction and orthotic devices have their indications, contraindications, and precautions that healthcare professionals must consider to ensure patient safety and treatment efficacy. The choice of intervention and the specific type of traction or orthotic device used should be based on the patient's individual condition, symptoms, and treatment goals. It is essential to tailor the treatment plan to the patient's specific needs and monitor their progress throughout the course of therapy.

The evidence supporting the use of cervical traction and orthotic devices in neck pain management is still evolving. While some studies have shown promising results, particularly for short-term pain relief and improved function, the long-term benefits of these interventions have not been well-established. More high-quality research is needed to confirm the efficacy of cervical traction and orthotic devices and to identify the most effective treatment protocols and devices for specific neck pain conditions.

In this chapter, we will explore the principles of cervical traction and various orthotic devices in greater detail, discuss their indications, contraindications, and precautions, and examine the current evidence supporting their use in neck pain treatment. We will also highlight the importance of a comprehensive, multimodal approach to neck pain management that incorporates cervical traction and orthotic devices as part of a broader treatment plan.

Cervical traction is a non-invasive therapy that has been used for decades to help alleviate neck pain by targeting the cervical spine's underlying structures. The fundamental principles of cervical traction involve gently stretching the cervical spine, decompressing the intervertebral discs, and reducing pressure on the nerves. This stretching and decompression can provide relief from pain, enhance blood circulation, and promote the healing of injured tissues. There are two primary types of cervical traction: mechanical and manual.

Mechanical cervical traction is administered using devices that apply a controlled force to stretch the neck muscles and ligaments. This form of traction can be continuous or intermittent, depending on the patient's needs and comfort level. Mechanical traction devices can be further divided into over-the-door and supine traction units. Over-the-door traction units are portable devices designed for home use, where the patient wears a head halter attached to a pulley system mounted on a door. The traction force is generated by adding weights to the system, and the treatment duration and frequency can be customized according to the clinician's recommendations. On the other hand, supine traction units allow patients to lie down during treatment, ensuring a more comfortable and controlled experience. These devices often feature built-in controls that enable the patient or the therapist to adjust the traction force and duration. Supine traction units can be used in clinical settings or at home, with some models designed for portable use.

Manual cervical traction is performed by a trained healthcare professional, such as a physical therapist or chiropractor, who uses their hands to apply a controlled force to the patient's neck. The therapist adjusts the traction force, direction, and duration based on the patient's symptoms and response to treatment. Manual cervical traction allows for greater customization of the treatment but requires regular visits to a healthcare professional.

One of the primary advantages of cervical traction is that it can be tailored to the specific needs of each patient. Factors such as the patient's age, overall health, and the severity of their neck pain can influence the type of cervical traction employed, as well as the frequency and duration of treatment sessions. Furthermore, cervical traction can be combined with other treatments, such as physical therapy, medication, and complementary therapies, to create a comprehensive and individualized treatment plan.

The effectiveness of cervical traction is supported by various scientific studies. Research has shown that it can provide short-term pain relief and improved function for patients with conditions such as cervical radiculopathy and herniated discs. However, more high-quality research is needed to confirm its long-term efficacy and establish optimal treatment protocols.

Cervical traction is a non-invasive therapy that offers a viable option for patients suffering from neck pain. By gently stretching the cervical spine and decompressing the intervertebral discs, cervical traction can relieve pain, improve blood circulation, and promote the healing of injured tissues. The choice between mechanical and manual cervical traction depends on the patient's needs, preferences, and the availability of trained healthcare professionals.

Mechanical cervical traction is a therapeutic approach that employs specially designed devices to apply controlled force to the cervical spine, gradually stretching the neck muscles and ligaments. This method of traction helps alleviate neck pain by decompressing the intervertebral discs, reducing pressure on the nerves, and promoting relaxation of the muscles. Mechanical cervical traction devices offer the advantage of being more precise and consistent compared to manual traction, as they allow for better control over the force, duration, and frequency of the applied traction.

Mechanical cervical traction can be applied either continuously or intermittently, depending on the patient's needs and therapeutic goals. Continuous traction involves applying a steady force to the cervical spine for an extended period, whereas intermittent traction applies the force in cycles, with periods of traction followed by periods of relaxation. The intensity of the traction force can be adjusted according to the patient's comfort level and the specific treatment objectives.

Mechanical traction devices can be broadly classified into two categories: over-the-door and supine traction units. Over-the-door traction units are simple, portable devices that can be easily set up at home. They consist of a head halter that fits around the patient's head and a pulley system mounted on a door. The traction force is generated by adding weights to the pulley system, and the force can be adjusted by changing the amount of weight used. Over-the-door traction units are relatively inexpensive and convenient for home use but may not provide the same level of control and precision as supine traction units.

Supine traction units, on the other hand, are more advanced devices that allow patients to lie down during the traction treatment, ensuring a more comfortable and controlled experience. These units often come with built-in electronic controls that enable the patient or the therapist to adjust the traction force, duration, and cycle settings. Some supine traction units also have additional features, such as heating elements, vibration, or infrared therapy, to enhance the therapeutic effects of the treatment.

Supine traction units can be used in clinical settings, such as physical therapy clinics or hospitals, as well as at home, with some models specifically designed for portable use. While supine traction units tend to be more expensive than over-the-door devices, they offer a higher level of precision, control, and comfort, making them a popular choice for both healthcare professionals and patients.

Mechanical cervical traction devices provide a non-invasive and controlled approach to alleviating neck pain by applying precise, adjustable force to the cervical spine. Both over-the-door and supine traction units have their advantages and limitations, and the choice between them depends on factors such as patient comfort, therapeutic goals, and budget. As part of a comprehensive neck pain treatment plan, mechanical cervical traction can complement other interventions, such as physical therapy, medication, and lifestyle modifications, to promote healing and restore normal function.

Over-the-door traction units have become popular for home use, as they offer an accessible and cost-effective solution for patients seeking relief from neck pain. These portable devices comprise a head halter, a pulley system, and a set of weights. The head halter is designed to cradle the patient's head securely, distributing the traction force evenly across the neck. The pulley system, which is mounted on a door, is responsible for translating the weight-induced force into vertical traction on the cervical spine.

To use an over-the-door traction unit, the patient should first consult with a healthcare professional to determine the appropriate traction force, treatment duration, and frequency. This information is crucial for customizing the treatment plan and ensuring that the patient experiences optimal benefits from the therapy while minimizing the risk of injury.

Once the patient has received their clinician's recommendations, they can set up the over-the-door traction unit at home by following the manufacturer's instructions. It is essential to ensure that the door is sturdy and securely closed to prevent accidents during treatment. The patient should then carefully adjust the head halter to fit comfortably and securely around their head, avoiding any unnecessary pressure on the jaw or face. The chin strap should be snug but not overly tight to allow for natural jaw movement and swallowing.

After adjusting the head halter, the patient can attach the pulley system to the door and connect the head halter to the pulley using the provided straps or hooks. The clinician-recommended weights can then be added to the traction system, which will create a vertical force that gently stretches the neck muscles and ligaments. It is essential to start with a lower traction force and gradually increase it over time, as tolerated.

During the treatment, the patient should be seated comfortably with their back supported and their feet flat on the floor. They should maintain a relaxed posture, with their head and neck aligned with the spine. The duration of each treatment session can vary depending on the healthcare professional's recommendations, but generally, sessions last between 15 and 30 minutes. The patient should monitor their symptoms and communicate any discomfort or adverse effects to their healthcare provider.

The effectiveness of over-the-door traction units for neck pain relief may vary depending on the individual patient's condition and the underlying cause of their pain. Some patients may experience significant relief from their symptoms, while others may require additional interventions such as physical therapy, medication, or alternative treatments. As with any therapy, it is essential for the patient to follow their healthcare professional's recommendations and adhere to the prescribed treatment plan to achieve the best results.

Supine traction units are designed to provide a more comfortable and controlled experience for patients, as they allow them to lie down during treatment. This position has several advantages over the sitting or standing positions used in other traction methods, such as over-the-door traction units. In the supine position, the patient's spine is in a more neutral alignment, which helps to distribute the traction force more evenly across the cervical spine. Additionally, this position allows for better relaxation of the neck muscles, which can enhance the effectiveness of the traction therapy.

These supine traction units often come equipped with built-in controls that enable the patient or the therapist to adjust the traction force and duration precisely. This customization is essential to provide the most effective treatment while minimizing the risk of injury or discomfort. The traction force can be gradually increased over time as the patient's tolerance improves, and the duration of each session can be adjusted according to the clinician's recommendations.

Supine traction units are versatile and can be used in various settings, including clinical environments and at home. In clinical settings, such as physical therapy clinics or rehabilitation centers, the therapist can closely monitor the patient's progress and make necessary adjustments to the traction parameters. They can also provide hands-on assistance and guidance to ensure proper positioning and technique.

For home use, some supine traction unit models are designed for portability, making them easy to set up and store. These home-based units often come with detailed instructions for safe and effective use. However, patients should consult their healthcare provider before starting a home traction program to ensure they receive appropriate guidance on the proper technique and treatment parameters.

In addition to the adjustable traction force and duration, some supine traction units offer advanced features, such as the ability to change the angle of traction. This functionality can target specific areas of the cervical spine more effectively and allows for the treatment of various neck pain conditions. Another feature found in some units is the use of pneumatic or electronic systems to control the traction force. These systems can offer more precise control over the traction parameters and may provide a smoother, more comfortable experience for the patient.

Despite the numerous benefits of supine traction units, it is essential to recognize that they may not be suitable for all patients or neck pain conditions. Certain contraindications and precautions, as mentioned earlier in this chapter, must be considered before using any cervical traction therapy. Patients should work closely with their healthcare provider to determine if supine traction is appropriate for their specific condition and to develop a customized treatment plan tailored to their individual needs.

Manual cervical traction is a therapeutic technique performed by trained healthcare professionals, such as physical therapists, chiropractors, or osteopathic physicians. This hands-on approach involves the application of a controlled force to the patient's neck to gently stretch the cervical spine, decompress the intervertebral discs, and alleviate pressure on the nerves. This technique aims to reduce pain, improve mobility, and enhance the healing process in patients with neck pain.

During a manual cervical traction session, the healthcare professional positions the patient comfortably, either seated or lying down, depending on the practitioner's preference and the patient's comfort. The therapist then uses their hands to stabilize the patient's head while applying a controlled force to the neck. The traction force can be directed longitudinally (along the length of the spine), laterally (toward the sides), or at a specific angle based on the patient's symptoms and anatomical considerations.

One of the benefits of manual cervical traction is the ability to customize the treatment according to the patient's needs. The therapist can adjust the traction force, direction, and duration based on the patient's symptoms, response to treatment, and overall comfort. Additionally, the therapist can monitor the patient's progress during the treatment, allowing for real-time adjustments and modifications as needed.

Manual cervical traction also enables the healthcare professional to incorporate other treatment modalities into the session, such as soft tissue mobilization, joint mobilization, or therapeutic exercises. This integrated approach allows for a more comprehensive treatment plan, targeting multiple aspects of the patient's neck pain and dysfunction.

Despite the advantages of manual cervical traction, there are some limitations to consider. One of the primary drawbacks is the requirement for regular visits to a healthcare professional, which may be challenging for patients with limited access to care or busy schedules. Additionally, the effectiveness of manual cervical traction may be influenced by the practitioner's skill and experience, potentially leading to variable outcomes.

As with any therapeutic intervention, the success of manual cervical traction depends on proper patient selection and adherence to treatment recommendations. Healthcare professionals must consider the patient's specific condition, any contraindications to traction, and the patient's overall goals and preferences when determining the most appropriate treatment plan.

Manual cervical traction is a valuable treatment option for patients with neck pain, offering a customized, hands-on approach to care. Although it requires regular visits to a healthcare professional, the benefits of this technique, particularly when combined with other therapeutic interventions, can lead to significant improvements in pain, mobility, and overall quality of life for many patients.

Cervical traction is a valuable therapeutic option for patients experiencing various neck pain conditions. One such condition is cervical radiculopathy, which arises when nerve roots in the cervical spine become compressed or irritated. Cervical traction can alleviate the pressure on the nerve roots, thereby providing relief from pain, numbness, and weakness radiating to the arms or hands.

Another indication for cervical traction is cervical spondylosis, a degenerative condition characterized by the wear and tear of spinal discs and facet joints in the neck. Cervical traction can help reduce joint stiffness, decompress the affected spinal segments, and improve neck mobility in patients with spondylosis. Similarly, traction can be beneficial for patients with herniated or bulging cervical discs, as it can create space between the vertebrae and alleviate pressure on the affected discs.

Cervical traction can also be helpful for individuals with facet joint syndrome, a condition involving inflammation and pain in the facet joints of the cervical spine. By gently stretching the neck muscles and ligaments, traction can reduce muscle spasms, alleviate joint pain, and promote a more balanced alignment of the cervical spine. Patients with muscle spasms or strains and whiplash-associated disorders can also benefit from cervical traction, as it can help relieve pain and improve range of motion.

Despite the therapeutic benefits of cervical traction for various neck pain conditions, it is crucial to consider contraindications and precautions before initiating treatment. Cervical traction should be used with caution or avoided in cases of acute neck trauma or instability, as it may exacerbate the injury or compromise the structural integrity of the cervical spine.

Similarly, patients with rheumatoid arthritis or other inflammatory conditions affecting the cervical spine should exercise caution when considering cervical traction. Traction may potentially worsen inflammation, leading to increased pain and joint damage. Additionally, individuals with cervical spine malignancies or infections should avoid cervical traction, as it could contribute to the spread of cancer cells or infectious agents.

Vertebral artery insufficiency, a condition characterized by reduced blood flow to the brain due to narrowing or occlusion of the vertebral arteries, is another contraindication for cervical traction. Traction can exacerbate this condition by further reducing blood flow, thereby increasing the risk of stroke or other neurological complications.

Patients with osteoporosis or other bone-weakening conditions should also approach cervical traction with caution, as the increased force on the cervical spine may increase the risk of fractures or other injuries. Furthermore, individuals who have undergone prior cervical spine surgery should consult their healthcare provider before initiating cervical traction, as it may interfere with the healing process or compromise the surgical site.

While cervical traction can offer significant benefits for patients with various neck pain conditions, it is essential to consider the potential contraindications and precautions before initiating treatment. A thorough assessment by a healthcare professional is crucial to determine the appropriateness of cervical traction for each patient and to ensure safe and effective treatment outcomes.

Orthotic devices, often referred to as cervical collars or neck braces, play a crucial role in supporting and stabilizing the neck while restricting its movement, which in turn helps to alleviate pain. These devices serve several purposes, such as immobilizing the neck following trauma or

138

surgery, maintaining proper alignment during the healing process, and offering temporary pain relief during daily activities. Cervical orthotic devices can be broadly classified into three categories: soft, semi-rigid, and rigid collars.

Soft cervical collars provide a gentle support to the neck muscles and restrict excessive neck movement. They are made from foam or padded materials that are comfortable to wear. These collars are often prescribed for mild neck pain conditions, such as muscle strains or ligament sprains, and can offer temporary relief from discomfort. However, they are not designed for long-term use, as extended wear can lead to muscle weakness and a reduced range of motion in the neck. Soft collars are generally recommended for short periods, such as a few hours a day or as directed by a healthcare professional.

Semi-rigid cervical collars offer a higher level of support and immobilization compared to soft collars. They consist of a combination of rigid plastic components and soft padding, providing more restriction to neck movement while still ensuring comfort. These collars are suitable for patients with moderate neck pain or stiffness, and they can be used to provide post-operative support or during the healing process following a cervical injury. Like soft collars, long-term use of semi-rigid collars is not recommended, as it may contribute to muscle atrophy and decreased neck mobility.

Rigid cervical collars are designed to provide the maximum level of support and immobilization for the neck. These devices are constructed from rigid plastic or metal components and are specifically engineered to maintain the alignment of the cervical spine, limit movement, and stabilize the neck. Rigid collars are typically prescribed for patients with severe cervical injuries, to immobilize the neck following surgery, or to manage specific conditions such as cervical fractures or dislocations. Due to their restrictive nature, these collars are generally used for shorter durations or as directed by a healthcare professional to avoid the negative consequences of long-term immobilization.

When selecting a cervical orthotic device, several factors should be considered, including the patient's specific condition, the desired level of support and immobilization, and the duration of use. It is essential for the device to be properly fitted and adjusted according to the patient's individual anatomy and comfort level. An ill-fitting cervical collar can cause discomfort, skin irritation, or reduced effectiveness of the device. In addition, healthcare professionals should educate patients on the proper use of the orthotic device, including when and how long to wear it, and the importance of engaging in appropriate exercises and rehabilitation to maintain neck strength and mobility.

While cervical orthotic devices can be helpful in managing neck pain, they should not be relied upon as the sole treatment modality. A comprehensive approach to neck pain treatment typically includes other conservative interventions such as physical therapy, medication management, and lifestyle modifications. The combination of these interventions, along with the appropriate use of orthotic devices, can help to alleviate pain, promote healing, and restore function for patients with neck pain.

Soft cervical collars, commonly known as foam collars, are designed to provide gentle support and stability to the neck. They are typically made from lightweight and breathable materials such as foam or padded fabric, which offer comfort and cushioning to the cervical spine. These collars function by restricting excessive neck movement, helping to alleviate pain and discomfort associated with muscle strains, ligament sprains, or mild cervical radiculopathy. By limiting motion, soft cervical collars allow the injured structures to rest and recover, reducing inflammation and promoting the healing process.

The design of soft cervical collars often includes an adjustable closure mechanism, such as Velcro, which allows for a customized fit based on the patient's neck size and comfort level. The collar should be snug enough to provide support but not too tight as to restrict blood flow or cause discomfort. Proper fitting of the collar is essential to ensure its effectiveness and minimize the risk of skin irritation or pressure sores.

In addition to providing support, soft cervical collars may also serve as a helpful reminder for patients to maintain proper posture and avoid abrupt or forceful neck movements that could exacerbate their symptoms. The proprioceptive feedback provided by the collar can help patients become more aware of their neck positioning and encourage the adoption of healthier postural habits.

While soft cervical collars can provide temporary relief for patients experiencing neck pain, they are not intended for long-term use. Prolonged immobilization of the neck can lead to muscle atrophy, joint stiffness, and reduced range of motion. Consequently, healthcare professionals typically recommend that soft cervical collars be worn only for short periods, such as during particularly painful episodes or specific activities that may aggravate the patient's symptoms.

It is essential for patients to follow their healthcare provider's guidance regarding the appropriate duration and frequency of soft collar use. In many cases, the use of a soft cervical collar will be complemented by other conservative treatment measures, such as physical therapy, pain medication, and lifestyle modifications. These interventions can help to address the underlying causes of neck pain and improve the patient's overall functional ability, reducing the need for long-term reliance on a cervical collar.

Soft cervical collars can play a valuable role in the management of acute neck pain by providing gentle support, restricting excessive movement, and promoting healing. However, their use should be limited to short periods and implemented alongside other treatment strategies to address the root causes of neck pain and prevent complications associated with long-term immobilization.

Semi-rigid cervical collars are a type of orthotic device that combines the benefits of soft and rigid collars. They offer a higher degree of support and immobilization compared to soft collars, while still maintaining a certain level of comfort for the patient. The design of these collars incorporates a combination of rigid plastic materials and soft padding, striking a balance between support and comfort.

The primary function of semi-rigid cervical collars is to restrict neck movement, which can help alleviate pain and discomfort associated with moderate neck pain, stiffness, or cervical injuries. By limiting motion in the affected area, semi-rigid collars provide stability and support to the cervical spine, promoting the healing process and preventing further injury.

In addition to their use in cases of moderate neck pain or stiffness, semi-rigid cervical collars can also serve as post-operative support for patients who have undergone cervical spine surgery. In these cases, the collar helps maintain the alignment and stability of the cervical spine, allowing the patient to safely perform daily activities while recovering from the procedure.

However, it is crucial to consider the potential drawbacks of semi-rigid cervical collar use. Similar to soft collars, long-term reliance on semi-rigid collars is not recommended, as it may lead to muscle atrophy and reduced neck mobility. Prolonged use of these collars can cause the neck muscles to weaken, which may exacerbate neck pain and stiffness in the long run. To avoid this, healthcare professionals should carefully monitor the patient's progress and adjust the collar-wearing schedule accordingly.

It is also essential for patients to be educated on the proper use and fit of semi-rigid cervical collars. Inaccurate sizing or improper positioning can lead to discomfort, skin irritation, or reduced effectiveness of the device. Patients should consult with their healthcare provider to ensure the correct fit and follow any recommended adjustments to the collar over time.

Semi-rigid cervical collars can be an effective tool in the management of moderate neck pain or stiffness, as well as post-operative support and during the healing process after a cervical injury. However, their use should be carefully monitored, and patients should follow the guidance of their healthcare provider to ensure the optimal outcome. Additionally, it is important to remember that semi-rigid collars should be employed as part of a comprehensive treatment plan, which may also include other interventions such as physical therapy, medication management, and lifestyle modifications.

Rigid cervical collars are an essential orthotic device in the management of severe cervical injuries and conditions requiring maximum support and immobilization. These collars are designed with the primary aim of maintaining cervical spine alignment, restricting movement, and stabilizing the neck to allow for healing and recovery.

Rigid cervical collars consist of two main parts: an anterior (front) and a posterior (back) shell made of rigid plastic or metal components. The shells are lined with padding or foam to ensure patient comfort and proper fit. The two halves are secured together using adjustable straps, buckles, or Velcro, which allows for customization of fit and immobilization according to the patient's needs and the treating healthcare professional's recommendations.

One of the primary indications for rigid cervical collars is the management of severe cervical injuries, such as fractures or dislocations. In these cases, the collar helps to maintain spinal alignment, reduce the risk of further injury, and promote healing by immobilizing the affected vertebrae. Rigid cervical collars can also be used to provide post-surgical immobilization following procedures such as cervical fusion or discectomy. In this context, the collar helps to maintain proper alignment of the spine, protect the surgical site, and reduce the risk of complications during the healing process.

Rigid cervical collars may also be prescribed for patients with specific conditions that require maximum support, such as severe cervical spondylosis or advanced degenerative disc disease. In these cases, the collar helps to limit movement, alleviate pain, and prevent further damage to the cervical spine. It is important to note, however, that the use of a rigid cervical collar should always be accompanied by a comprehensive treatment plan that addresses the underlying cause of the patient's condition.

While rigid cervical collars provide the highest level of immobilization, their use is not without potential drawbacks. Prolonged immobilization can lead to muscle atrophy, joint stiffness, and reduced range of motion. Therefore, it is essential that the duration of collar use be carefully determined by the treating healthcare professional based on the patient's condition, progress, and individual needs. In some cases, a gradual transition to a semi-rigid or soft collar may be recommended as the patient's condition improves.

Moreover, proper sizing and fitting of the rigid cervical collar are crucial to ensure patient comfort and optimal immobilization. An improperly fitted collar can cause discomfort, skin irritation, and even compromise the effectiveness of the device. Healthcare professionals must take accurate measurements of the patient's neck circumference and height, and make necessary adjustments to the collar to achieve an appropriate fit.

Rigid cervical collars play a critical role in the management of severe cervical injuries and conditions requiring maximum support and immobilization. By maintaining cervical spine alignment, limiting movement, and stabilizing the neck, these collars can promote healing and recovery. However, it is essential to consider the potential risks and drawbacks associated with prolonged immobilization and to ensure proper sizing and fitting of the device for optimal patient outcomes.

Cervical orthotic devices, such as cervical collars, can be beneficial in various situations. For instance, they are often used in the management of acute neck strains or sprains, as they provide support and restrict movement to prevent further injury. Additionally, cervical orthotic devices are helpful in the treatment of whiplash-associated disorders, which result from sudden acceleration-deceleration forces acting on the neck. These devices can help limit excessive motion, reduce inflammation, and promote healing in the affected soft tissues.

Orthotic devices are also commonly used to provide post-surgical support and immobilization following cervical spine surgery. They help maintain the proper alignment of the spine, protecting the surgical site and allowing the tissues to heal without disruption. Moreover, cervical orthotic devices can be used in cases of cervical radiculopathy, a condition characterized by nerve compression at the neck level, leading to pain, numbness, or weakness radiating into the arm. By limiting neck movement, these devices can alleviate pressure on the affected nerve roots and decrease pain. Similarly, they can be employed in the management of cervical spondylosis, a degenerative condition affecting the cervical spine's joints and discs. Cervical collars can help provide temporary relief from pain and discomfort by reducing the strain on the cervical spine structures.

However, certain contraindications or precautions must be considered when using cervical orthotic devices. Inappropriate sizing or fit can lead to discomfort, skin irritation, or reduced effectiveness of the device. It is essential to ensure that the device is properly fitted and adjusted by a healthcare professional to prevent complications and achieve optimal therapeutic results.

Another important consideration is the potential for muscle weakness and reduced range of motion resulting from long-term use of cervical collars. Patients should follow the recommended wearing schedule provided by their healthcare professional to minimize the risk of these complications. Typically, the use of cervical orthotic devices should be limited to short periods, and the patient should gradually wean off the device as their condition improves. In some cases, healthcare professionals may prescribe neck strengthening exercises or physical therapy to promote muscle strength and flexibility during or after the use of a cervical collar.

In cases of severe cervical instability or spinal cord compression, a rigid cervical collar may not provide sufficient immobilization, and other interventions may be necessary. Such situations may require more aggressive treatment approaches, such as surgery or external fixation devices, to ensure adequate stabilization and protect the spinal cord from further injury. Healthcare professionals must carefully evaluate the patient's condition and determine the most appropriate course of action based on the individual's needs and clinical presentation.

The evidence supporting the effectiveness of cervical traction and orthotic devices in neck pain treatment is still evolving, with varying results reported in different studies. Despite their widespread use in clinical practice, further research is needed to solidify their efficacy and determine the best application methods for various neck pain conditions.

In the case of cervical traction, several studies have reported short-term benefits for patients with cervical radiculopathy and herniated discs. For instance, a randomized controlled trial by Fritz et al. (2014) demonstrated that cervical traction combined with exercise and manual therapy resulted in improved pain and functional outcomes for patients with cervical radiculopathy compared to a control group receiving only exercise and manual therapy. However, the long-term benefits of cervical traction remain less clear, with limited research examining the durability of these positive effects over time. Therefore, more high-quality, long-term studies are needed to establish the role of cervical traction in neck pain treatment definitively.

The use of cervical orthotic devices, such as cervical collars, has also shown mixed results in the management of neck pain. Some studies suggest that soft cervical collars, when used in combination with other conservative treatments like physical therapy and medication, can provide temporary pain relief and improved function. For example, a systematic review by Bono et al. (2007) found that cervical collars could be beneficial for short-term pain relief in patients with acute whiplash-associated disorders. However, the same review noted that there was insufficient evidence to support the use of cervical collars for chronic neck pain.

Conversely, other studies have reported no significant benefits or even detrimental effects associated with cervical collar use. A randomized controlled trial by Kuijper et al. (2009) found that patients with cervical radiculopathy who wore a semi-rigid collar for three weeks had no significant improvement in pain or functional outcomes compared to those who did not wear a collar. Furthermore, long-term use of cervical collars has been associated with negative consequences such as muscle weakness and reduced range of motion. Therefore, the application of cervical collars should be carefully considered and should be limited to short-term use in specific situations.

Overall, the evidence supporting the use of cervical traction and orthotic devices is still developing, and more high-quality research is needed to confirm their efficacy in neck pain management. It is crucial to consider the individual patient's condition and employ these supportive aids as part of a comprehensive, multimodal treatment plan that also includes other conservative interventions such as physical therapy, medication management, and lifestyle modifications.

Cervical traction and orthotic devices have proven to be valuable tools in the management of neck pain. By providing non-invasive and supportive treatment options, these devices can alleviate pain, promote healing, and restore function in the cervical spine. However, the effectiveness of these interventions may vary depending on the individual patient's condition, highlighting the importance of tailoring the treatment plan to the specific needs of each patient.

Healthcare professionals need to take into account the indications, contraindications, and precautions associated with cervical traction and orthotic devices to ensure patient safety and treatment efficacy. For instance, patients with severe cervical instability, inflammatory conditions, or prior cervical surgery may require alternative treatments or special considerations when using cervical traction or orthotic devices.

Patient adherence to the recommendations of their healthcare provider is crucial for the success of any treatment plan involving cervical traction or orthotic devices. This includes following the prescribed wearing schedule or traction protocol, as well as attending regular follow-up appointments to monitor progress and make necessary adjustments. Moreover, patients should be educated about the potential risks of long-term use of cervical collars, such as muscle weakness and reduced range of motion. This emphasizes the importance of maintaining neck mobility and strength through appropriate exercises and rehabilitation programs.

In the context of a comprehensive treatment plan, cervical traction and orthotic devices should be employed as part of a multimodal approach. This approach incorporates other conservative interventions, such as physical therapy, medication management, and lifestyle modifications, to address the underlying causes of neck pain effectively. Physical therapy, for example, can help patients develop better posture, improve muscle strength and flexibility, and learn techniques for pain management. In conjunction, medication management can address inflammation, pain, and muscle spasms, while lifestyle modifications, such as ergonomic improvements and stress management techniques, can reduce the likelihood of recurrent neck pain.

Ongoing research plays a significant role in enhancing our understanding of the role of cervical traction and orthotic devices in neck pain treatment. As scientific knowledge advances, clinicians can make more informed decisions about the use of these supportive aids, optimizing their effectiveness for individual patients. Additionally, advances in technology and materials science may lead to the development of more effective and comfortable devices in the future. For instance, improvements in cervical traction equipment may allow for more precise control over the traction force, duration, and direction, enhancing the overall therapeutic experience.

In conclusion, cervical traction and orthotic devices can be effective tools in the comprehensive treatment of neck pain when used judiciously and as part of a multimodal approach. By continually refining our understanding of these supportive aids and incorporating them into

147

personalized treatment plans, healthcare professionals can help patients with neck pain achieve optimal outcomes and improved quality of life.

Chapter 7

Medication Management

Analgesics, Anti-Inflammatories, and Muscle Relaxants

Neck pain is a prevalent issue that affects millions of people worldwide, significantly impacting their quality of life and daily functioning. Various factors can contribute to neck pain, including poor posture, muscle strain, degenerative conditions, nerve compression, and injuries. Medication management is a cornerstone of treatment for neck pain, often employed in combination with other conservative therapies such as physical therapy, lifestyle modifications, and complementary and alternative medicine.

The primary goals of medication management for neck pain include pain relief, reduction of inflammation, and facilitation of muscle relaxation. To achieve these goals, healthcare providers must consider the underlying cause of the neck pain, the severity and duration of symptoms, and any relevant patient factors such as age, medical history, and potential contraindications. By tailoring medication regimens to the individual patient, healthcare providers can optimize pain relief and functional improvement while minimizing the risk of side effects and complications.

Medication management for neck pain involves a wide range of pharmaceutical agents, each with its unique mechanisms of action, indications, and potential side effects. Some common medication classes used in the management of neck pain include analgesics, nonsteroidal anti-inflammatory drugs (NSAIDs), corticosteroids, muscle relaxants, antidepressants, and anticonvulsants. These medications may be used alone or in combination, depending on the specific needs of the patient and the nature of their neck pain.

In addition to understanding the various types of medications available for neck pain management, healthcare providers and patients must also be aware of the potential side effects and interactions associated with these drugs. This knowledge enables informed decision-making and ensures the safe and effective use of medications. Furthermore, it is crucial to recognize that medication management is often just one component of a comprehensive treatment plan for neck pain. Integrating medications with other conservative therapies, such as physical therapy, exercise, and posture modification, can help patients achieve optimal pain relief and long-term functional improvement.

Medication management is an essential aspect of neck pain treatment, encompassing a diverse array of pharmaceutical agents designed to alleviate pain, reduce inflammation, and promote muscle relaxation. By understanding the various medications available, their mechanisms of action, and potential side effects, healthcare providers and patients can work together to develop safe and effective treatment plans tailored to the individual's specific needs. Combining medication management with other conservative therapies can help patients achieve the best possible outcomes in their journey toward improved neck health and reduced pain.

Acetaminophen, also known as paracetamol, is a widely used over-the-counter (OTC) analgesic and antipyretic medication. As one of the most common pain-relief medications, it is often the first line of treatment for mild to moderate neck pain. The widespread use of acetaminophen can be attributed to its safety profile, ease of access, and low cost.

150

The precise mechanism of action of acetaminophen remains unclear. However, it is believed to involve the inhibition of prostaglandin synthesis in the central nervous system. Prostaglandins are lipid compounds that play a crucial role in inflammation and pain perception. They are responsible for sensitizing pain receptors, and inhibiting their synthesis can effectively reduce pain perception. This inhibition is thought to occur primarily in the central nervous system, with minimal impact on peripheral prostaglandin production, which distinguishes acetaminophen from nonsteroidal anti-inflammatory drugs (NSAIDs).

Acetaminophen is generally considered safe when used as directed, with a low incidence of side effects. The most common side effects are usually mild and include nausea and headache. However, long-term use or excessive doses can lead to hepatotoxicity (liver damage) and, in rare cases, acute liver failure. This risk is particularly concerning when daily doses exceed 4,000 milligrams (mg) for adults or when acetaminophen is combined with other medications that also contain acetaminophen, such as cold and flu remedies. To minimize the risk of liver damage, it is essential for patients to follow the recommended dosing guidelines and be cautious when using multiple medications containing acetaminophen.

Furthermore, individuals with pre-existing liver disease, chronic alcohol consumption, or who are using medications that induce liver enzymes, such as some anticonvulsants and tuberculosis drugs, may be at a higher risk of developing hepatotoxicity with acetaminophen use. In these cases, a lower maximum daily dose may be recommended, and close monitoring of liver function is essential.

Patients should also be aware of the potential for drug interactions with acetaminophen. For instance, the blood-thinning effect of warfarin, an anticoagulant medication, can be enhanced by the concurrent use of acetaminophen. As a result, it is crucial for individuals taking warfarin or similar medications to consult with their healthcare provider before using acetaminophen.

Acetaminophen is a widely used analgesic that can provide effective relief for mild to moderate neck pain. However, it is essential for patients to adhere to the recommended dosing guidelines and be vigilant for potential drug interactions and the risk of hepatotoxicity. As with any medication, it is crucial to consult with a healthcare professional before starting, stopping, or changing any medication regimen for neck pain.

Nonsteroidal anti-inflammatory drugs (NSAIDs) are a widely utilized class of medications that offer both analgesic and anti-inflammatory effects, making them particularly useful for addressing neck pain. NSAIDs work by inhibiting the activity of cyclooxygenase (COX) enzymes, which play a vital role in the production of prostaglandins. Prostaglandins are lipid compounds that contribute to inflammation and pain. By inhibiting COX enzymes, NSAIDs reduce prostaglandin synthesis, leading to a decrease in inflammation and pain.

There are two main types of COX enzymes: COX-1 and COX-2. COX-1 is responsible for the production of prostaglandins that protect the stomach lining and support blood clotting, while COX-2 is responsible for producing prostaglandins that cause inflammation and pain. Traditional NSAIDs, such as ibuprofen, naproxen, and aspirin, inhibit both COX-1 and COX-2 enzymes, providing pain relief and anti-inflammatory effects.

Selective COX-2 inhibitors, such as celecoxib, specifically target the COX-2 enzyme, resulting in a reduction of inflammation and pain without impacting the protective functions of COX-1. This selectivity may result in fewer gastrointestinal side effects compared to traditional NSAIDs. However, selective COX-2 inhibitors have been associated with an increased risk of cardiovascular events, necessitating careful consideration of patient risk factors when prescribing these medications.

NSAIDs can be effective for short-term relief of acute neck pain, particularly when inflammation is present. They can be used for various causes of neck pain, including muscle strains, ligament sprains, and degenerative conditions such as osteoarthritis. Over-the-counter NSAIDs are typically the first line of treatment, while prescription-strength NSAIDs may be considered for more severe or persistent pain.

While NSAIDs can provide significant relief for neck pain sufferers, their long-term use carries potential risks. One of the primary concerns with prolonged NSAID use is the increased risk of gastrointestinal (GI) complications. These complications can range from mild gastritis to more severe issues such as peptic ulcers and GI bleeding. This risk is particularly heightened in elderly patients, those with a history of GI issues, and individuals taking concomitant medications that can irritate the stomach lining, such as corticosteroids or anticoagulants.

In addition to GI complications, long-term use of NSAIDs has been associated with other potential side effects, including renal impairment, cardiovascular risks, and increased blood pressure. NSAIDs can reduce blood flow to the kidneys, potentially leading to acute kidney injury, particularly in patients with pre-existing kidney disease or those taking medications that affect renal blood flow, such as angiotensin-converting enzyme (ACE) inhibitors or diuretics. The cardiovascular risks associated with NSAIDs vary depending on the specific medication and patient population, but can include an increased risk of heart attack, stroke, and heart failure. These risks should be carefully weighed against the potential benefits of NSAID use, particularly in patients with known cardiovascular risk factors.

To minimize the risks associated with NSAIDs, healthcare providers should follow a patient-centered approach that focuses on using the lowest effective dose for the shortest duration possible. Additionally, patients should be closely monitored for potential side effects, and alternative pain management strategies should be considered in cases where the risks of NSAID use outweigh the benefits.

Opioid analgesics are a potent class of medications used to manage moderate to severe pain, including neck pain. These medications act on the mu, delta, and kappa opioid receptors in the central nervous system. By binding to these receptors, opioids reduce pain perception, provide relief, and, in some cases, induce a sense of euphoria.

Some commonly prescribed opioids for neck pain include hydrocodone (Vicodin, Lortab), oxycodone (OxyContin, Percocet), and tramadol (Ultram). These medications are available in various formulations, including immediate-release, extended-release, and combination products with other analgesics such as acetaminophen or NSAIDs. The choice of opioid and formulation depends on factors such as the severity and duration of pain, individual patient response, and the presence of any contraindications or potential drug interactions.

While opioids can be effective for short-term relief of severe neck pain, their use is associated with significant risks. One of the primary concerns with opioid use is the potential for dependence, which can develop even when the medication is used as prescribed. Dependence occurs when the body becomes accustomed to the presence of the drug, leading to withdrawal symptoms if the drug is abruptly discontinued.

In addition to dependence, opioids carry a risk of addiction. Addiction is a complex, chronic brain disease characterized by compulsive drug-seeking behavior despite negative consequences. Factors that can contribute to the development of opioid addiction include genetics, environmental influences, and individual psychological factors such as a history of substance abuse or mental health disorders.

The risk of overdose is another significant concern with opioid use. Overdose can occur when a patient takes too much of the medication, either intentionally or unintentionally, resulting in respiratory depression and, in severe cases, death. The risk of overdose is higher in patients who combine opioids with other central nervous system depressants, such as benzodiazepines or alcohol.

Due to these risks, opioids should be reserved for cases in which other pain management strategies have been ineffective or are contraindicated. When prescribing opioids for neck pain, healthcare providers should carefully assess the patient's risk factors for abuse, including personal and family history of substance abuse, mental health disorders, and previous history of opioid misuse. Providers should also consider using risk mitigation strategies, such as prescription drug monitoring programs and patient-provider agreements, to minimize the potential for misuse and diversion.

When initiating opioid therapy for neck pain, the lowest effective dose should be used for the shortest duration necessary to achieve pain relief and functional improvement. Healthcare providers should closely monitor the patient's progress and adjust the dose as needed, taking into consideration factors such as pain severity, functional status, and the presence of any adverse effects. If a decision is made to discontinue opioid therapy, the dose should be tapered gradually to minimize withdrawal symptoms.

It is also essential for patients and healthcare providers to be aware of the potential drug interactions between opioids and other medications, as well as any contraindications to opioid use. Some common drug interactions include the combination of opioids with benzodiazepines, which can increase the risk of respiratory depression, and the use of opioids with certain antidepressants, which can lead to a potentially life-threatening condition called serotonin syndrome.

Opioids can be an effective option for managing severe neck pain in select cases when used judiciously and with appropriate caution. Healthcare providers should carefully weigh the potential risks and benefits of opioid therapy and employ strategies to minimize the risk of dependence, addiction, and overdose. Patients should be educated about the proper use, storage, and disposal of opioids, as well as the signs and symptoms of overdose and the availability of naloxone, an opioid antagonist that can reverse the effects of an opioid overdose in emergency situations.

In some cases, alternative opioid formulations or routes of administration may be considered for managing neck pain, particularly when oral opioids are not effective or well-tolerated. Transdermal opioid formulations, such as the fentanyl patch, can provide sustained pain relief for patients with chronic neck pain who require continuous opioid therapy. The transdermal route bypasses the gastrointestinal system, which can reduce the risk of side effects such as nausea and constipation. However, transdermal opioids are not suitable for patients with acute or rapidly fluctuating pain, as the onset of action is slow and the duration of effect is prolonged.

Another alternative route of administration for opioids is the intranasal route, which involves the administration of a medication, such as butorphanol, via a nasal spray. Intranasal opioids can provide rapid pain relief and may be useful for patients with breakthrough pain or difficulty swallowing oral medications. However, intranasal opioids are associated with their own set of side effects, such as nasal irritation and congestion, and their use should be carefully monitored by a healthcare provider.

Opioid rotation refers to the practice of switching from one opioid to another in order to maintain effective pain relief while minimizing side effects and the risk of dependence or addiction. This strategy can be useful in patients who develop tolerance to a particular opioid or experience unacceptable side effects. When conducting an opioid rotation, it is important to calculate the equianalgesic dose of the new opioid to avoid underdosing or overdosing the patient.

In some cases, combination therapy with opioids and other analgesic medications may be necessary to achieve optimal pain relief. For example, a patient with neck pain and inflammation may benefit from the addition of an NSAID to their opioid regimen, as the two medications work through different mechanisms to provide additive or synergistic pain relief. Similarly, the combination of an opioid and an adjuvant medication, such as an antidepressant or anticonvulsant, may be effective for patients with neuropathic neck pain.

Patient education and counseling are critical components of opioid therapy for neck pain. Patients should be informed about the potential risks and benefits of opioid use, as well as the importance of adhering to their prescribed dosing regimen and monitoring for side effects. They should also be educated about the proper storage and disposal of opioids to minimize the risk of accidental exposure or diversion.

In addition, patients should be counseled on non-pharmacologic pain management strategies, such as physical therapy, relaxation techniques, and lifestyle modifications, which can help improve their overall pain and functional status. By providing comprehensive education and support, healthcare providers can empower patients to take an active role in their pain management and make informed decisions about their treatment options.

The use of opioids for neck pain management requires a careful and individualized approach, taking into consideration the potential risks and benefits of therapy, as well as the patient's unique medical history and circumstances. With appropriate patient selection, monitoring, and education, opioids can be a valuable tool for managing severe neck pain in select cases.

Corticosteroids are a class of anti-inflammatory medications that can be used to manage neck pain, particularly when it is associated with significant inflammation or an autoimmune component. These medications work by mimicking the action of cortisol, a naturally occurring hormone produced by the adrenal glands. Corticosteroids help reduce inflammation by suppressing the immune response, inhibiting the production of inflammatory mediators, and decreasing the expression of pro-inflammatory genes.

Corticosteroids can be administered in several ways, depending on the severity and location of the inflammation. Oral corticosteroids, such as prednisone, are typically used for short-term relief of severe inflammation. They are often prescribed in a tapering dosage regimen, starting with a high dose and gradually reducing the dose over time to minimize side effects and allow the body to adjust.

In some cases, healthcare providers may administer corticosteroid injections directly into the affected area to provide targeted relief of inflammation and pain. These injections, also known as epidural steroid injections, can be particularly helpful for patients with neck pain caused by conditions such as herniated discs, spinal stenosis, or radiculopathy. By delivering the medication directly to the site of inflammation, corticosteroid injections can provide rapid relief with fewer systemic side effects compared to oral corticosteroids.

Topical corticosteroids, such as creams or gels, are less commonly used for neck pain but may be beneficial in specific cases, such as localized inflammation due to an underlying skin condition or superficial soft tissue inflammation. These formulations can provide targeted anti-inflammatory effects with minimal systemic absorption, reducing the risk of side effects.

Despite their potential benefits, corticosteroids should be used judiciously due to their potential side effects, particularly when used for prolonged periods. Short-term side effects can include weight gain, fluid retention, hypertension, mood changes, and hyperglycemia. Long-term use of corticosteroids is associated with more severe side effects, such as osteoporosis, increased susceptibility to infections, adrenal insufficiency, and Cushing's syndrome.

To minimize the risks associated with corticosteroid use, healthcare providers should carefully consider the patient's medical history, potential contraindications, and the severity of their neck pain. When prescribing corticosteroids, the lowest effective dose should be used for the shortest duration necessary to achieve the desired therapeutic effect. In addition, patients should be monitored closely for any signs of side effects or complications.

Patients using corticosteroids should also be educated about the potential risks and benefits of the medication, as well as the importance of adhering to their prescribed regimen. If a patient experiences side effects or if the corticosteroid therapy is no longer effective, the healthcare provider may consider alternative treatment options or adjust the dosage to minimize risks while maintaining adequate pain relief.

Benzodiazepines are a class of medications that act on gamma-aminobutyric acid (GABA) receptors in the central nervous system, promoting muscle relaxation and sedation. GABA is the primary inhibitory neurotransmitter in the brain, and when benzodiazepines bind to its receptors, they enhance the inhibitory effects of GABA, leading to muscle relaxation and reduced muscle spasms. Some commonly prescribed benzodiazepines for neck pain include diazepam and clonazepam. These medications can be helpful for patients experiencing neck pain due to muscle spasms or tension, as well as those with underlying anxiety disorders that may exacerbate muscle tension.

The efficacy of benzodiazepines in treating muscle-related neck pain varies depending on the specific medication, dosage, and duration of treatment. In general, short-term use of benzodiazepines may provide significant relief for patients with acute muscle spasms, while long-term use is less likely to be beneficial and may even worsen pain in some cases due to the development of tolerance and dependence.

While benzodiazepines can provide relief for muscle-related neck pain, their use is associated with potential risks, including dependence, tolerance, and withdrawal. Dependence occurs when the body becomes accustomed to the presence of the medication, and stopping or reducing the dosage may lead to withdrawal symptoms such as increased anxiety, insomnia, and muscle pain. Tolerance refers to the reduced effectiveness of the medication over time, requiring higher doses to achieve the same therapeutic effect. These risks are particularly concerning in patients with a history of substance abuse or those taking other medications with sedative effects, such as opioids or alcohol.

Furthermore, benzodiazepines have several potential side effects, including drowsiness, dizziness, impaired coordination, and cognitive impairment. These side effects can pose risks to patient safety, particularly in elderly individuals or those with pre-existing balance or cognitive issues.

Due to these risks, benzodiazepines should be used with caution and under the guidance of a healthcare professional. When initiating treatment with benzodiazepines, the lowest effective dose should be used, and the duration of treatment should be kept as short as possible to minimize the risk of dependence and tolerance. When discontinuing benzodiazepines, it is crucial to taper the dose gradually under the supervision of a healthcare professional to minimize withdrawal symptoms and reduce the risk of rebound muscle spasms.

In some cases, alternative muscle relaxants, such as non-benzodiazepine muscle relaxants or antispasmodic medications, may be more appropriate for treating muscle-related neck pain due to their lower risk of dependence and withdrawal. However, the choice of muscle relaxant should be tailored to the individual patient, considering factors such as the severity and duration of pain, the presence of underlying medical conditions, and the potential for drug-drug interactions.

Non-benzodiazepine muscle relaxants are a diverse group of medications that work through various mechanisms to promote muscle relaxation and relieve pain. These medications are typically prescribed for short-term use to alleviate muscle-related neck pain caused by muscle spasms, strains, or tension.

Cyclobenzaprine, a commonly prescribed non-benzodiazepine muscle relaxant, is thought to act centrally within the brainstem to reduce muscle tone. This action makes it particularly useful for short-term relief of muscle spasms associated with neck pain. While cyclobenzaprine is generally well-tolerated, some potential side effects include drowsiness, dizziness, and dry mouth. Additionally, cyclobenzaprine can interact with other medications, particularly monoamine oxidase inhibitors (MAOIs), so it is essential to discuss any potential drug interactions with a healthcare provider.

Baclofen is another non-benzodiazepine muscle relaxant that acts on GABA-B receptors to inhibit the release of excitatory neurotransmitters, leading to decreased muscle tone and spasticity. This mechanism of action makes baclofen particularly useful in treating muscle-related neck pain that involves spasticity, such as that caused by certain neurological conditions. Baclofen can be administered orally or, in more severe cases, intrathecally (directly into the spinal fluid) via an implanted pump. Potential side effects of baclofen include drowsiness, dizziness, and weakness. Long-term use of baclofen may lead to dependence, and abrupt discontinuation can cause withdrawal symptoms, so it is crucial to taper the medication gradually under a healthcare provider's supervision.

Tizanidine is an alpha-2 adrenergic agonist that works by inhibiting the release of norepinephrine, resulting in decreased muscle tone and spasm. Tizanidine is typically prescribed for short-term management of muscle-related neck pain and is particularly useful in cases where muscle spasms are the primary cause of discomfort. However, tizanidine can cause side effects such as drowsiness, dizziness, and dry mouth. It is also associated with potential liver toxicity, so regular liver function monitoring is recommended during treatment. Tizanidine has the potential to interact with various other medications, including certain blood pressure medications and fluoroquinolone antibiotics, so discussing potential drug interactions with a healthcare provider is essential.

While non-benzodiazepine muscle relaxants can be effective in relieving muscle-related neck pain, their use is associated with potential side effects and risks. These medications should be used with caution in patients with a history of liver or kidney impairment and those taking other medications with sedative effects. It is essential to discuss the potential benefits and risks of non-benzodiazepine muscle relaxants with a healthcare provider to determine the most appropriate treatment for an individual's specific needs. When using these medications, it is crucial to follow the prescribed dosing regimen and monitor for any potential side effects or interactions with other medications.

Antidepressants have demonstrated efficacy in providing relief for some patients with chronic neck pain, particularly when the pain has a neuropathic component. Among the various classes of antidepressants, tricyclic antidepressants (TCAs) and selective serotonin-norepinephrine reuptake inhibitors (SNRIs) are the most commonly prescribed for pain management. These medications are thought to exert their analgesic effects by modulating pain perception in the central nervous system.

Tricyclic antidepressants (TCAs) are an older class of antidepressant medications that have shown potential in providing pain relief for some cases of chronic neck pain, especially when it is neuropathic. Commonly prescribed TCAs for neck pain management include amitriptyline, nortriptyline, and desipramine. The analgesic effects of TCAs are primarily attributed to their ability to inhibit the reuptake of serotonin and norepinephrine, neurotransmitters that play a crucial role in pain modulation.

Despite their potential effectiveness in relieving neck pain, the use of TCAs is associated with several side effects. Some common side effects include sedation, dry mouth, constipation, urinary retention, and orthostatic hypotension. Moreover, TCAs can potentially interact with other medications, leading to adverse effects or reduced efficacy. As a result, they should be used with caution, especially in elderly patients and those with pre-existing cardiovascular, liver, or kidney conditions. Healthcare providers must carefully consider the risk-benefit profile of TCAs and initiate treatment with low doses, gradually titrating the dose based on patient response and tolerability.

Selective serotonin-norepinephrine reuptake inhibitors (SNRIs) are a newer class of antidepressants that have demonstrated potential in providing relief for some patients with chronic neck pain. Like TCAs, SNRIs are thought to exert their analgesic effects by inhibiting the reuptake of serotonin and norepinephrine, thereby modulating pain perception in the central nervous system. Some commonly prescribed SNRIs for neck pain management include duloxetine and venlafaxine.

In comparison to TCAs, SNRIs tend to have a more favorable side effect profile, with fewer anticholinergic side effects and less sedation. However, they can still cause side effects such as dizziness, nausea, dry mouth, and increased blood pressure. SNRIs should be used with caution in patients with a history of liver or kidney impairment, as well as those taking other medications that can interact with these drugs.

The choice between TCAs and SNRIs for neck pain management should be based on individual patient factors, potential side effects, drug-drug interactions, and the specific clinical context. In some cases, a combination of antidepressants and other medications, such as analgesics, anti-inflammatory drugs, or muscle relaxants, may be necessary to achieve optimal pain relief and functional improvement. It is essential to involve the patient in shared decision-making and regularly monitor their progress and tolerability to ensure the safe and effective use of these medications in neck pain management.

Selective serotonin-norepinephrine reuptake inhibitors (SNRIs) have emerged as a promising class of antidepressant medications for the management of chronic neck pain. These medications have demonstrated efficacy in treating various chronic pain conditions, including neuropathic pain, fibromyalgia, and musculoskeletal pain. The use of SNRIs for neck pain is supported by their ability to modulate pain perception in the central nervous system through the inhibition of serotonin and norepinephrine reuptake.

Duloxetine is a commonly prescribed SNRI for neck pain management. It has been approved by the US Food and Drug Administration (FDA) for the treatment of chronic musculoskeletal pain, including chronic low back pain and osteoarthritis pain. Several clinical trials have demonstrated the effectiveness of duloxetine in reducing pain and improving function in patients with chronic neck pain. The recommended starting dose for duloxetine in treating chronic pain is typically 30 mg daily, with a gradual increase to a maintenance dose of 60 mg daily as tolerated.

Venlafaxine is another SNRI that has been used off-label for the treatment of chronic neck pain. While it has not received specific FDA approval for this indication, some clinical studies have suggested that venlafaxine may be effective in reducing pain and improving function in patients with chronic neck pain, particularly when the pain is neuropathic in nature. The recommended starting dose for venlafaxine in treating chronic pain is usually 37.5 mg daily, with a gradual increase to a maintenance dose of 75-225 mg daily as tolerated.

Compared to TCAs, SNRIs generally have a more favorable side effect profile, with fewer anticholinergic side effects such as dry mouth, constipation, urinary retention, and blurred vision. They also tend to cause less sedation, which can be an advantage for patients who require daytime pain relief. However, SNRIs can still cause side effects such as dizziness, nausea, dry mouth, and increased blood pressure. In some cases, SNRIs may also cause sweating, sexual dysfunction, and insomnia.

It is important to use SNRIs with caution in patients with a history of liver or kidney impairment, as these conditions may affect the metabolism and excretion of the medications, leading to increased risk of side effects. Additionally, SNRIs should be used cautiously in patients taking other medications that can interact with these drugs, such as monoamine oxidase inhibitors (MAOIs), other serotonergic medications, or medications that affect the metabolism of SNRIs through the cytochrome P450 system.

When initiating treatment with an SNRI for chronic neck pain, healthcare providers should closely monitor the patient's response to the medication and adjust the dose as needed to balance pain relief with the risk of side effects. It is also important to educate patients about the potential side effects and the need for gradual dose titration to minimize the risk of adverse reactions. When discontinuing SNRIs, the dose should be tapered gradually to reduce the risk of withdrawal symptoms.

Anticonvulsant medications, originally developed for the treatment of epilepsy, have gained recognition for their effectiveness in managing various forms of chronic pain, including neck pain, especially when the pain is neuropathic in nature. Neuropathic pain arises from the dysfunction or damage of the nervous system and is often characterized by symptoms such as burning, tingling, or shooting sensations. Anticonvulsants, such as gabapentin and pregabalin, have shown promise in alleviating these symptoms by modulating pain perception in the central nervous system.

Gabapentin, initially developed as an antiepileptic drug, has become a popular choice for the treatment of neuropathic neck pain. Gabapentin's exact mechanism of action is not completely understood; however, it is

163

thought to bind to the alpha-2-delta subunit of voltage-gated calcium channels, reducing the release of excitatory neurotransmitters like glutamate, substance P, and calcitonin gene-related peptide. This reduction in neurotransmitter release leads to a decrease in neuronal excitability and, subsequently, a decrease in pain perception.

Gabapentin is typically administered in oral form, with the dosage titrated up slowly to minimize side effects. The drug's effectiveness is often dose-dependent, with higher doses generally providing more significant pain relief. However, it is essential to balance the need for pain relief with the potential for side effects.

Pregabalin, a structural analog of gabapentin, is another anticonvulsant commonly prescribed for neuropathic neck pain. Like gabapentin, pregabalin is thought to bind to the alpha-2-delta subunit of voltage-gated calcium channels, reducing the release of excitatory neurotransmitters and modulating pain perception. Pregabalin has demonstrated effectiveness in treating various neuropathic pain conditions, including postherpetic neuralgia and diabetic peripheral neuropathy, and has been shown to provide relief for some patients with chronic neck pain.

Compared to gabapentin, pregabalin has a more predictable pharmacokinetic profile, allowing for more consistent dosing and a faster onset of action. Pregabalin is also administered orally and should be titrated slowly to minimize side effects.

While anticonvulsants such as gabapentin and pregabalin can be effective in relieving neuropathic neck pain, their use is associated with potential side effects. Common side effects include dizziness, drowsiness, fatigue, and peripheral edema. Less common but more severe side effects can include mood changes, suicidal ideation, and hypersensitivity reactions.

These medications should be used with caution in patients with a history of liver or kidney impairment, as impaired organ function may lead to decreased drug clearance and an increased risk of side effects. Furthermore, caution is advised when using anticonvulsants alongside other medications with sedative effects or those that can interact with these drugs, as this may lead to additive side effects or altered drug efficacy.

When prescribing anticonvulsants for neuropathic neck pain, it is essential to educate patients about the potential side effects, the importance of adhering to the prescribed dosing regimen, and the need for regular monitoring. Patients should be instructed to report any new or worsening side effects to their healthcare provider promptly. Additionally, patients should be monitored for changes in pain levels, functional status, and the development of any new symptoms or side effects. This monitoring will help ensure that the medication is providing adequate pain relief while minimizing the risk of adverse effects.

In some cases, anticonvulsants may be used in combination with other medications or non-pharmacological treatment options to achieve optimal pain relief and functional improvement for patients with chronic neck pain. Combining anticonvulsants with analgesics, anti-inflammatory drugs, muscle relaxants, or antidepressants may provide a synergistic effect and improve overall pain management. However, when using combination therapy, it is crucial to monitor patients closely for potential drug-drug interactions and additive side effects.

Future research in the field of anticonvulsants for neck pain may focus on identifying new therapeutic targets and developing novel medications with improved efficacy and tolerability. Additionally, further studies are needed to determine the most effective dosing regimens and to identify specific patient populations that may benefit the most from anticonvulsant therapy for neck pain.

Anticonvulsant medications, such as gabapentin and pregabalin, have demonstrated effectiveness in managing neuropathic neck pain for some patients. These medications work by binding to voltage-gated calcium channels and modulating pain perception in the central nervous system. While anticonvulsants can provide significant pain relief, their use is associated with potential side effects, and caution should be exercised in patients with liver or kidney impairment or those taking other medications that can interact with these drugs. Healthcare providers should closely monitor patients on anticonvulsant therapy for changes in pain levels, functional status, and the development of any new symptoms or side effects. Combination therapy with other medications or non-pharmacological treatments may be necessary in some cases to achieve optimal pain relief and functional improvement.

Medication management is a vital aspect of neck pain treatment, offering a range of options to address the diverse causes and symptoms associated with this common condition. The judicious use of medications, such as analgesics, anti-inflammatory drugs, muscle relaxants, antidepressants, and anticonvulsants, can significantly improve patients' quality of life by providing pain relief, reducing inflammation, and promoting muscle relaxation. However, navigating the complex landscape of medication management requires careful consideration of several factors, including the potential risks and benefits of each drug, individual patient characteristics, and appropriate dosing and monitoring.

One of the primary concerns in medication management for neck pain is balancing efficacy with safety. Each medication class carries its unique set of potential side effects and contraindications, which must be weighed against the anticipated benefits. For example, while NSAIDs and opioids can be highly effective in relieving pain, their use is associated with an increased risk of gastrointestinal complications, dependence, and addiction, respectively. Therefore, healthcare providers must carefully assess each patient's medical history, concurrent medications, and potential risk factors before prescribing these drugs.

Another crucial aspect of medication management is tailoring treatment to the specific needs of individual patients. Each patient's unique medical history, symptoms, and underlying causes of neck pain must be taken into account when selecting the most appropriate medication or combination of medications. For example, patients with neuropathic neck pain may benefit more from antidepressants or anticonvulsants than from traditional analgesics, whereas patients with muscle spasms may find relief with muscle relaxants. Furthermore, some patients may require a combination of medications to achieve optimal pain relief and functional improvement, underscoring the importance of a personalized approach to treatment.

Appropriate dosing and monitoring are also critical components of successful medication management for neck pain. Healthcare providers must be vigilant in prescribing the lowest effective dose for the shortest duration necessary to minimize the risk of side effects and complications. This is particularly important when using medications with a narrow therapeutic window, such as opioids or benzodiazepines. Additionally, regular monitoring of patients' progress and medication adherence is essential to ensure the ongoing effectiveness and safety of the prescribed treatment regimen.

Finally, it is important to recognize that medication management is often only one part of a comprehensive treatment plan for neck pain. In many cases, medications should be used in conjunction with other conservative therapies, such as physical therapy, manual therapy, and lifestyle modifications, to address the multifaceted nature of neck pain and promote long-term improvement. Moreover, patients should be encouraged to maintain open communication with their healthcare providers and report any concerns or side effects related to their medications promptly.

In conclusion, medication management plays a crucial role in the treatment of neck pain, offering a wide array of options to address various symptoms and underlying causes. By carefully considering the potential risks and benefits of each medication, individual patient factors, and the need for appropriate dosing and monitoring, healthcare providers can help patients achieve optimal pain relief and functional improvement while minimizing potential complications. As always, patients should consult with their healthcare providers before starting, stopping, or changing any medication regimen for neck pain.

168

Chapter 8

Interventional Pain Management

Cervical Epidural Steroid Injections to Cervical Spinal Cord Stimulation and Dorsal Root Ganglion Stimulation

Interventional pain management techniques have emerged as a crucial component of modern pain medicine, addressing the limitations of conservative treatments for chronic neck pain. Neck pain is a widespread condition that can significantly impact an individual's quality of life, often resulting from various factors such as poor posture, muscle strain, nerve compression, and degenerative changes in the cervical spine. When conservative treatments like medication, physical therapy, and lifestyle modifications fail to provide adequate relief, interventional pain management techniques offer an alternative approach to alleviate discomfort and improve functionality.

These minimally invasive procedures are designed to diagnose and treat the underlying causes of chronic pain by directly targeting the affected anatomical structures and pain pathways. By focusing on the source of pain, these techniques can provide more effective and longer-lasting relief compared to conservative treatments, which often address only the symptoms of pain. Additionally, the minimally invasive nature of these procedures reduces the risk of complications and promotes faster recovery times, making them a desirable option for many patients.

Interventional pain management techniques encompass a wide array of approaches, including epidural steroid injections, nerve blocks, and radiofrequency ablation, among others. Epidural steroid injections involve the administration of anti-inflammatory medication into the epidural space surrounding the spinal cord, reducing inflammation and providing relief from conditions such as radiculopathy and spinal stenosis. Nerve blocks, on the other hand, involve the injection of local anesthetic agents near specific nerves or nerve plexuses, temporarily interrupting the transmission of pain signals and providing diagnostic information about the source of pain. Radiofrequency ablation uses heat generated by radiofrequency energy to disrupt pain signals transmitted by targeted nerves, offering long-lasting relief for conditions like facet joint pain and neuropathic pain.

In recent years, advancements in medical technology have led to the development of innovative interventional pain management techniques, such as spinal cord stimulation and regenerative medicine therapies. These cutting-edge approaches leverage the body's natural healing mechanisms and the latest understanding of pain neurophysiology to provide more targeted and personalized pain relief. As research in this field continues to progress, interventional pain management techniques will likely play an increasingly important role in the comprehensive management of chronic neck pain, offering hope to those who have exhausted other treatment options.

Facet joints, also known as zygapophyseal joints, are small joints located between each vertebra in the spine. These synovial joints play a crucial role in providing stability and flexibility to the spinal column, allowing it to bend, twist, and extend. Each facet joint is composed of two opposing surfaces of cartilage, which are enclosed within a capsule filled with synovial fluid. This fluid helps to lubricate and cushion the joint, facilitating smooth movement.

Facet joint injections are a minimally invasive interventional pain management technique used to treat neck pain arising from various conditions that affect these joints. The procedure typically involves the administration of a combination of anesthetic and corticosteroid medications directly into the affected facet joint. The anesthetic provides immediate pain relief, while the corticosteroid helps to reduce inflammation and swelling in the long term.

Facet joint injections can be used to treat a variety of conditions that cause neck pain, such as facet joint arthritis or degeneration, spondylosis, and whiplash injuries. These conditions can lead to inflammation, irritation, or compression of the nerves that transmit pain signals from the facet joints to the brain, resulting in chronic neck pain and stiffness.

The facet joint injection procedure is performed under the guidance of fluoroscopy, a real-time X-ray imaging technique that allows the physician to accurately visualize the target joint and ensure proper placement of the needle. Once the target joint has been identified, the skin and underlying tissue are numbed using a local anesthetic. A thin needle is then carefully advanced through the skin and into the facet joint under fluoroscopic guidance. Once the needle is correctly positioned, the physician injects the medication mixture into the joint space.

The effectiveness of facet joint injections varies from person to person, with some patients experiencing significant pain relief that lasts for several months, while others may only have a temporary or partial improvement. In some cases, multiple injections may be required to achieve optimal pain relief. Facet joint injections are often used as part of a comprehensive treatment plan that includes physical therapy, medication management, and lifestyle modifications.

It is important to note that while facet joint injections can provide significant pain relief, they do not address the underlying cause of the pain. Therefore, it is essential to work closely with healthcare providers to develop a personalized treatment plan that addresses the root cause of the pain and promotes long-term healing and improved quality of life.

A cervical epidural steroid injection is a minimally invasive interventional pain management technique used to alleviate neck pain associated with various spinal conditions. These conditions include cervical radiculopathy, spinal stenosis, and disc herniation, among others. This procedure involves injecting a corticosteroid medication into the epidural space surrounding the spinal cord in the neck region to reduce inflammation, relieve pain, and promote healing in the affected area.

Cervical radiculopathy refers to the irritation or compression of nerve roots in the cervical spine, often causing pain, numbness, and weakness that may radiate down the arms. Spinal stenosis is a narrowing of the spinal canal, which can compress the spinal cord and nerve roots, leading to pain and other neurological symptoms. Disc herniation occurs when the soft, gel-like center of an intervertebral disc pushes through the outer layer, potentially compressing nearby nerves and causing pain.

The cervical epidural steroid injection procedure typically begins with the patient lying face down or sitting, depending on the physician's preference and the patient's comfort. The skin over the injection site is cleaned and numbed using a local anesthetic. Using fluoroscopy, a type of real-time X-ray imaging, the physician guides a thin needle through the skin and deeper tissues, reaching the epidural space in the cervical spine. Once the needle is in the correct location, a contrast dye may be injected to confirm the proper placement. Finally, the corticosteroid medication, often mixed with a local anesthetic, is injected into the epidural space.

The corticosteroid medication works by decreasing the inflammatory response in the affected area, which can provide relief from pain and promote healing. The local anesthetic provides immediate pain relief, while the steroid's effects may take several days to become apparent. The duration of pain relief varies from patient to patient, with some experiencing relief for weeks to months. In some cases, the procedure may need to be repeated if the pain returns or does not improve sufficiently.

Cervical epidural steroid injections are generally considered safe and well-tolerated, with a low risk of complications. However, potential risks and side effects may include infection, bleeding, nerve injury, allergic reactions, headache, and increased pain. It is crucial for patients to discuss their medical history and any medications they are taking with their physician before undergoing the procedure to minimize these risks.

Cervical epidural steroid injections can be an effective treatment option for patients experiencing neck pain due to conditions such as cervical radiculopathy, spinal stenosis, or disc herniation. By injecting corticosteroid medication into the epidural space, this procedure aims to reduce inflammation, relieve pain, and promote healing in the affected area. While generally safe and well-tolerated, patients should be aware of the potential risks and side effects and consult with their healthcare provider to determine if this treatment is appropriate for their specific needs.

The cervical transforaminal epidural steroid injection (CTESI) is an advanced interventional pain management technique that has been proven effective in providing relief from neck pain associated with conditions such as cervical radiculopathy and herniated discs. This procedure differs from the standard cervical epidural steroid injection in that it allows for a more targeted delivery of medication, leading to better outcomes for certain patients.

CTESI is performed under fluoroscopic guidance, a real-time X-ray imaging technique that ensures accurate needle placement. The patient is positioned lying face down or on their side, and a local anesthetic is applied to numb the skin and tissues at the injection site. The physician then inserts a thin needle through the skin and advances it into the targeted foramen, which is the opening through which the spinal nerve exits. The needle's position is confirmed using a contrast dye injection, visualized through fluoroscopy.

Once the needle's position has been verified, the physician injects a combination of a corticosteroid and a local anesthetic into the epidural space near the nerve root. The corticosteroid works to reduce inflammation around the affected nerve, while the local anesthetic provides immediate pain relief. This dual-action medication can alleviate symptoms caused by nerve compression, such as radiating pain, numbness, or weakness in the arms or hands.

CTESI offers several advantages over traditional cervical epidural steroid injections. The targeted approach allows for a more precise delivery of medication, which can result in more effective and longer-lasting pain relief. Additionally, the procedure can help physicians pinpoint the exact source of pain, leading to better-informed treatment decisions.

As with any medical procedure, there are potential risks and side effects associated with CTESI. Some of the most common side effects include temporary pain at the injection site, headache, and facial flushing. More severe but rare complications can include infection, bleeding, nerve damage, or an allergic reaction to the injected medications. The risk of complications can be minimized by selecting experienced physicians and following proper post-procedure care instructions.

The cervical transforaminal epidural steroid injection is a valuable tool in the arsenal of interventional pain management techniques for treating neck pain caused by nerve root compression. This targeted approach can provide significant relief for patients suffering from conditions such as cervical radiculopathy and herniated discs. However, as with any medical procedure, it is essential to carefully weigh the potential benefits against the risks and to consult with a qualified healthcare professional to determine the most appropriate course of treatment for each individual patient.

The cervical sympathetic block is an interventional pain management technique that targets the sympathetic nervous system, a part of the autonomic nervous system responsible for the body's "fight or flight" response. The sympathetic nervous system is also involved in the transmission of pain signals, particularly in chronic pain conditions such as complex regional pain syndrome (CRPS) and nerve-related neck pain. The cervical sympathetic block procedure aims to disrupt the transmission of these pain signals by injecting a local anesthetic into the sympathetic nerves located in the neck region.

The sympathetic nerves in the neck region include the stellate ganglion and the cervical sympathetic chain. The stellate ganglion is a collection of nerve cell bodies situated near the junction of the C7 and T1 vertebrae, while the cervical sympathetic chain is a series of interconnected ganglia that run along the length of the cervical spine. These structures are responsible for transmitting pain signals from the upper extremities, head, and neck to the spinal cord and brain.

174

The cervical sympathetic block is typically performed under fluoroscopic guidance, a real-time X-ray imaging technique, to ensure accurate placement of the needle and anesthetic. The patient is placed in a comfortable position, and the skin over the injection site is cleaned and numbed with a local anesthetic. A thin needle is then carefully advanced towards the targeted sympathetic nerves under fluoroscopic guidance. Once the needle is correctly positioned, the local anesthetic is injected, temporarily blocking the transmission of pain signals in the sympathetic nerves.

The effects of a cervical sympathetic block can be immediate, with patients reporting significant pain relief shortly after the procedure. In addition to pain relief, patients may also experience improved blood flow to the affected area, as the sympathetic nervous system plays a role in regulating blood vessel constriction. This improved blood flow may promote healing and reduce inflammation in the affected tissues. However, it is essential to note that the pain relief provided by a cervical sympathetic block is temporary, lasting from a few hours to several weeks, depending on the individual patient and the underlying condition being treated.

In some cases, patients may require a series of cervical sympathetic blocks to achieve optimal pain relief. For patients with chronic pain who experience significant relief from the procedure, additional treatments may be considered to provide more long-lasting pain relief. These treatments can include radiofrequency ablation of the sympathetic nerves or implantation of a spinal cord stimulator, which can modulate the pain signals transmitted by the sympathetic nerves.

Overall, the cervical sympathetic block is a valuable diagnostic and therapeutic tool in the management of chronic pain conditions involving the sympathetic nervous system. By providing temporary pain relief and improved blood flow, this procedure can help guide further treatment decisions and improve the quality of life for patients suffering from debilitating neck pain.

Cervical radiofrequency neurotomy, also known as radiofrequency ablation, is a minimally invasive procedure that provides relief for patients suffering from chronic neck pain. This technique is particularly useful in cases where conservative treatments have been ineffective, and the source of pain can be traced back to the medial branch nerves that innervate the facet joints in the cervical spine.

The procedure begins with the patient lying face down on a specialized table, and the skin over the treatment area is thoroughly cleansed and prepped. Local anesthesia is administered to numb the area and reduce discomfort during the procedure. Sedation may also be provided to help the patient remain relaxed and calm throughout the process.

Under the guidance of fluoroscopy, a type of real-time X-ray imaging, the physician carefully inserts a thin, needle-like probe through the skin and advances it toward the targeted medial branch nerves. This allows the physician to precisely target the affected nerves while minimizing the risk of damage to surrounding structures. Once the probe is in position, a small electrical current is passed through it to ensure proper placement and verify that the targeted nerve is responsible for the pain.

When the correct nerve has been identified, radiofrequency energy is delivered through the probe, generating heat that creates a small lesion on the nerve tissue. This lesion disrupts the transmission of pain signals from the affected nerves to the brain, providing relief from neck pain. The probe is then carefully removed, and a small bandage is applied to the skin. The entire procedure typically takes about 30 to 60 minutes, depending on the number of nerves being treated.

Following the procedure, patients may experience some soreness or discomfort in the treated area, which can usually be managed with over-the-counter pain medications and ice packs. Most patients can return to their normal activities within a few days, although strenuous activities and heavy lifting should be avoided for several weeks.

The effectiveness of cervical radiofrequency neurotomy can vary depending on the individual patient and the specific cause of their neck pain. In general, this procedure has been shown to provide significant pain relief for up to one to two years in many patients. However, it is important to note that nerve tissue has the ability to regenerate over time, which may result in the return of pain. In such cases, the procedure can be repeated if necessary.

As with any medical procedure, there are potential risks and complications associated with cervical radiofrequency neurotomy. These may include infection, bleeding, nerve damage, or temporary numbness in the treated area. It is essential to discuss the potential benefits and risks with a qualified healthcare professional to determine if cervical radiofrequency neurotomy is an appropriate treatment option for an individual's specific needs.

The medial branch block is a diagnostic procedure that aims to determine if a specific facet joint is the source of pain, particularly in cases of chronic neck or back pain. Facet joints are small joints located between each vertebra, allowing the spine to bend and twist. Pain originating from these joints can be caused by various factors, such as arthritis, degeneration, or injury. The medial branch nerves are responsible for transmitting pain signals from the facet joints to the brain.

The medial branch block procedure involves injecting a local anesthetic, sometimes in combination with a corticosteroid, near the medial branch nerves. This injection temporarily numbs the targeted nerves, interrupting the transmission of pain signals. The procedure is typically performed under fluoroscopic guidance, a type of real-time X-ray imaging, to ensure accurate placement of the needle.

Before the procedure, the patient's skin is cleaned and numbed with a local anesthetic at the injection site. A thin needle is then inserted through the skin, guided by fluoroscopy, and positioned close to the medial branch nerves. The anesthetic, and sometimes a corticosteroid, is then injected, numbing the targeted nerves.

Following the procedure, the patient is monitored for a brief period to assess the response to the injection. If the patient experiences significant pain relief, it may confirm that the facet joint is the pain source. In such cases, further treatment options such as radiofrequency neurotomy can be considered to provide long-term pain relief. It is important to note that the degree and duration of pain relief can vary among individuals, and multiple medial branch blocks may be necessary to accurately diagnose the pain source.

However, the medial branch block is not without potential risks or complications. Some patients may experience temporary discomfort or soreness at the injection site. There is also a risk of infection, bleeding, or allergic reaction to the medications used in the procedure. In rare cases, nerve damage may occur. Therefore, it is crucial to discuss the potential risks and benefits of the procedure with a qualified healthcare professional before undergoing the medial branch block.

The medial branch block is a valuable diagnostic tool that can help determine if a specific facet joint is the source of chronic neck or back pain. By temporarily numbing the medial branch nerves, the procedure can provide important information about the pain source, guiding further treatment options and potentially improving the patient's quality of life.

Spinal cord stimulation (SCS) is an advanced interventional pain management technique that has been used for decades to treat chronic pain, including neck pain. The treatment involves the implantation of a small, battery-powered device called a spinal cord stimulator beneath the skin, typically in the lower back or buttock region. This device is connected to thin, flexible wires called leads, which are placed in the epidural space of the spine, close to the spinal cord.

The spinal cord stimulator works by delivering low-voltage electrical impulses to the spinal cord through the leads. These electrical impulses help to modulate the transmission of pain signals from the spinal cord to the brain. By interfering with these pain signals, SCS can provide significant pain relief for patients who have not responded to more conservative treatments such as medications, physical therapy, or injections.

Before undergoing the implantation procedure, patients are typically required to undergo a trial period with a temporary external stimulator to determine if SCS is effective in reducing their pain. This trial usually lasts between three and seven days, and if the patient experiences significant pain relief, they may proceed with the permanent implantation of the spinal cord stimulator.

The implantation procedure is performed by a pain management specialist or neurosurgeon under local anesthesia and, in some cases, mild sedation. The process involves making a small incision in the skin to insert the leads into the epidural space and to create a pocket for the stimulator device. Once the leads and stimulator are in place, the device is tested to ensure proper functioning, and the incisions are closed.

One of the benefits of spinal cord stimulation is its adaptability. The therapy can be customized to the individual's needs by adjusting the frequency, intensity, and location of the electrical impulses. Furthermore, as the patient's pain levels or patterns change over time, the settings of the stimulator can be adjusted to maintain its effectiveness. Additionally, the device can be turned on or off as needed, giving the patient control over their pain management.

SCS has been proven effective in reducing pain for many patients with chronic neck pain, including those with failed back surgery syndrome, complex regional pain syndrome (CRPS), and neuropathic pain. However, it is important to note that SCS is not a cure for neck pain; rather, it is a management tool that helps to alleviate pain and improve the patient's quality of life. Potential risks associated with spinal cord stimulation include infection, bleeding, lead migration, and device malfunction. Therefore, it is crucial to discuss the benefits, risks, and alternatives with a qualified pain management specialist before considering this treatment option.

Dorsal root ganglion stimulation (DRG) is an innovative and more targeted form of neuromodulation therapy, which has emerged as an alternative to traditional spinal cord stimulation (SCS) for the treatment of chronic pain. The dorsal root ganglion is a bundle of sensory neurons located outside the spinal cord, functioning as a relay station for transmitting pain signals from peripheral nerves to the central nervous system. In certain chronic pain conditions, these ganglia can become sensitized, leading to amplified pain signals and increased pain perception.

DRG stimulation involves the surgical implantation of a small device, consisting of a pulse generator and a thin, flexible lead with electrodes. The pulse generator, typically implanted beneath the skin in the buttock or lower abdomen, generates electrical impulses, which are transmitted through the electrodes to the targeted dorsal root ganglion. The electrical impulses modulate the pain signals before they reach the spinal cord, effectively altering the perception of pain and providing relief to the patient. The stimulation parameters, such as intensity and frequency, can be customized to the individual's needs and adjusted over time to maintain optimal pain relief.

This technique has demonstrated effectiveness in treating chronic pain conditions that have proven to be resistant to more conservative treatments or traditional spinal cord stimulation. Among these conditions are complex regional pain syndrome (CRPS) and postherpetic neuralgia, both of which can cause severe neck pain. DRG stimulation offers several advantages over traditional SCS, including a more precise targeting of the affected nerves, potentially resulting in fewer side effects and improved pain relief.

Clinical studies have shown that DRG stimulation can provide significant and sustained pain reduction in a majority of patients, often leading to improvements in function, quality of life, and reduced reliance on pain medications. However, it is essential to note that DRG stimulation is not a cure for chronic pain but rather a management tool to help alleviate pain and improve overall well-being. As with any medical procedure, there are potential risks and complications associated with DRG stimulation, such as infection, lead migration, or device malfunction. Therefore, a thorough evaluation by a pain specialist is necessary to determine if a patient is an appropriate candidate for this treatment.

Dorsal root ganglion stimulation is a promising and targeted form of neuromodulation therapy that has shown potential in treating various chronic pain conditions, including those that cause severe neck pain. As research continues to advance our understanding of the mechanisms underlying chronic pain and the development of new technologies, DRG stimulation and other interventional pain management techniques will continue to evolve, offering hope to those suffering from debilitating neck pain.

Trigger point injections are a minimally invasive treatment option aimed at addressing myofascial pain syndrome, a condition characterized by painful knots of muscle fibers known as trigger points. These trigger points can cause localized or referred pain, often leading to neck pain, stiffness, and restricted range of motion.

The etiology of trigger points is not entirely understood but is believed to be associated with muscle overuse, injury, poor posture, stress, and underlying medical conditions that affect muscle and nerve function. These painful knots can be classified as active or latent. Active trigger points cause pain at rest and during movement, while latent trigger points cause discomfort only when palpated or pressed.

The procedure for trigger point injections is relatively straightforward. The clinician first identifies the location of the trigger point by palpating the affected muscle and locating the area of maximal tenderness. Once identified, the skin over the trigger point is cleaned and sterilized to minimize the risk of infection. A fine needle is then inserted through the skin and into the trigger point. The injection typically contains a local anesthetic, such as lidocaine or bupivacaine, to numb the area and alleviate pain. Sometimes, a corticosteroid is added to the injection to help reduce inflammation and promote healing.

The needle insertion itself can disrupt the tight muscle fibers, while the anesthetic helps to relax the muscle and improve blood flow to the area. The combination of these effects can provide significant pain relief and improve the range of motion in the neck. Some patients may experience immediate relief after the procedure, while others may require multiple sessions to achieve optimal results.

It is essential to note that trigger point injections are not a standalone treatment for chronic neck pain but are commonly used in conjunction with other therapies, such as physical therapy, stretching exercises, and massage. These complementary treatments help address underlying muscle imbalances and poor posture that may contribute to the development of trigger points and neck pain.

While trigger point injections are generally considered safe, there are potential risks and side effects. Some patients may experience temporary pain or soreness at the injection site, while others may have an allergic reaction to the anesthetic or corticosteroid. In rare cases, there is a risk of infection or nerve damage from the needle. It is crucial to discuss these risks with your healthcare provider and ensure that the procedure is performed by a qualified and experienced professional.

Trigger point injections can be an effective treatment option for managing neck pain caused by myofascial trigger points. They can provide targeted pain relief and improve the range of motion, especially when combined with other therapies that address the root causes of pain. By offering a minimally invasive and targeted approach, trigger point injections can improve the quality of life for patients suffering from chronic neck pain.

Stem cell and platelet-rich plasma (PRP) therapy are emerging regenerative medicine techniques that harness the body's innate healing capabilities to promote tissue repair and reduce inflammation in the affected areas. These therapies have shown potential in addressing neck pain caused by various conditions, such as degenerative disc disease and facet joint arthritis.

Stem cell therapy focuses on the use of undifferentiated cells with the ability to differentiate into various specialized cell types, aiding in tissue repair and regeneration. In the context of neck pain treatment, stem cells are typically harvested from the patient's bone marrow or adipose tissue. Once harvested, these cells are processed and then injected into the damaged area, where they can potentially regenerate damaged tissues, reduce inflammation, and promote the healing process. Studies have indicated that stem cell therapy may help alleviate pain, improve function, and even slow down the progression of degenerative conditions affecting the cervical spine.

Platelet-rich plasma (PRP) therapy, on the other hand, utilizes the growth factors and other bioactive proteins found in the patient's blood to stimulate the body's natural healing response. To obtain PRP, a small sample of the patient's blood is drawn and placed in a centrifuge to separate the platelet-rich plasma from the other blood components. The isolated PRP, which contains a high concentration of platelets, is then injected into the injured site. These platelets release growth factors and other bioactive molecules that promote tissue repair, reduce inflammation, and recruit additional healing cells to the area. PRP therapy has been used for various musculoskeletal conditions, including neck pain arising from soft tissue injuries, whiplash, and degenerative changes in the cervical spine.

While both stem cell and PRP therapies have shown promise in treating neck pain and other musculoskeletal conditions, it is essential to note that these treatments are still relatively new and require further research to establish their long-term effectiveness and safety. Clinical trials are ongoing to determine the optimal protocols for stem cell and PRP therapy, including the ideal concentration of stem cells or platelets, the frequency of injections, and the combination with other treatments. As more evidence becomes available, these regenerative therapies may become a valuable addition to the arsenal of interventional pain management techniques for neck pain, providing patients with more options for relief and improved quality of life.

In conclusion, interventional pain management techniques have emerged as a vital component of modern pain management, offering an array of minimally invasive options for diagnosing and treating chronic neck pain. These innovative procedures have significantly improved the quality of life for many patients who have not experienced sufficient relief from conservative treatments such as medication, physical therapy, and lifestyle modifications.

One of the key advantages of interventional pain management techniques is their ability to be tailored to the specific needs of each patient. By targeting the source of pain with precision, these procedures can effectively address various underlying conditions that contribute to neck pain, such as degenerative disc disease, facet joint arthritis, and nerve compression. This personalized approach ensures that patients receive the most appropriate treatment for their unique circumstances, maximizing the chances of a successful outcome.

The development and refinement of interventional pain management techniques have been driven by advances in our understanding of the mechanisms underlying chronic pain, as well as technological innovations that enable greater precision and control during procedures. For example, the use of fluoroscopy and ultrasound guidance has facilitated more accurate needle placement, while innovations in neuromodulation technologies, such as spinal cord and dorsal root ganglion stimulation, have allowed for more targeted and effective disruption of pain signals.

Moreover, the field of interventional pain management is witnessing a growing interest in regenerative medicine approaches, such as stem cell and platelet-rich plasma (PRP) therapy. These treatments harness the body's natural healing capabilities to promote tissue repair and reduce inflammation, offering a promising avenue for addressing the root cause of neck pain rather than merely managing its symptoms. As our understanding of the complex interplay between cellular and molecular processes involved in tissue regeneration and repair continues to grow, it is anticipated that these therapies will become more refined and effective.

While interventional pain management techniques have already demonstrated significant success in alleviating chronic neck pain, ongoing research and development are crucial to further improve these treatments and expand their applicability. This includes not only refining existing techniques and identifying new therapeutic targets but also enhancing our understanding of the diverse factors that contribute to the development and persistence of chronic pain. By unraveling the intricate relationships between genetic, environmental, and lifestyle factors, researchers will be better equipped to develop targeted and personalized interventional pain management strategies.

In summary, interventional pain management techniques offer a valuable and expanding toolbox for diagnosing and treating chronic neck pain, providing hope and improved quality of life for those suffering from debilitating pain. As research and technological advancements continue to drive innovation in this field, it is anticipated that even more effective and targeted treatments will become available, transforming the landscape of pain management and offering lasting relief to those in need.

Chapter 9

Neuromodulation

Spinal Cord Stimulation (SCS), Dorsal Root Ganglion Stimulation (DRG) and Peripheral Nerve Stimulation

Neuromodulation is a therapeutic approach that aims to alleviate chronic pain by modulating the nervous system's activity, thus reducing the perception of pain. This chapter will provide an in-depth examination of three advanced neuromodulation techniques utilized in the treatment of cervical spine and upper extremity pain: spinal cord stimulation (SCS), dorsal root ganglion stimulation (DRG), and peripheral nerve stimulation (PNS). We will delve into the underlying principles, procedural details, indications, and outcomes for each technique while highlighting the latest developments in the field.

Spinal cord stimulation (SCS) is a minimally invasive, reversible, and adjustable therapy that aims to alleviate chronic pain by modulating the spinal cord's neural activity. The technique is based on the gate control theory, which was proposed by Melzack and Wall in 1965. This theory suggests that non-painful electrical stimuli can inhibit the transmission of pain signals to the brain, essentially "closing the gate" on pain perception. The gate control theory posits that the activation of large-diameter, non-nociceptive (A-beta) nerve fibers can suppress the transmission of pain signals carried by smaller-diameter nociceptive (A-delta and C) fibers in the spinal cord.

SCS involves the implantation of an electrode array, also known as a lead, in the epidural space, close to the spinal cord's dorsal columns. The lead typically contains multiple electrodes that can be programmed independently to deliver electrical impulses to specific areas of the spinal cord. This allows for precise targeting of pain pathways and enables adjustments to the stimulation parameters based on the patient's individual needs and response to therapy.

The lead is connected to an implantable pulse generator (IPG) or a rechargeable battery, which is responsible for generating the electrical impulses that modulate spinal cord activity. The IPG is typically implanted in a subcutaneous pocket in the patient's abdomen, buttock, or chest area, depending on the patient's body habitus and physician's preference. The IPG can be programmed wirelessly using an external programmer, allowing for non-invasive adjustments to the stimulation settings.

The electrical impulses delivered by the SCS system create a sensation known as paresthesia, which is described as a tingling or buzzing sensation. This paresthesia is believed to compete with or override the pain signals being transmitted to the brain, leading to pain reduction. However, recent advances in SCS technology have led to the development of high-frequency and burst stimulation paradigms that can provide pain relief without the production of paresthesia. These newer stimulation techniques are thought to modulate pain pathways through different neural mechanisms, although the exact processes are still being investigated.

SCS is a dynamic and adaptable therapy, as the stimulation parameters can be adjusted over time to optimize pain relief and accommodate changes in the patient's pain patterns. In addition to altering the amplitude, frequency, and pulse width of the electrical impulses, physicians can also modify the specific electrode combinations used for stimulation. This allows for the targeting of specific spinal cord regions and the fine-tuning of therapy based on the patient's unique pain experience.

Spinal cord stimulation (SCS) is primarily indicated for the treatment of chronic, intractable pain when other conservative and interventional treatments have been unsuccessful. It is most commonly utilized for conditions such as failed back surgery syndrome (FBSS), which refers to persistent or recurrent pain following one or more spinal surgeries, complex regional pain syndrome (CRPS), a chronic pain condition characterized by severe pain, swelling, and changes in the skin, and cervical radiculopathy, a condition arising from nerve root compression in the cervical spine, which can cause pain, weakness, or numbness in the neck, shoulder, or arm.

The SCS procedure consists of two distinct stages, beginning with a trial period to assess the effectiveness of the therapy, followed by permanent implantation if the trial is successful. The trial period is a crucial step in determining whether SCS will provide adequate pain relief and functional improvement for the patient.

During the trial period, the patient is typically administered local anesthesia and sedation to ensure comfort. The physician then inserts a temporary electrode lead into the epidural space, which is the area surrounding the spinal cord, using fluoroscopic guidance. This imaging technique allows the physician to visualize the lead placement in real-time, ensuring accurate positioning near the dorsal columns of the spinal cord. Once the lead is in place, it is connected to an external stimulator that delivers electrical impulses to the targeted area.

The trial period usually lasts for about a week, during which the patient evaluates the degree of pain relief and functional improvement provided by the spinal cord stimulation. Regular communication with the physician during this time allows for adjustments to the stimulation parameters, optimizing the therapy for the individual patient. Success during the trial phase is generally defined as a 50% or greater reduction in pain, coupled with improved functionality and a positive impact on the patient's quality of life.

If the trial period is deemed successful, the patient proceeds to the second stage of the SCS procedure, which involves the permanent implantation of the electrode lead and pulse generator. This procedure is typically performed under twilight sedation with local anesthetic, however general anesthesia may also be used with intraoperative neuromonitoring. The surgeon creates a small incision to insert the implantable pulse generator (IPG) beneath the skin, usually in the lower back or buttock area. The electrode lead, which remains in the epidural space from the trial period, is then connected to the IPG. The incisions are closed, and the IPG is programmed to deliver the optimal stimulation parameters determined during the trial phase.

It is essential to note that while spinal cord stimulation has proven effective for many patients experiencing chronic, intractable pain, the outcomes may vary between individuals. Careful patient selection, precise lead placement, and thorough follow-up care are critical factors in achieving successful pain relief and improved functionality with SCS therapy.

Spinal cord stimulation (SCS) has proven to be a promising treatment option for patients with chronic cervical and upper extremity pain. Many individuals who undergo this therapy report significant reductions in pain intensity, improvements in daily function, and a decreased reliance on pain medications. These positive outcomes can lead to a better quality of life for patients who previously struggled to manage their chronic pain. However, it is important to note that the efficacy of SCS can vary among individuals, and not all patients achieve satisfactory pain relief.

Another advancement in SCS technology is the emergence of high-frequency (10 kHz) Spinal cord stimulation. In contrast to traditional SCS, which typically operates at frequencies between 40 and 60 Hz, high-frequency (10 kHz) therapy delivers electrical pulses at a much higher frequency of 10,000 Hz. Research has shown that high-frequency (10 kHz) therapy can provide superior pain relief and a more extensive area of paresthesia coverage compared to traditional SCS. This is particularly beneficial for patients with chronic pain conditions that are difficult to treat or who have not responded well to conventional SCS.

Recent technological advances have expanded the capabilities of SCS, leading to the development of novel stimulation paradigms that may offer improved outcomes for certain patients. One such advance is the introduction of burst stimulation. Burst stimulation differs from traditional SCS in that it delivers closely spaced groups of electrical pulses, or "bursts," followed by a period of no stimulation.

This pattern is thought to more closely mimic the natural firing patterns of neurons, potentially leading to a more effective modulation of pain signals by activating both the medial and lateral pathways which stimulates different areas of the brain essentially treating both the pain and the suffering. Clinical studies have shown that burst stimulation can provide similar or improved pain relief compared to traditional SCS, with some patients experiencing a reduction in paresthesia, a tingling sensation commonly associated with SCS.

Closed-loop stimulation is a further development in SCS technology that aims to personalize and optimize therapy for individual patients. In closed-loop systems, the stimulator continuously monitors the patient's neural activity and adjusts the stimulation parameters accordingly. This adaptive approach allows the system to respond to changes in the patient's pain levels or neural activity, potentially providing more effective and efficient pain relief. Early clinical studies of closed-loop SCS have shown promising results, with patients reporting improvements in pain intensity and functional outcomes.

In summary, advancements in SCS technology, such as burst stimulation, high-frequency therapy, and closed-loop stimulation, have expanded the therapeutic options available to patients with chronic cervical and upper extremity pain. These novel stimulation paradigms have the potential to improve patient outcomes by offering more effective pain relief, reduced paresthesia, and personalized therapy. Further research is needed to optimize these technologies, identify the patients who will benefit most from each approach, and refine patient selection criteria to maximize the potential benefits of spinal cord stimulation.

Dorsal root ganglion stimulation (DRG) is a targeted neuromodulation technique designed to alleviate chronic pain by focusing on the dorsal root ganglia, which are clusters of nerve cell bodies situated just outside the spinal cord. The dorsal root ganglia are critical components of the peripheral nervous system, serving as the connection point between peripheral nerves and the spinal cord. Sensory neurons within the dorsal root ganglia are responsible for transmitting pain signals from the body to the central nervous system.

The primary objective of DRG stimulation is to modulate the activity of these specific sensory neurons, thereby interrupting the transmission of pain signals and ultimately providing pain relief. The rationale behind DRG stimulation is based on the concept that electrical stimulation of the neurons in the dorsal root ganglia can disrupt the neuronal activity responsible for pain perception. This disruption is achieved by generating electrical impulses that alter the pain signals' transmission, effectively "masking" or "blocking" the perception of pain.

Unlike traditional spinal cord stimulation (SCS), DRG stimulation directly targets the dorsal root ganglia, providing more focal stimulation. This targeted approach can potentially lead to a reduction in unwanted side effects that may be associated with traditional SCS, such as paresthesia in non-painful areas or stimulation-induced discomfort. By honing in on the specific sensory neurons within the dorsal root ganglia, DRG stimulation allows for a more precise modulation of the pain signals, resulting in better pain relief with fewer side effects.

DRG stimulation achieves this targeted effect by utilizing specially designed electrode leads that are placed adjacent to the dorsal root ganglia. These leads deliver electrical impulses to the sensory neurons, altering their activity and disrupting the transmission of pain signals to the spinal cord and brain. The intensity, frequency, and duration of the electrical impulses can be adjusted and tailored to the individual patient's needs, allowing for a personalized approach to pain management.

Recent advances in DRG stimulation technology have enabled the development of multi-contact leads, which can target specific neuronal populations within the dorsal root ganglia with increased precision. These multi-column leads can deliver spatially selective stimulation, further enhancing the focal nature of DRG stimulation and improving the therapy's efficacy while minimizing potential side effects.

In summary, dorsal root ganglion stimulation is a targeted neuromodulation technique that focuses on modulating the activity of sensory neurons within the dorsal root ganglia to block the transmission of pain signals. This direct targeting approach offers a more focal stimulation compared to traditional spinal cord stimulation, potentially reducing unwanted side effects and improving pain relief. With ongoing advances in technology and a better understanding of pain mechanisms, DRG stimulation continues to evolve as an effective treatment option for chronic pain management.

Dorsal root ganglion stimulation (DRG) has shown significant promise in treating various focal, neuropathic pain conditions. It is particularly effective in managing complex regional pain syndrome (CRPS), postherpetic neuralgia, and nerve injury-related pain. DRG stimulation is especially beneficial for patients who have very focal pain symptoms or they have not experienced adequate pain relief with conventional therapies, including medications, physical therapy, and spinal cord stimulation (SCS).

The procedure for DRG stimulation consists of a trial period followed by permanent implantation, similar to the process used for SCS implantation. The trial period allows the patient and medical team to assess the effectiveness of the stimulation before committing to a permanent implant. The trial typically lasts for about a week, during which the patient's pain relief and functional improvement are closely monitored.

During the trial, the patient is given local anesthesia and sedation to ensure comfort throughout the procedure. The physician then inserts a specially designed electrode lead into the epidural space using fluoroscopic guidance. This imaging technique allows for precise placement of the lead near the targeted dorsal root ganglion, ensuring optimal stimulation of the affected nerve fibers. The lead is then connected to an external stimulator, which delivers electrical impulses to the DRG to modulate its activity and alleviate pain.

Throughout the trial phase, the patient and medical team closely evaluate the effectiveness of the DRG stimulation in providing pain relief and improving function. If the trial is deemed successful, typically defined as a 50% or greater reduction in pain, the patient proceeds to the second stage of the procedure, involving permanent implantation of the electrode lead and implantable pulse generator (IPG). The physician, at this point would remove the trial leads and schedule the permanent implant approximately 2-4 weeks later.

During the permanent implantation procedure, the patient is again given local anesthesia and sedation. The Physician then places the permanent leads. These leads are carefully positioned near the targeted DRG using fluoroscopic guidance, ensuring optimal stimulation. The leads are then connected to the IPG, which is typically implanted under the skin in the patient's lower back or buttock area.

The IPG delivers electrical impulses to the DRG through the electrode lead, modulating the activity of the targeted nerve fibers and providing pain relief. The stimulation parameters, such as pulse width, frequency, and amplitude, can be adjusted to optimize the therapy's effectiveness and minimize side effects. The patient can control the IPG using a handheld remote, allowing for adjustments to the stimulation intensity and other settings as needed.

Dorsal root ganglion stimulation is a proven therapy for focal, neuropathic pain conditions, offering significant benefits for patients who have focal neuropathic pain or if they have not found adequate pain relief with conventional treatments. The DRG stimulation procedure involves a trial period followed by permanent implantation, allowing patients to evaluate the therapy's effectiveness before committing to a long-term solution. With its targeted approach and adjustable settings, DRG stimulation holds considerable potential for improving the lives of patients suffering from chronic pain.

Dorsal root ganglion (DRG) stimulation has emerged as a proven treatment option for patients suffering from focal, neuropathic pain conditions. Studies have shown that DRG stimulation can lead to significant reductions in pain intensity, improved functionality, and a better overall quality of life for many patients. As with spinal cord stimulation (SCS), the efficacy of DRG stimulation can vary among individuals, with some experiencing more substantial pain relief than others.

Clinical trials and real-world evidence have demonstrated that DRG stimulation can be particularly effective for conditions such as complex regional pain syndrome (CRPS), postherpetic neuralgia, and post-surgical pain or causalgia. For instance, a multicenter controlled trial conducted reported that DRG stimulation provided superior pain relief and greater treatment success in patients with CRPS compared to traditional SCS. Furthermore, DRG stimulation has been shown to offer sustained pain relief, with some studies reporting long-term benefits lasting up to three years or more.

Recent advancements in DRG stimulation technology have focused on enhancing the precision and effectiveness of the therapy, while minimizing potential side effects. One such innovation is the development of multi-contact leads which allow for more refined control of the stimulation field, enabling clinicians to target specific DRG neurons more accurately. This enhanced targeting can result in improved pain relief and a reduction in side effects, such as paresthesia or discomfort caused by unwanted stimulation of neighboring neural structures.

Another advancement in DRG stimulation is the development of spatially selective stimulation techniques. These methods involve the use of advanced algorithms and stimulation patterns to optimize the delivery of electrical impulses to specific DRG neurons. Spatially selective stimulation can help to minimize the spread of the stimulation field to surrounding tissues, further reducing potential side effects and improving the therapy's overall efficacy.

In addition to hardware and software advancements, ongoing research in DRG stimulation is focused on understanding the underlying mechanisms of action, as well as identifying potential biomarkers to predict treatment responsiveness. This knowledge could help to refine patient selection, optimize stimulation parameters, and personalize therapy to achieve better outcomes for a broader range of patients.

In summary, DRG stimulation has demonstrated proven results in providing targeted pain relief for patients with focal, neuropathic pain conditions. Recent advancements in technology, such as highly specialized leads and selective stimulation techniques, have further enhanced the therapy's efficacy and minimized potential side effects. As our understanding of the underlying pain mechanisms and DRG stimulation continues to grow, it is expected that further innovations and refinements will emerge, offering improved pain management and a better quality of life for patients suffering from chronic pain.

Peripheral nerve stimulation (PNS) is a neuromodulation technique that directly targets peripheral nerves to modulate their activity and alleviate pain. The underlying principle of PNS is based on the premise that electrical stimulation of peripheral nerves can disrupt the transmission of pain signals to the spinal cord and brain, thus providing pain relief. This mechanism involves the interplay of various components, such as the electrode lead, the implantable pulse generator or external stimulator, and the targeted peripheral nerve.

The electrode lead plays a crucial role in the PNS system, as it is responsible for delivering the electrical stimulation to the targeted peripheral nerve. These leads are designed to be flexible and thin to minimize tissue damage during implantation and provide optimal contact with the nerve. The leads can be implanted either percutaneously or surgically, depending on the specific nerve targeted and the patient's individual needs.

The implantable pulse generator (IPG) or external stimulator serves as the power source for the PNS system. It generates electrical impulses that are transmitted through the electrode lead to the targeted peripheral nerve. The IPG is typically implanted subcutaneously in a location that is easily accessible for adjustments and battery replacements. Alternatively, an external stimulator can be used, which is connected to the electrode lead through a temporary extension cable. This option is generally reserved for trial periods or situations where a fully implantable system is not feasible.

The electrical impulses generated by the IPG or external stimulator can be adjusted in terms of frequency, amplitude, and pulse width to achieve the desired level of pain relief. This customization allows the stimulation parameters to be fine-tuned for each patient, optimizing pain relief while minimizing potential side effects such as muscle twitching or discomfort. The electrical impulses interact with the targeted peripheral nerve, disrupting the transmission of pain signals to the spinal cord and brain. The precise mechanism by which PNS provides pain relief is not yet fully understood, but it is thought to involve a combination of direct inhibition of pain signal transmission and the activation of endogenous pain modulation systems, such as the release of endorphins and the activation of descending inhibitory pathways.

PNS has been shown to be effective for various types of chronic pain, including neuropathic pain, post-surgical pain, and complex regional pain syndrome. The therapy's success is thought to be linked to its ability to directly target the peripheral nerves involved in pain transmission, which can be more effective than modulating pain signals at the spinal cord level, as seen in spinal cord stimulation. However, further research is needed to fully elucidate the specific mechanisms by which PNS provides pain relief and to optimize the therapy for various pain conditions.

Peripheral nerve stimulation (PNS) is an effective treatment option for various neuropathic pain conditions. It is particularly beneficial for patients experiencing peripheral nerve injuries, post-surgical neuralgia, and phantom limb pain, among other chronic pain disorders. PNS is often considered when other treatments such as medication, physical therapy, or more invasive procedures have failed to provide adequate pain relief or are not suitable for the patient.

The PNS implantation process typically begins with a trial period, during which the patient and physician assess the effectiveness of the therapy in managing the patient's pain. The trial period is a crucial step, as it helps to determine whether the patient will benefit from the permanent implantation of the PNS system. During this stage, the physician inserts the electrode lead near the targeted peripheral nerve, using either ultrasound or fluoroscopic guidance for accurate placement.

To ensure patient comfort and minimize discomfort, the procedure is carried out under local anesthesia. Once the electrode lead is in place, it is connected to an external stimulator. The external stimulator delivers electrical impulses to the targeted peripheral nerve, modulating its activity to disrupt the transmission of pain signals. The patient is closely monitored during the trial period, typically lasting for about a week, to evaluate the therapy's effectiveness in managing their pain.

If the trial is successful, which usually means a significant reduction in pain intensity and improved functional capacity, the trial lead is removed and the patient proceeds to the next stage of the PNS implantation or the permanent implant of the electrode lead and the pulse generator. The pulse generator is a small, battery-powered device responsible for generating the electrical impulses required for PNS therapy.

During the permanent implantation procedure, the physician implants the pulse generator under the skin, usually in the patient's buttock, abdomen, or chest. The newly implanted electrode lead is then connected to the pulse generator, completing the PNS system. Once the system is fully operational, the electrical impulses delivered to the targeted peripheral nerve can be adjusted and programmed by the physician to optimize pain relief for the patient.

It is important to note that, although PNS has shown significant potential in managing various neuropathic pain conditions, its effectiveness varies among individuals. Factors such as the cause of pain, the targeted peripheral nerve, and the patient's overall health can impact the success of the therapy. Therefore, a thorough evaluation and careful patient selection are crucial in determining the most appropriate candidates for PNS treatment.

Peripheral nerve stimulation (PNS) has shown positive outcomes in the management of various neuropathic pain conditions, including post-surgical neuralgia, peripheral nerve injuries, and phantom limb pain. Many patients who undergo PNS report significant pain reduction, improved function, and a better quality of life. These improvements can translate into increased independence, greater ability to participate in daily activities, and reduced reliance on pain medications.

Despite its potential benefits, the efficacy of PNS varies among individuals. Factors that may contribute to this variability include the underlying pain condition, the targeted nerve's location, and the patient's response to electrical stimulation. Furthermore, some patients may experience temporary pain relief that diminishes over time, necessitating adjustments to stimulation parameters or additional interventions. It is essential to carefully select and assess patients before PNS to maximize the likelihood of successful outcomes.

Recent advancements in PNS technology have aimed to improve the therapy's effectiveness, safety, and convenience. One such development is the emergence of wireless systems, which eliminate the need for implanted pulse generators. Instead, these systems use an external transmitter to wirelessly deliver electrical stimulation to the implanted electrode. This approach reduces the invasiveness of the procedure and the risk of complications associated with implanted devices, such as infection or device migration.

Closed-loop PNS systems represent another innovative advancement in the field. These systems continually monitor the patient's neural activity and adjust stimulation parameters in real-time, tailoring the therapy to the individual's needs. By adapting to changes in the patient's pain levels and neural activity, closed-loop PNS has the potential to provide more personalized and effective pain relief. Additionally, this adaptive approach may prolong the device's battery life and reduce the need for frequent adjustments by healthcare providers.

Research is ongoing to further refine and expand the applications of PNS. For example, studies are investigating the optimal stimulation parameters, such as pulse width, frequency, and amplitude, to maximize pain relief and minimize side effects. Other areas of investigation include the development of more biocompatible and durable electrode materials, the use of computational models to predict patient responses to stimulation, and the combination of PNS with other therapies, such as regenerative medicine or pharmacological interventions.

Peripheral nerve stimulation has demonstrated promising results in the management of various neuropathic pain conditions, with recent technological advancements aimed at improving the therapy's effectiveness, safety, and convenience. As research continues to enhance our understanding of PNS and its potential applications, this neuromodulation technique may offer hope to many patients suffering from chronic pain who have not found relief with other treatment options.

Spinal cord stimulation, dorsal root ganglion stimulation, and peripheral nerve stimulation are advanced neuromodulation techniques that have shown promise in treating various painful conditions of the cervical spine and upper extremities. Each technique offers a unique approach to pain management by targeting different aspects of the nervous system, such as the spinal cord, dorsal root ganglia, or peripheral nerves.

While these therapies have demonstrated positive outcomes for many patients, their effectiveness varies among individuals. This variability may be attributed to factors such as the underlying pain mechanisms, patient response to electrical stimulation, and the precision of electrode placement. As a result, further research is needed to optimize their application, develop better patient selection criteria, and enhance the overall efficacy of neuromodulation therapies.

Technological advancements in neuromodulation continue to evolve, offering the potential for improved pain management and a better quality of life for patients suffering from chronic pain. Burst stimulation, for example, has shown superior pain relief and a more extensive area of paresthesia coverage compared to traditional spinal cord stimulation. This innovation allows for more effective neural modulation without the tingling sensation often associated with conventional stimulation, potentially enhancing patient comfort and satisfaction.

The development of specialized leads in dorsal root ganglion stimulation has enabled more precise targeting of specific sensory neurons. By allowing for spatially selective stimulation, these leads can enhance the therapy's efficacy while minimizing side effects and unwanted stimulation of adjacent neural structures. This level of precision could lead to more consistent and reliable outcomes for patients with focal, neuropathic pain conditions.

Closed-loop systems represent another significant advancement in neuromodulation technology. These systems use feedback from the patient's neural activity to adjust stimulation parameters in real-time, resulting in more personalized and adaptive therapies. By continuously monitoring and responding to the patient's pain levels and neural signals, closed-loop systems have the potential to optimize pain relief, reduce side effects, and improve overall treatment outcomes.

In conclusion, spinal cord stimulation, dorsal root ganglion stimulation, and peripheral nerve stimulation have proven to be valuable tools in the management of various painful conditions affecting the cervical spine and upper extremities. However, the efficacy of these therapies varies among individuals, necessitating ongoing research and development to optimize their application. Technological advancements, such as high-frequency stimulation, multi-column leads, and closed-loop systems, hold promise for enhancing the effectiveness of neuromodulation therapies, leading to improved pain management and a better quality of life for patients suffering from chronic pain.

As our understanding of pain mechanisms and neuromodulation techniques continues to grow, the field of chronic pain management is ripe for innovation. Researchers are exploring new therapeutic approaches and refining existing ones to improve patient outcomes, leading to the emergence of several promising areas of investigation.

One such area is the development of personalized neuromodulation strategies. By taking into account the patient's unique pain characteristics, genetic factors, and neural activity, it may be possible to enhance the effectiveness of therapies like SCS, DRG stimulation, and PNS. For instance, machine learning algorithms can be employed to analyze neural signals and optimize stimulation parameters, enabling a more tailored approach to pain management. Moreover, incorporating genetic information into treatment planning may help identify patients who are more likely to respond to specific neuromodulation techniques, further personalizing the therapeutic process.

Combining neuromodulation techniques with other treatments is another area of interest. Investigating the optimal timing, sequence, and combination of therapies can help tailor treatment plans to individual needs and maximize pain relief. For example, integrating pharmacological interventions or behavioral therapies with neuromodulation may offer synergistic benefits for some patients. By understanding how various treatments interact and complement one another, healthcare providers can develop more comprehensive and effective pain management strategies.

The emerging field of bioelectronic medicine holds great promise for the future of neuromodulation. This discipline aims to treat various medical conditions by modulating the activity of specific neural circuits using electrical or other forms of energy. As researchers continue to uncover the intricacies of neural pathways and their role in pain perception, bioelectronic medicine has the potential to expand the scope of neuromodulation therapies and improve their specificity. This approach could enable the targeting of not only pain but also other symptoms and comorbidities associated with chronic pain conditions, offering a more holistic approach to patient care.

Regenerative medicine techniques, such as stem cell therapy or tissue engineering, have the potential to revolutionize pain management by addressing the underlying causes of pain. By repairing or replacing damaged neural tissues, these therapies can provide more long-lasting pain relief and functional improvement for patients. Combining neuromodulation with regenerative medicine strategies could create synergistic effects that enhance overall treatment outcomes, providing a more comprehensive approach to chronic pain management.

Lastly, non-invasive neuromodulation techniques are being explored as potential alternatives to implanted devices for certain pain conditions. Methods such as transcranial magnetic stimulation (TMS) and transcranial direct current stimulation (tDCS) offer less invasive and more accessible pain management options. These techniques can be especially beneficial for patients who are not candidates for implantable devices or prefer to avoid surgery. As research continues to advance our understanding of non-invasive neuromodulation, it may become an increasingly viable option for a broader range of pain conditions.

In conclusion, the future of chronic pain management lies in the integration of technological advances, personalized approaches, and interdisciplinary collaboration. By exploring these promising areas of investigation, researchers and healthcare providers can unlock the full potential of neuromodulation and other innovative therapies, ultimately transforming the lives of patients living with chronic pain.

Chapter 10

Minimally Invasive Spine Surgery

Advanced Techniques to Preserve Healthy Tissue

Minimally invasive spine surgery (MISS) has transformed the field of spinal surgery by introducing methods that minimize the disruption of surrounding tissues while still effectively addressing spinal disorders. The preservation of healthy tissue is a key aspect of MISS, as it leads to less post-operative pain, reduced blood loss, shorter hospital stays, and faster recovery times. The growing popularity of MISS can be attributed to the advancements in technology and surgical instrumentation, which have enabled surgeons to treat various spinal conditions with remarkable precision and minimal collateral damage.

The primary objective of MISS is to minimize the trauma to muscles, ligaments, and other soft tissues surrounding the spine. This approach significantly differs from traditional open surgery, where larger incisions and the cutting or stripping of muscles were necessary to access the spine. In MISS, advanced surgical techniques are employed to access the spine through smaller incisions, thereby reducing tissue damage and promoting faster healing.

One such advanced technique is muscle dilation, which involves the gentle separation of muscle fibers using dilators to create a pathway to the spine without cutting or tearing the muscle tissue. This method allows the surgeon to access the spinal column with minimal disruption to the surrounding muscles, resulting in reduced postoperative pain and a quicker recovery process.

Another essential component of MISS is the use of tubular retractors, which hold the separated muscle fibers apart and maintain the pathway created by muscle dilation. Tubular retractors provide a clear view of the surgical site and protect the surrounding tissues during the procedure. These retractors come in various sizes and shapes, enabling surgeons to choose the most appropriate tool for the specific surgery being performed.

Advanced imaging techniques, such as intraoperative fluoroscopy, endoscopy, and navigation systems, play a critical role in MISS by providing real-time guidance and visualization. These imaging tools allow the surgeon to perform complex procedures with a high degree of accuracy, ensuring that healthy tissues remain unaffected. Additionally, preoperative imaging studies, such as magnetic resonance imaging (MRI) and computed tomography (CT) scans, help in planning the surgery and determining the most suitable approach for each patient.

The development and implementation of specialized surgical instruments have also contributed to the advancement of MISS. These instruments are designed to be used through small incisions, allowing for precise manipulation and control while minimizing tissue damage. Examples of such instruments include microsurgical tools, endoscopic devices, and laser technologies, which offer improved precision and reduced collateral damage compared to conventional surgical tools.

It is important to note that while MISS offers numerous advantages in terms of preserving healthy tissue and promoting faster recovery, not all patients are suitable candidates for these procedures. A thorough evaluation of a patient's medical history, physical examination, and imaging studies is necessary to determine whether MISS is the most appropriate treatment option. In some cases, traditional open surgery may still be the best choice based on the patient's specific condition and overall health.

In conclusion, the advanced techniques employed in minimally invasive spine surgery have revolutionized the treatment of spinal disorders by preserving healthy tissue and minimizing collateral damage. The combination of muscle dilation, tubular retractors, advanced imaging, and specialized surgical instruments has allowed surgeons to perform complex procedures with greater precision and less trauma to the patient. As technology and surgical techniques continue to evolve, the benefits of MISS are expected to become even more pronounced, offering improved outcomes for a broader range of patients.

Minimally invasive spine surgery (MISS) is a versatile approach to treating a variety of spinal conditions. The selection of patients for MISS is based on a comprehensive assessment that includes a thorough evaluation of medical history, physical examination, and imaging studies such as magnetic resonance imaging (MRI), computed tomography (CT) scans, and X-rays.

Degenerative disc disease is a common indication for MISS. This condition occurs when the intervertebral discs lose their integrity and structural support, leading to chronic pain and potential neurological symptoms. MISS can address degenerative disc disease by removing damaged disc material or by fusing affected vertebrae to stabilize the spine.

Herniated discs, another common indication for MISS, occur when the inner gel-like substance of an intervertebral disc protrudes through the outer fibrous ring, causing pressure on nearby nerves and resulting in pain, numbness, or weakness. MISS techniques, such as microdiscectomy, can remove the herniated portion of the disc, alleviating pressure on the affected nerve and providing symptom relief.

Spinal stenosis, a narrowing of the spinal canal, can cause compression of the spinal cord or nerve roots, leading to pain and neurological symptoms. MISS techniques, including laminectomy and laminotomy, can create more space for the spinal cord or nerve roots by removing parts of the bone or other structures contributing to the narrowing.

Spondylolisthesis, a condition in which one vertebra slips forward over the one below it, can cause instability and pressure on nerves. MISS techniques, such as transforaminal lumbar interbody fusion (TLIF), can stabilize the affected vertebrae and relieve pressure on the spinal nerves.

Compression fractures, often caused by osteoporosis or trauma, can result in severe pain and spinal deformity. MISS techniques, such as kyphoplasty or vertebroplasty, involve injecting bone cement into the affected vertebra to stabilize the fracture and restore the vertebral height.

Spinal deformities, such as scoliosis, which involve an abnormal curvature of the spine, can also be treated with MISS. In some cases, percutaneous pedicle screw fixation and other fusion techniques can correct the deformity and provide spinal stability.

Despite the versatility of MISS, not all patients are suitable candidates for these procedures. Contraindications may include severe spinal instability that requires extensive reconstruction, which may be better addressed through traditional open surgery. Active infections, such as discitis or osteomyelitis, may also contraindicate MISS, as these conditions need to be treated and resolved before any surgical intervention.

Morbid obesity is another potential contraindication, as excessive body weight can increase the risk of complications and make it challenging to access the spine using minimally invasive techniques. Weight loss and lifestyle modifications may be necessary before a patient can be considered for MISS.

The presence of extensive scar tissue from previous surgeries may also complicate MISS, as it can make it difficult to visualize and access the spine without causing further damage. In such cases, traditional open surgery may be a more appropriate option based on the patient's specific condition and overall health.

Ultimately, the decision to pursue minimally invasive spine surgery depends on a thorough evaluation of each patient's unique circumstances. By carefully considering the potential benefits and risks, surgeons can determine the most appropriate treatment approach for each individual.

Minimally invasive spine surgery is founded on three key principles that differentiate it from traditional open surgery. These principles include muscle dilation, the use of tubular retractors, and advanced imaging techniques.

Muscle dilation is a fundamental aspect of minimally invasive spine surgery that significantly reduces the disruption of surrounding soft tissues. In traditional open surgery, accessing the spine often requires cutting through or stripping away muscles, which can lead to increased pain, blood loss, and longer recovery times. MISS, on the other hand, employs a technique known as muscle dilation to minimize tissue damage and facilitate faster healing.

During the muscle dilation process, the surgeon uses a series of progressively larger dilators to gently separate muscle fibers without cutting or tearing them. By gradually expanding the space between muscle fibers, a clear and stable pathway is created, allowing access to the spine with minimal tissue damage. This approach preserves the integrity of the surrounding soft tissues, leading to less postoperative pain, reduced inflammation, and quicker recovery times.

One of the benefits of muscle dilation is that it helps to maintain the normal anatomical structure and function of the muscles surrounding the spine. By preserving the muscles, the risk of postoperative complications, such as muscle atrophy, weakness, or scarring, is significantly reduced. In addition, muscle dilation contributes to a decreased risk of infection, as the limited tissue disruption results in a smaller surgical wound.

Overall, the principle of muscle dilation is a cornerstone of minimally invasive spine surgery, providing a less invasive alternative to traditional open surgery while maintaining the efficacy of the procedure. This approach ensures that patients can benefit from reduced postoperative pain, faster recovery times, and a lower likelihood of complications, ultimately leading to improved outcomes and a better quality of life.

Tubular retractors have revolutionized minimally invasive spine surgery by facilitating access to the surgical site while minimizing soft tissue disruption. They play a critical role in preserving the muscle dilation pathway created by the surgeon during the initial stages of the procedure. By holding the separated muscle fibers apart, tubular retractors provide a clear and unobstructed view of the spine, enabling the surgeon to perform complex procedures with high precision and reduced risk of complications.

These retractors are cylindrical tubes made of medical-grade stainless steel or other biocompatible materials. The tubular design ensures that the pressure exerted on the surrounding tissue is evenly distributed, preventing damage to the delicate muscle fibers, blood vessels, and nerves in the vicinity of the surgical site. This not only minimizes postoperative pain and swelling but also reduces the risk of tissue injury and scarring, which can contribute to faster recovery times and improved long-term outcomes for patients.

One of the key advantages of tubular retractors is their modularity. They come in various sizes, lengths, and diameters, allowing surgeons to select the most appropriate tool for a specific procedure. Some tubular retractors also feature expandable designs, which can be adjusted intraoperatively to accommodate changes in the surgical field or facilitate the insertion of larger surgical instruments. The adaptability of tubular retractors contributes to their versatility, making them suitable for a wide range of minimally invasive spine surgeries, including discectomies, laminectomies, and spinal fusions.

In addition to providing a clear view of the surgical site, tubular retractors can also be used in conjunction with advanced imaging techniques, such as intraoperative fluoroscopy, endoscopy, or computer-assisted navigation systems. These technologies enhance visualization and guidance, enabling the surgeon to navigate complex anatomical structures with greater accuracy and confidence. By combining the benefits of tubular retractors with state-of-the-art imaging systems, minimally invasive spine surgery can be performed with exceptional precision, leading to better surgical outcomes and reduced postoperative complications.

While tubular retractors have undoubtedly improved the field of minimally invasive spine surgery, their use requires specialized training and experience. Surgeons must be adept at working within the limited confines of the retractor, as well as handling the unique challenges associated with minimally invasive techniques. Mastery of these skills is crucial for ensuring the safety and effectiveness of the procedure, as well as achieving optimal patient outcomes.

Tubular retractors are indispensable tools in minimally invasive spine surgery, offering numerous benefits, such as improved visualization, reduced soft tissue disruption, and increased precision. Their versatility and compatibility with advanced imaging technologies further enhance their utility, making them an essential component of modern spine surgery. As the field continues to evolve and new techniques emerge, the role of tubular retractors in minimally invasive spine surgery is expected to remain integral to achieving optimal patient outcomes.

High-quality imaging plays a vital role in the success of minimally invasive spine surgery. By providing real-time guidance and visualization, advanced imaging techniques allow surgeons to perform complex procedures with precision and minimal tissue disruption. The integration of intraoperative fluoroscopy, endoscopy, and navigation systems has revolutionized spinal surgery, enabling more accurate and less invasive interventions.

Intraoperative fluoroscopy is a widely used imaging modality in minimally invasive spine surgery. It utilizes continuous X-ray imaging to provide real-time visualization of the spine during surgery, allowing the surgeon to monitor the position of surgical instruments and implanted devices, such as screws and cages. This real-time guidance is particularly valuable when inserting hardware into the spine, as it helps ensure proper placement and minimizes the risk of complications. However, the use of fluoroscopy exposes both the patient and surgical team to ionizing radiation. Therefore, it is essential to follow appropriate safety measures, such as using protective shielding and limiting exposure time, to minimize radiation risks.

Endoscopy is another essential imaging technique in minimally invasive spine surgery. It involves inserting a thin, flexible tube called an endoscope through a small incision to visualize the surgical site. The endoscope is equipped with a camera and a light source, providing high-resolution images that can be displayed on a monitor in the operating room. Endoscopic spine surgery offers several advantages over traditional open surgery, including better visualization of the surgical site, reduced soft tissue disruption, and smaller incisions. Endoscopic techniques have been successfully applied to various spinal procedures, such as microdiscectomies, laminectomies, and foraminotomies.

Navigation systems have become increasingly important in minimally invasive spine surgery. These systems use preoperative imaging data, such as MRI or CT scans, to create a three-dimensional model of the patient's spine, which is then used to guide the surgeon during the procedure. Some navigation systems also incorporate intraoperative imaging, allowing real-time updates to the 3D model as the surgery progresses. Navigation systems enhance surgical accuracy and safety by providing precise guidance for instrument placement, reducing the risk of complications, and minimizing the need for repeat surgeries.

Preoperative imaging studies, including magnetic resonance imaging (MRI) and computed tomography (CT) scans, are essential for planning minimally invasive spine surgery. MRI scans provide detailed information about the soft tissues surrounding the spine, such as muscles, ligaments, and intervertebral discs, while CT scans offer high-resolution images of the bony structures. Together, these imaging modalities help surgeons identify the underlying cause of the patient's symptoms, determine the most suitable surgical approach, and plan the procedure in detail.

Advanced imaging techniques are critical to the success of minimally invasive spine surgery. Intraoperative fluoroscopy, endoscopy, and navigation systems provide real-time guidance and visualization, enabling surgeons to perform complex procedures with precision and minimal tissue disruption. Preoperative imaging studies, such as MRI and CT scans, play a crucial role in planning the surgery and selecting the most appropriate approach. As imaging technology continues to advance, it will further enhance the safety, accuracy, and effectiveness of minimally invasive spine surgery.

Minimally invasive spine surgery techniques have revolutionized the treatment of various spinal conditions, reducing recovery time and minimizing complications compared to traditional open surgery. In this section, we will delve deeper into one of the most common procedures, microdiscectomy, and discuss its indications, techniques, and potential benefits.

Microdiscectomy is a minimally invasive procedure primarily utilized for the treatment of lumbar disc herniations causing radicular pain, commonly known as sciatica, and neurological symptoms. Disc herniations occur when the inner gel-like nucleus pulposus of the intervertebral disc protrudes through a tear in the outer annulus fibrosus, compressing nerve roots or the spinal cord. This compression leads to pain, numbness, tingling, and muscle weakness, affecting the patient's quality of life.

The primary goal of microdiscectomy is to remove the herniated portion of the disc, relieving pressure on the affected nerve root and alleviating symptoms. The procedure is typically indicated for patients who have not responded to conservative treatment measures, such as pain medication, physical therapy, and epidural steroid injections, or for those experiencing progressive neurological deficits.

During a microdiscectomy, the patient is placed in the prone position on the operating table under general anesthesia. The surgeon makes a small incision, usually 1-2 inches in length, over the affected disc level. Using muscle dilation techniques and tubular retractors, the surgeon creates a minimally invasive working channel that provides direct access to the spine while minimizing disruption to the surrounding soft tissues.

Once the operative field is exposed, the surgeon uses a microscope or endoscope for enhanced visualization of the surgical site. Specialized instruments, such as a high-speed drill or Kerrison rongeur, are used to carefully remove a small portion of the lamina and ligamentum flavum, providing access to the affected nerve root and herniated disc material. The nerve root is gently retracted, and the herniated portion of the disc is removed using microsurgical techniques. Throughout the procedure, the surgeon is careful to preserve the integrity of the remaining disc and spinal structures.

209

Following the removal of the herniated disc material, the nerve root is inspected to ensure adequate decompression. The tubular retractors are then carefully removed, allowing the muscle fibers to return to their original position. The incision is closed using sutures or surgical staples, and a sterile dressing is applied.

One of the main advantages of microdiscectomy over traditional open discectomy is the reduced damage to the surrounding muscles and soft tissues. This minimally invasive approach often results in less postoperative pain, a lower risk of complications, and faster recovery. Most patients can return to light activities within a few weeks, and full recovery generally occurs within 6-8 weeks. However, the specific timeline for recovery depends on the individual patient and the extent of the surgery.

It is important to note that while microdiscectomy can provide significant relief from pain and neurological symptoms, it may not completely eliminate all discomfort. Furthermore, there is a small risk of recurrent disc herniation, which may require additional treatment or surgery. Nevertheless, microdiscectomy remains a highly effective and widely used minimally invasive spine surgery technique for the treatment of lumbar disc herniations.

Laminectomy and laminotomy are spinal decompression surgeries designed to alleviate pressure on the spinal cord or nerve roots caused by various conditions, such as spinal stenosis, herniated discs, or degenerative disc disease. While both procedures aim to provide relief from pain and other neurological symptoms, the specific techniques involved in each differ in the extent of lamina removal.

A laminectomy involves the complete removal of the lamina, the bony arch that forms the posterior part of the vertebral bone. This removal creates more space for the spinal cord and nerve roots, reducing compression and associated symptoms. In contrast, a laminotomy entails the removal of only a portion of the lamina, maintaining more of the vertebral bone's structural integrity. The choice between the two procedures depends on the patient's specific condition, the extent of the spinal cord or nerve root compression, and the surgeon's preference.

Minimally invasive techniques have revolutionized the approach to laminectomy and laminotomy, allowing for less disruption to surrounding tissues and resulting in faster recovery times. The surgeon accesses the spine through a small incision, typically measuring just a few centimeters in length. This minimally invasive approach reduces blood loss, minimizes the risk of infection, and causes less postoperative pain compared to traditional open surgery.

Once the incision is made, the surgeon uses tubular retractors to separate the muscles surrounding the spine. This technique, known as muscle dilation, minimizes the need for cutting or stripping muscle tissue, resulting in less postoperative pain and a quicker return to normal function. The tubular retractors hold the separated muscle fibers apart, providing a clear view of the surgical site while minimizing soft tissue disruption.

Advanced imaging techniques, such as intraoperative fluoroscopy or endoscopy, are crucial in minimally invasive laminectomy and laminotomy. These technologies allow the surgeon to visualize the spine in real-time, ensuring precise and accurate removal of the lamina or portions of it. In addition, computer-assisted navigation systems may be employed to guide the surgeon throughout the procedure, further enhancing precision and reducing the risk of complications.

Once the lamina has been removed, the surgeon can address the underlying cause of spinal cord or nerve root compression. This may involve removing bone spurs, herniated disc material, or other structures contributing to the pressure. Once the compression is relieved, the retractors are removed, allowing the muscle fibers to return to their original position. The incision is then closed using sutures or surgical staples.

The recovery process following minimally invasive laminectomy or laminotomy is typically faster than that of traditional open surgery. Patients may experience less postoperative pain and can often return to daily activities more quickly. However, the specific recovery timeline depends on the individual patient, the procedure performed, and the underlying spinal condition. Physical therapy is usually recommended to help restore strength, flexibility, and mobility in the spine, further enhancing the recovery process.

Minimally invasive laminectomy and laminotomy are effective surgical techniques for relieving pressure on the spinal cord or nerve roots, resulting in reduced pain and improved function for patients with various spinal conditions. These minimally invasive approaches minimize tissue damage and promote faster recovery compared to traditional open surgery. However, it is essential for patients to carefully discuss the potential benefits, risks, and alternatives with their healthcare team to make an informed decision about their treatment options.

Anterior Cervical Discectomy and Fusion (ACDF) is a well-established minimally invasive procedure used to address cervical disc herniations, degenerative disc disease, and spinal stenosis in the neck region. The primary goal of the ACDF surgery is to relieve pain and neurological symptoms caused by the compression of nerve roots or the spinal cord, while stabilizing the cervical spine to prevent further degeneration.

The ACDF procedure is typically performed under general anesthesia. To access the cervical spine, the surgeon makes a small incision, usually 1 to 2 inches long, in the front of the neck. This anterior approach allows the surgeon to work through the natural planes between the neck muscles and tissues, minimizing disruption to the surrounding structures. Additionally, this approach avoids the need to manipulate the spinal cord directly, reducing the risk of nerve damage.

Once the cervical spine is accessed, the surgeon carefully removes the damaged intervertebral disc, taking care not to disturb the adjacent nerve roots and spinal cord. This process, called discectomy, creates a space between the two adjacent vertebrae. To maintain the natural alignment and curvature of the cervical spine, the surgeon inserts a bone graft or synthetic spacer into the empty disc space. This implant serves as a scaffold to promote fusion between the adjacent vertebrae over time, ultimately restoring the stability of the cervical spine.

To further secure the implant and provide immediate stability, the surgeon attaches a small metal plate to the front of the vertebrae using screws. The plate serves as an internal brace, holding the vertebrae in the correct position while the fusion process occurs. In some cases, the surgeon may use additional hardware, such as posterior cervical screws and rods, to enhance stability, particularly in patients with more complex spinal conditions.

Compared to traditional open surgery, minimally invasive ACDF offers several advantages. The smaller incision and reduced disruption of soft tissues can result in less postoperative pain and swelling, facilitating a quicker recovery. Furthermore, the MISS approach often leads to reduced blood loss during surgery and a lower risk of infection. Patients who undergo minimally invasive ACDF typically have shorter hospital stays and can return to their daily activities more quickly than those who have traditional open surgery.

However, it is essential to recognize that ACDF is not suitable for all patients with cervical spine conditions. The procedure is most effective for treating patients with single or multi-level disc herniations, degenerative disc disease, or spinal stenosis that predominantly affects the front part of the spine. For patients with more extensive spinal cord compression or spinal instability involving the posterior elements, other surgical approaches may be more appropriate.

As with any surgery, there are potential risks and complications associated with ACDF, such as infection, bleeding, nerve injury, nonunion (failure of the vertebrae to fuse), or hardware failure. However, when performed by an experienced spine surgeon using minimally invasive techniques, ACDF has a high success rate, providing significant relief from pain and neurological symptoms for many patients.

Transforaminal Lumbar Interbody Fusion (TLIF) is a minimally invasive spine surgery that addresses various spinal conditions, including degenerative disc disease, spondylolisthesis, and spinal stenosis. The procedure aims to provide stability, correct spinal alignment, and alleviate pain by fusing two vertebrae together. This fusion eliminates motion at the targeted spinal segment, reducing irritation and inflammation of the surrounding nerves.

TLIF is performed using a posterior approach, meaning that the surgeon accesses the spine through a small incision in the lower back. To minimize muscle disruption, the surgeon employs tubular retractors that create a tunnel-like pathway to the affected area, keeping muscle fibers separated and preserving the surrounding tissue. This approach leads to reduced blood loss, postoperative pain, and faster recovery compared to traditional open surgery.

Once the surgeon gains access to the spine, specialized instruments are used to remove the damaged disc, decompressing the affected nerves. The removal of the disc creates a void between the adjacent vertebrae, which needs to be filled to promote fusion. An interbody cage, typically made of metal, plastic, or a combination of materials, is used to fill this space. The cage is packed with bone graft material, which can be harvested from the patient's own body (autograft), a donor (allograft), or synthetic bone substitutes.

The bone graft material stimulates the body's natural bone growth, ultimately leading to fusion between the adjacent vertebrae over time. This process may take several months to a year, and the rate of successful fusion varies among patients. Factors that may influence fusion success include the patient's age, overall health, smoking habits, and the presence of other medical conditions.

In addition to the interbody cage, pedicle screws and rods are used to provide immediate stability and support to the spine. The screws are placed through the pedicles of the adjacent vertebrae, with rods connecting the screws, forming a rigid construct. This hardware acts as an internal brace, maintaining the correct spinal alignment while the fusion process occurs.

Postoperative care for patients undergoing TLIF includes pain management, early mobilization, and a customized physical therapy program. Pain management strategies may involve a combination of medications, such as opioids, nonsteroidal anti-inflammatory drugs (NSAIDs), and muscle relaxants. Patients are encouraged to walk and engage in light activities within hours of surgery to promote circulation and prevent blood clots. Physical therapy plays a vital role in the recovery process, helping patients regain strength, flexibility, and mobility in the spine.

Potential risks and complications associated with TLIF include infection, bleeding, nerve injury, hardware failure, nonunion (failure of the vertebrae to fuse), and adjacent segment degeneration (the development of degeneration in spinal segments adjacent to the fusion site). Despite these risks, TLIF has been shown to be a safe and effective minimally invasive treatment option for various spinal conditions, leading to significant improvements in pain, function, and quality of life for many patients.

Percutaneous pedicle screw fixation is an essential component of minimally invasive spine surgery that provides crucial stabilization to the spine in various clinical scenarios, such as trauma, spinal deformities, or as an adjunct to other spinal fusion procedures. This technique has gained popularity due to its ability to provide adequate spinal fixation while minimizing soft tissue damage, leading to reduced postoperative pain and faster recovery times.

The fundamental principle of percutaneous pedicle screw fixation involves the insertion of pedicle screws into the vertebral bodies using a minimally invasive approach. The procedure typically starts with the patient in the prone position under general anesthesia. Surgeons use fluoroscopic guidance, a real-time imaging technique, to visualize the spine's anatomy and accurately place the screws.

Before the screw placement, the surgeon makes small skin incisions, approximately 1-2 centimeters in length, over the targeted pedicles. These incisions are strategically placed to minimize tissue damage and blood loss. The surgeon then uses specialized instruments called Jamshidi needles to create a pathway to the pedicles while avoiding critical structures such as nerves and blood vessels. Once the pathway is established, the surgeon inserts a guidewire through the Jamshidi needle, which serves as a guide for screw placement.

Subsequently, the surgeon uses a cannulated pedicle screw, which is designed to fit over the guidewire, ensuring precise and controlled insertion into the pedicle. This process is repeated for each screw, with the number of screws depending on the specific spinal condition and the extent of stabilization required. Throughout the procedure, the surgeon relies on fluoroscopic guidance to confirm proper screw placement and avoid potential complications.

After the pedicle screws have been inserted, the surgeon connects them using rods, which provide structural support and stability to the spine. The rods are introduced through the same small incisions and secured to the screws using specialized connectors known as tulip heads and locking caps. This assembly ensures a robust fixation system that can withstand the forces exerted on the spine during normal activities.

The percutaneous pedicle screw fixation procedure has several advantages over traditional open surgery, including less muscle dissection, reduced blood loss, decreased postoperative pain, and shorter hospital stays. Additionally, the fluoroscopic guidance utilized during the procedure ensures accurate screw placement, reducing the risk of complications such as nerve injury or malpositioned screws.

However, it is essential to recognize that percutaneous pedicle screw fixation is not without potential risks and complications. These may include infection, bleeding, screw loosening or breakage, and, although rare, injury to nerves or blood vessels. To minimize these risks, surgeons must exercise meticulous technique and adhere to established safety guidelines.

Percutaneous pedicle screw fixation represents a significant advancement in minimally invasive spine surgery, offering a safe and effective means of stabilizing the spine while minimizing tissue damage and promoting faster recovery. As technology and surgical techniques continue to evolve, this approach is expected to play an increasingly vital role in the treatment of various spinal conditions.

Following minimally invasive spine surgery, a comprehensive postoperative care plan is essential to optimize the recovery process. Patients typically experience reduced postoperative pain, shorter hospital stays, and a faster return to daily activities compared to traditional open surgery. However, the specific recovery timeline depends on the individual patient, the procedure performed, and the underlying spinal condition.

Postoperative care for minimally invasive spine surgery begins with effective pain management. Surgeons may prescribe a combination of medications to control pain, including opioids, non-steroidal anti-inflammatory drugs (NSAIDs), and muscle relaxants. It is crucial to balance the need for pain relief with the potential side effects and risks associated with these medications. As the patient's pain subsides, the medication regimen can be adjusted accordingly.

216

Another essential component of postoperative care is early mobilization. Patients are typically encouraged to start walking within hours of surgery, as tolerated, to promote circulation and prevent blood clots. Early mobilization also helps reduce stiffness, minimize muscle atrophy, and improve overall function. The healthcare team will monitor the patient's progress and provide guidance on appropriate activities during the recovery process.

Physical therapy plays a crucial role in postoperative care and recovery. A customized physical therapy program helps restore strength, flexibility, and mobility in the spine, further enhancing the recovery process. The program may include a combination of stretching exercises, strengthening exercises, and low-impact aerobic activities, tailored to the patient's specific needs and abilities. The physical therapist will work closely with the patient to establish appropriate goals and monitor progress throughout the recovery process.

In addition to pain management, early mobilization, and physical therapy, postoperative care for minimally invasive spine surgery also involves monitoring for potential complications. These may include infection, bleeding, nerve injury, spinal fluid leakage, or failure to relieve symptoms. Regular follow-up appointments with the surgeon are essential to assess the patient's progress, address any concerns, and identify potential complications early. Imaging studies, such as X-rays or CT scans, may be used to evaluate the surgical site and monitor the healing process.

Nutrition also plays a role in the recovery process following minimally invasive spine surgery. A well-balanced diet rich in protein, vitamins, and minerals can support tissue repair, promote bone healing, and boost the immune system. In some cases, patients may benefit from nutritional supplements to ensure they receive adequate nutrients for optimal recovery.

Patients should also receive guidance on how to care for their surgical incision. This may include instructions on how to clean the incision site, signs of infection to watch for, and when to change the dressing. Proper incision care is crucial in preventing infection and promoting optimal healing.

Emotional well-being is another important aspect of recovery following minimally invasive spine surgery. It is not uncommon for patients to experience feelings of anxiety, depression, or frustration during the recovery process. Support from friends, family, and healthcare providers can help alleviate these feelings and promote a positive mindset. In some cases, patients may benefit from psychological counseling or participation in support groups.

The recovery process following minimally invasive spine surgery can vary significantly between patients. Factors such as age, overall health, the specific procedure performed, and the patient's commitment to postoperative care can all influence the recovery timeline. By closely adhering to their healthcare team's recommendations and engaging in a comprehensive postoperative care plan, patients can optimize their recovery and achieve the best possible outcomes.

As with any surgery, there are potential risks and complications associated with minimally invasive spine surgery. Despite the generally lower risk of complications compared to traditional open surgery, it is essential for patients to understand and consider these potential issues when making informed decisions about their treatment options.

One potential complication is infection, which may occur at the site of the incision or within the deeper tissues surrounding the spine. Surgeons take precautions to minimize the risk of infection, such as maintaining a sterile environment and administering prophylactic antibiotics. However, if an infection does occur, it may require additional treatments such as antibiotics or, in severe cases, further surgical intervention to remove infected tissue.

Bleeding is another possible complication, although blood loss is typically less in minimally invasive spine surgery compared to open procedures. In rare instances, excessive bleeding may require blood transfusions or additional surgical intervention to control. Careful surgical technique and patient monitoring can help minimize the risk of bleeding complications.

Nerve injury is a potential risk in any spinal surgery. While minimally invasive techniques aim to reduce the likelihood of nerve damage by minimizing tissue disruption, there is still a possibility that nerves may be injured during the procedure. Nerve injuries can result in pain, numbness, weakness, or loss of function in the affected area. In some cases, these symptoms may be temporary, while in others, they may be permanent.

Spinal fluid leakage, also known as a cerebrospinal fluid (CSF) leak, can occur if the protective membrane surrounding the spinal cord, called the dura mater, is inadvertently punctured during surgery. A CSF leak may cause headaches, dizziness, or other neurological symptoms. In many cases, the leak resolves on its own with conservative management, such as bed rest and hydration. However, in some instances, further intervention, such as a blood patch or additional surgery, may be necessary to repair the leak.

Failure to relieve symptoms is another potential complication of minimally invasive spine surgery. Although many patients experience significant improvement in their symptoms after surgery, some may not experience the desired level of relief. This could be due to various factors, such as incomplete decompression of the affected nerves, the development of scar tissue, or the persistence of the underlying spinal condition. In some cases, additional procedures or treatments may be necessary to address the ongoing symptoms.

Lastly, the possibility of additional surgery may be necessary if the initial procedure does not achieve the desired outcome or if complications arise. Factors such as patient age, overall health, and the complexity of the spinal condition can influence the likelihood of needing further intervention. It is essential for patients to maintain open communication with their healthcare team and follow postoperative care instructions to minimize the risk of complications and optimize their surgical outcomes.

While minimally invasive spine surgery offers numerous advantages over traditional open surgery, it is not without potential risks and complications. Patients should be fully informed about these possibilities and engage in shared decision-making with their healthcare team to determine the most appropriate treatment option for their specific situation.

The field of minimally invasive spine surgery (MISS) is continuously evolving, fueled by the rapid development of new technologies and techniques that aim to further improve patient outcomes. In this section, we will explore some of the most promising advancements in the realm of MISS, including robotic-assisted surgery, regenerative medicine, and other novel approaches.

Robotic-assisted surgery is a groundbreaking advancement in the field of MISS. By utilizing robotic systems, surgeons can achieve increased precision, control, and stability during surgical procedures. These systems often incorporate 3D imaging and navigation, allowing for accurate preoperative planning and real-time guidance during surgery. The enhanced precision provided by robotic assistance may lead to reduced complications, improved surgical results, and faster patient recovery times. As robotic technology continues to advance, it is expected to play an increasingly significant role in MISS, offering potential benefits such as reduced operative time and radiation exposure for both patients and surgical teams.

Regenerative medicine is an emerging field that seeks to harness the body's natural healing capabilities to repair and regenerate damaged tissues. In the context of MISS, regenerative medicine approaches, including stem cell therapies and tissue engineering, may offer promising alternatives to traditional spinal fusion procedures.

Stem cell therapies, for example, involve the use of pluripotent stem cells or mesenchymal stem cells to promote tissue repair and regeneration. In spinal surgery, these cells may be injected or implanted at the site of injury or degeneration to encourage the growth of new, healthy tissue. Although still in the early stages of clinical development, stem cell therapies have shown promise in preclinical studies and small clinical trials for treating degenerative disc disease, spinal cord injury, and other spinal conditions.

Tissue engineering, on the other hand, involves the creation of biological substitutes for damaged tissues using a combination of cells, scaffolds, and growth factors. In the field of MISS, tissue-engineered constructs could potentially be used to replace damaged intervertebral discs or augment spinal fusion procedures, leading to improved long-term outcomes and reduced need for additional surgeries.

As MISS continues to evolve, researchers and surgeons are developing new surgical approaches and materials to further improve patient outcomes and reduce complications. For example, novel spinal implants made from advanced biomaterials, such as 3D-printed porous titanium or bioresorbable polymers, are being explored for their potential to enhance fusion rates, reduce implant-related complications, and promote bone growth.

Additionally, emerging surgical techniques such as endoscopic spinal surgery, which utilizes small, flexible endoscopes to access the spine, may offer even less invasive options for treating certain spinal conditions. Endoscopic techniques are particularly promising for the treatment of lumbar disc herniations and spinal stenosis, as they allow for direct visualization of the affected structures while minimizing tissue disruption and preserving spinal stability.

As technology and surgical techniques continue to advance, minimally invasive spine surgery is expected to play an increasingly significant role in the treatment of spinal disorders. The ongoing development of new tools, materials, and techniques will further improve patient outcomes, reduce complications, and expand the range of conditions that can be effectively treated using minimally invasive approaches. While many of these emerging technologies and approaches are still in the early stages of development, they hold great promise for revolutionizing the field of MISS and ultimately improving the quality of life for countless patients suffering from spinal conditions.

Patient selection is a vital step in determining the appropriateness of minimally invasive spine surgery (MISS) for each individual. Several factors can influence the decision, including the patient's overall health, the specific spinal condition being treated, and the presence of contraindications. A comprehensive evaluation of the patient's medical history, physical examination, and imaging studies, such as magnetic resonance imaging (MRI), computed tomography (CT) scans, and X-rays, will assist in determining the most suitable treatment approach.

The patient's overall health is an essential factor in the decision-making process. Patients with comorbidities, such as diabetes, cardiovascular disease, or compromised immune systems, may face increased risks during and after surgery. Furthermore, factors like obesity, advanced age, and a history of multiple spinal surgeries can impact the success of MISS and may necessitate a more conservative approach or traditional open surgery.

The specific spinal condition being treated is another crucial factor in patient selection. While MISS has proven effective in treating various spinal disorders, some cases may be too complex or severe for minimally invasive techniques. For example, patients with significant spinal instability or deformity, extensive scarring from previous surgeries, or active infections may not be suitable candidates for MISS.

Shared decision-making is an essential component of the treatment process, as it involves collaboration between the patient and their healthcare team to arrive at the most appropriate treatment plan. The surgeon should provide detailed information about the potential benefits, risks, and alternatives to minimally invasive spine surgery. This discussion should include the expected outcomes, recovery process, and potential complications associated with MISS.

During the shared decision-making process, patients should be encouraged to ask questions and express their concerns or preferences regarding the proposed treatment. It is essential for the patient to understand the implications of choosing MISS over other treatment options, such as conservative therapies, traditional open surgery, or even no intervention at all. A clear understanding of the risks and benefits associated with each option will empower the patient to make an informed decision that best aligns with their individual needs and circumstances.

In some cases, patients may benefit from seeking a second opinion or consulting with a multidisciplinary team of healthcare professionals, including physiatrists, pain management specialists, and physical therapists. This collaborative approach can help ensure that all potential treatment options are thoroughly explored and that the chosen course of action is tailored to the patient's unique needs.

Careful patient selection and shared decision-making are critical aspects of the treatment process for minimally invasive spine surgery. By considering the patient's overall health, the specific spinal condition being treated, and any contraindications, healthcare professionals can ensure that

MISS is the most appropriate option for each patient. Engaging in open and honest communication throughout the decision-making process will empower patients to make informed choices about their treatment, leading to better outcomes and greater satisfaction with their care.

In conclusion, minimally invasive spine surgery (MISS) has revolutionized the treatment of various spinal conditions by offering numerous benefits over traditional open surgery. The primary advantage of MISS is the reduced disruption of surrounding tissues, which leads to decreased postoperative pain, shorter hospital stays, and faster recovery times. As technology and surgical techniques continue to advance, the range of conditions that can be treated using minimally invasive approaches is expected to expand, leading to improved patient outcomes and increased satisfaction.

In recent years, the development of advanced imaging techniques, such as intraoperative fluoroscopy, endoscopy, and navigation systems, has played a crucial role in the success of minimally invasive spine surgery. These technologies enable surgeons to visualize the surgical site in real-time, ensuring precise and accurate placement of instruments while minimizing the risk of complications. Additionally, the ongoing evolution of surgical instruments, such as tubular retractors and specialized tools, has further refined the MISS techniques, leading to increasingly better outcomes for patients.

Despite the numerous advantages of minimally invasive spine surgery, it is essential to recognize that it may not be the best option for every patient. Some individuals may have contraindications or anatomical variations that make traditional open surgery a more appropriate choice. As a result, careful patient selection is of paramount importance in ensuring optimal results.

Shared decision-making between the patient and their healthcare team is a critical aspect of the treatment process. The surgeon should discuss the potential benefits, risks, and alternatives to minimally invasive spine surgery, helping the patient make an informed decision about their treatment. By understanding the expected outcomes, recovery process, and potential complications, patients can make the best choice for their individual situation.

Furthermore, the field of minimally invasive spine surgery is continuously evolving, with new technologies and techniques emerging that promise even better outcomes for patients. For example, robotic-assisted surgery offers increased precision and control for the surgeon, potentially reducing complications and enhancing surgical results. Similarly, advances in regenerative medicine, such as stem cell therapies and tissue engineering, may offer promising alternatives to spinal fusion in the future.

Ultimately, the success of minimally invasive spine surgery relies on a combination of factors, including appropriate patient selection, advanced technology, and the expertise of the surgical team. By remaining informed about the latest developments in the field and engaging in shared decision-making with their healthcare providers, patients can make the best possible choices for their unique circumstances, ensuring the highest likelihood of successful treatment and a swift return to a pain-free, active life.

Chapter 11

Cervical Disc Replacement

Surgical Options for Persistent Neck Pain

Cervical disc replacement is a surgical procedure designed to address severe and persistent neck pain that arises from various cervical spine pathologies, such as degenerative disc disease, herniated discs, and other issues. This innovative approach to treating neck pain involves the removal of the damaged disc and its replacement with an artificial one that closely replicates the movement and function of a natural disc.

Cervical disc replacement, commonly known as cervical arthroplasty, has gained considerable attention and popularity over the past few years. One reason for this increasing interest is the potential advantages that cervical disc replacement offers over traditional fusion surgery. Some of the benefits include the preservation of the natural range of motion and the reduction of stress on adjacent spinal segments, which can lead to a decreased risk of adjacent segment degeneration.

In traditional fusion surgery, the damaged disc is removed, and the adjacent vertebrae are fused together using bone grafts, screws, and plates. This approach limits the range of motion at the treated level, which can place additional stress on the adjacent spinal segments, potentially leading to further degeneration over time. In contrast, cervical disc replacement aims to maintain the natural biomechanics of the cervical spine by inserting an artificial disc that allows for smooth, pain-free movement in multiple directions.

Furthermore, cervical disc replacement has shown promising results in terms of patient outcomes, with many individuals experiencing significant improvements in pain relief, functional recovery, and quality of life. As a result, cervical disc replacement has emerged as a viable alternative to fusion surgery for patients with persistent neck pain that has not responded to conservative treatments.

The development of advanced artificial disc designs and materials has played a crucial role in the success of cervical disc replacement. These state-of-the-art devices are engineered to mimic the biomechanical properties of natural discs, providing support, flexibility, and shock absorption to the spinal column. The artificial discs are designed to move in multiple directions, allowing for flexion, extension, lateral bending, and axial rotation, thereby closely replicating the natural range of motion in the cervical spine.

Moreover, cervical disc replacement has demonstrated a lower risk of complications and a faster recovery period when compared to traditional fusion surgery. Patients undergoing cervical disc replacement often experience a quicker return to their normal activities, with less postoperative pain and a reduced need for long-term pain medication. This contributes to the growing interest in cervical disc replacement as an effective and less invasive solution for persistent neck pain.

Cervical disc replacement offers a promising and increasingly popular surgical option for patients suffering from severe and persistent neck pain due to degenerative disc disease, herniated discs, or other cervical spine pathologies. By preserving the natural range of motion and reducing stress on adjacent spinal segments, cervical disc replacement has the potential to improve patient outcomes and provide a more effective alternative to traditional fusion surgery.

Cervical disc replacement is typically considered for patients who have not responded to conservative treatments such as medication, physical therapy, and epidural injections. The primary indications for this surgery include cervical radiculopathy and cervical myelopathy.

Cervical radiculopathy occurs when the cervical nerve roots are compressed, which can result in pain, numbness, or weakness in the arms. This condition can be caused by various factors such as herniated discs, bone spurs, or spinal stenosis. Cervical myelopathy, on the other hand, is a more severe condition that involves the compression of the spinal cord, leading to neurological deficits and potential disability. This can be caused by spinal stenosis, degenerative disc disease, or ossification of the posterior longitudinal ligament (OPLL).

However, not all patients with neck pain are suitable candidates for cervical disc replacement. There are several contraindications for this procedure that may exclude certain individuals from being eligible candidates. Advanced age or poor bone quality are factors that may increase the risk of complications and poor outcomes. In such cases, the patient's bone structure may not provide adequate support for the artificial disc, potentially leading to implant failure or migration.

Spinal instability, which can be caused by trauma, ligamentous injury, or severe facet joint degeneration, may also preclude a patient from being a suitable candidate for disc replacement. In these instances, spinal fusion surgery may be a more appropriate treatment option to stabilize the affected spinal segments.

Multilevel cervical pathology presents another contraindication for cervical disc replacement. This procedure is typically limited to one or two levels of the spine, and patients with more extensive degeneration may require alternative surgical approaches, such as a combination of disc replacement and fusion surgery or a multilevel laminoplasty, depending on the specific pathology and individual patient factors.

Lastly, certain conditions may preclude the use of cervical disc replacement altogether. Spinal infections, tumors, or significant deformity, such as severe scoliosis or kyphosis, may necessitate alternative treatments or more extensive surgical procedures to address the underlying pathology. In these cases, a comprehensive evaluation by a spine surgeon is crucial to determine the most appropriate treatment plan for the patient's unique needs.

The preoperative evaluation and planning phase for cervical disc replacement is a critical step in ensuring the success of the procedure. This process enables the surgeon to determine the patient's suitability for the surgery and make informed decisions about the most appropriate surgical approach, implant type, and level(s) for disc replacement.

The first step in the preoperative evaluation is a comprehensive medical history and physical examination. During this phase, the surgeon will gather information about the patient's overall health, the duration and severity of neck pain, any previous treatments or surgeries, and any underlying medical conditions that may impact the outcome of the surgery. The physical examination will focus on assessing the patient's neurological function, including muscle strength, reflexes, and sensation, as well as the range of motion and alignment of the cervical spine.

Imaging studies play a crucial role in the preoperative evaluation, providing detailed information about the patient's cervical spine anatomy and the extent of the underlying pathology. X-rays can reveal any bony abnormalities, such as bone spurs or vertebral body degeneration, and help assess spinal alignment. Magnetic resonance imaging (MRI) is particularly useful for visualizing soft tissue structures, such as the intervertebral discs, spinal cord, and nerve roots, allowing the surgeon to identify disc herniation, spinal stenosis, or other causes of nerve compression. Computed tomography (CT) scans may also be used to obtain high-resolution images of the bony anatomy and assist in surgical planning.

In some cases, the surgeon may perform diagnostic nerve blocks or selective nerve root injections as part of the preoperative evaluation. These procedures involve injecting a local anesthetic and/or corticosteroid medication near the suspected source of neck pain, typically under fluoroscopic guidance. If the patient experiences significant pain relief following the injection, this can help confirm the specific spinal level responsible for the symptoms and provide valuable information about the potential success of the surgery.

228

Once the patient is deemed an appropriate candidate for cervical disc replacement, the surgeon will carefully consider various factors to select the most suitable artificial disc. These factors include the patient's anatomy, such as the size and shape of the intervertebral space and the presence of any anatomical variations, as well as the desired range of motion and the specific surgical technique to be used. The choice of implant may also be influenced by the surgeon's experience and familiarity with different artificial disc designs, as well as any available clinical data on the safety and efficacy of the implants.

Cervical disc replacement is performed using a variety of surgical techniques and artificial disc designs, each with its unique features and considerations. The most common surgical approach for cervical disc replacement is the anterior cervical discectomy and arthroplasty (ACDA), which involves accessing the cervical spine through an incision in the front of the neck. This approach allows the surgeon to directly visualize the affected disc and surrounding structures, resulting in a more precise and controlled dissection. Additionally, the anterior approach minimizes the risk of damage to the spinal cord, nerve roots, and surrounding muscles, leading to better postoperative outcomes and fewer complications.

Alternative approaches, such as the posterior or lateral approaches, are less commonly used in cervical disc replacement due to the increased risk of complications and technical difficulties. The posterior approach requires the surgeon to navigate around the spinal cord and nerve roots, which can increase the risk of neurological injury. The lateral approach, while providing good access to the intervertebral disc space, can be technically challenging and may require more extensive dissection of the surrounding tissues, resulting in increased postoperative pain and longer recovery times.

When it comes to implant types, artificial cervical discs can be broadly categorized into two groups: constrained and unconstrained designs. Constrained discs typically feature a ball-and-socket or a pivoting hinge mechanism, which allows for limited motion in multiple directions. These types of discs are designed to provide stability and support while maintaining some degree of flexibility to closely mimic the natural motion of the cervical spine. Examples of constrained artificial discs include the Prestige LP and the Mobi-C.

Unconstrained discs, on the other hand, feature a more flexible design, with separate components that can move independently to replicate the natural motion of the cervical spine. These types of discs generally consist of a central core, usually made of a highly resilient polymer, sandwiched between two metal endplates that attach to the adjacent vertebrae. The unconstrained design allows for a greater range of motion, potentially reducing stress on the adjacent spinal segments and decreasing the risk of adjacent segment degeneration. Examples of unconstrained artificial discs include the ProDisc-C and the Bryan Cervical Disc.

The choice of implant depends on several factors, such as the surgeon's preference, the patient's anatomy, and the desired range of motion. Additionally, the choice may be influenced by the patient's age, overall health, and the extent of the cervical spine pathology. It is important for the surgeon and patient to discuss the various implant options and their potential benefits and risks in order to select the most appropriate artificial disc for the individual's needs and goals.

The cervical disc replacement procedure is a meticulous process involving several crucial steps. Initially, patients are placed under general anesthesia to ensure they remain unconscious and pain-free throughout the surgery. Once anesthetized, the patient is positioned supine on the operating table, with their neck slightly extended. This position facilitates access to the cervical spine while minimizing the risk of damaging the spinal cord and nerve roots.

The surgeon then proceeds with the anterior cervical approach, making a small incision on the front of the neck, either to the right or left of the trachea. By carefully dissecting the tissue layers, the surgeon exposes the cervical spine. The anterior cervical approach is preferred because it minimizes the risk of damaging critical structures such as the spinal cord and nerve roots, as well as reducing the risk of postoperative complications.

Following the exposure of the cervical spine, the surgeon moves on to the disc removal step. The affected disc is cautiously removed using specialized instruments, with care taken to preserve the adjacent vertebral bodies and spinal ligaments. During this step, the surgeon may also remove any bone spurs or other structures that may be compressing the spinal cord or nerve roots, as these can contribute to the patient's pain and neurological symptoms.

After the damaged disc has been removed, the surgeon proceeds to the implant sizing and trial phase. During this stage, the intervertebral space is measured, and an appropriately sized trial implant is selected to ensure proper fit and alignment. The trial implant is temporarily inserted between the vertebrae to confirm the correct size, placement, and range of motion. This trial phase is essential for preventing complications and ensuring the best possible outcome for the patient.

Once the appropriate implant size is confirmed, the surgeon inserts the artificial disc into the intervertebral space. This step requires careful attention to proper alignment and secure fixation to the adjacent vertebrae. The artificial disc is designed to allow for smooth, pain-free motion in multiple directions, replicating the natural function of the patient's cervical spine.

Finally, the surgical site is thoroughly irrigated to remove any debris or contaminants. The tissue layers are meticulously closed in layers using sutures or staples, ensuring proper healing and minimizing the risk of infection. A sterile dressing is applied to protect the incision site as the patient recovers from the procedure.

Overall, the cervical disc replacement procedure is a complex and precise surgical intervention that requires a skilled surgeon, state-of-the-art equipment, and a thorough understanding of the patient's unique anatomy and needs. By adhering to these detailed steps, the surgeon aims to alleviate the patient's pain, restore function, and improve their overall quality of life.

Following cervical disc replacement surgery, patients are carefully monitored in the recovery room for several hours. This period allows healthcare professionals to closely observe the patient's vital signs, neurological function, and pain levels, ensuring a smooth transition to the postoperative phase. Once stable, patients are transferred to a hospital room where they typically stay for 1-2 days to receive further care and begin their recovery process.

One of the key aspects of postoperative care is effective pain management. A multimodal approach is commonly employed, combining different types of medications to address various sources of pain. Opioids are prescribed to alleviate severe pain, while nonsteroidal anti-inflammatory drugs (NSAIDs) help reduce inflammation and provide additional pain relief. Muscle relaxants may also be used to minimize muscle spasms and discomfort. It is essential to administer these medications as prescribed and follow a gradual tapering plan to prevent dependency or adverse side effects.

Physical therapy plays a critical role in the recovery process, often commencing within the first 24 hours after surgery. A trained physical therapist will guide patients through specific exercises designed to restore mobility, strengthen neck muscles, and improve overall functionality. Early mobilization, such as walking and performing gentle range-of-motion exercises, is encouraged as soon as patients feel comfortable, as this helps prevent complications like blood clots and accelerates the healing process.

Surgeons provide detailed postoperative care instructions tailored to each patient's unique needs and recovery progress. These instructions include guidance on wound care, such as keeping the incision site clean and dry, as well as how to identify signs of infection, like increased redness, swelling, or discharge. Patients should promptly report any concerns to their healthcare team.

Activity restrictions are an essential aspect of postoperative care, as they allow the body to heal and prevent complications. Patients may be advised to wear a soft cervical collar for a short period, usually around 1-2 weeks, to support the neck during the initial healing phase. This collar helps stabilize the neck and minimize excessive movement, promoting a successful recovery.

Most patients can expect to return to work and engage in light activities within 2-4 weeks after surgery, provided they do not involve heavy lifting or strenuous movements. Surgeons will typically outline a gradual return-to-activity plan, allowing patients to progressively increase their activity levels as their recovery progresses. More strenuous activities, such as sports or heavy manual labor, may be restricted for 6-12 weeks or longer, depending on the patient's individual recovery and the surgeon's recommendations.

Regular follow-up appointments with the surgeon are scheduled throughout the recovery process to monitor healing, assess neurological function, and address any concerns or complications that may arise. These appointments provide an opportunity for the healthcare team to evaluate the patient's progress and adjust the postoperative care plan as needed, ensuring the best possible outcome.

Postoperative care and recovery after cervical disc replacement surgery involve a comprehensive approach to pain management, early mobilization through physical therapy, personalized activity restrictions, and close monitoring by the healthcare team. By adhering to these guidelines and maintaining open communication with their healthcare providers, patients can maximize their chances of a successful recovery and long-term pain relief.

Cervical disc replacement has been shown to provide significant pain relief and functional improvement for patients with cervical radiculopathy or myelopathy. Compared to traditional fusion surgery, cervical disc replacement offers the potential advantages of preserving the natural range of motion, reducing adjacent segment degeneration, and facilitating a faster recovery.

However, as with any surgical procedure, cervical disc replacement carries certain risks and complications. One potential complication is infection. Although rare, infections can occur at the surgical site or within the intervertebral space, necessitating further treatment with antibiotics or additional surgery. To minimize this risk, surgeons employ strict sterile techniques during the procedure, and patients may receive prophylactic antibiotics before and after surgery.

Another potential complication is implant failure or dislocation. The artificial disc may not function properly, become dislodged, or wear out over time, potentially requiring revision surgery. Factors that may contribute to implant failure include improper sizing or placement, patient noncompliance with postoperative restrictions, or mechanical issues with the implant itself. To mitigate these risks, surgeons carefully select and place the implant, and patients are advised to follow postoperative instructions closely.

Nerve or spinal cord injury is another possible complication of cervical disc replacement, although it is uncommon. Damage to the nerves or spinal cord can occur during surgery, resulting in pain, weakness, or loss of function. To minimize this risk, surgeons utilize meticulous surgical techniques and advanced intraoperative monitoring to protect neural structures during the procedure.

In some cases, patients may continue to experience pain or neurological symptoms after surgery, potentially due to incomplete decompression, scar tissue formation, or other factors. To address these issues, surgeons strive to achieve optimal decompression during the procedure, and patients may be advised to participate in postoperative physical therapy to manage scar tissue and promote healing.

Despite these risks, cervical disc replacement has emerged as a viable and effective treatment option for patients with persistent neck pain resulting from cervical spine pathology. Long-term studies have demonstrated favorable outcomes, with the majority of patients reporting significant improvements in pain and function, as well as high satisfaction rates with the procedure. By carefully selecting appropriate candidates for cervical disc replacement and employing advanced surgical techniques, surgeons can minimize complications and maximize patient outcomes.

As the field of spine surgery continues to evolve, there are several areas of development and innovation that have the potential to improve patient outcomes and reduce complications in cervical disc replacement procedures.

One promising area of research is the development of improved implant materials and designs. Ongoing studies are exploring new biomaterials and implant designs that aim to increase the durability, functionality, and biocompatibility of artificial cervical discs. Advancements in this area could potentially extend the lifespan of the implants, reducing the need for revision surgeries, and further enhance the range of motion and stability offered by the artificial disc. Researchers are also investigating novel surface coatings and materials that may promote better osseointegration and reduce the risk of implant migration or failure.

Another significant advancement in cervical disc replacement surgery is the development of minimally invasive surgical techniques. By utilizing smaller incisions and specialized instruments, these approaches may reduce tissue trauma, blood loss, and recovery time while maintaining comparable clinical outcomes to traditional open surgery. Minimally invasive techniques also have the potential to minimize postoperative pain and scarring, shorten hospital stays, and enable a quicker return to daily activities for patients. As these techniques continue to be refined and optimized, it is anticipated that they will become more widely adopted in cervical disc replacement procedures.

The use of patient-specific implants and 3D printing is another exciting development in the field of cervical disc replacement. By designing implants based on individual patient anatomy and biomechanics, surgeons can ensure a more precise fit and alignment, potentially leading to better clinical outcomes. The growing field of 3D printing offers the possibility to fabricate customized implants tailored to each patient's unique spinal anatomy. As 3D printing technology advances and becomes more cost-effective, it is expected that the use of patient-specific implants will become more prevalent in cervical disc replacement procedures.

Furthermore, the integration of robotic-assisted surgery and intraoperative navigation systems has the potential to revolutionize the field of spine surgery. These technologies can provide surgeons with real-time feedback and enhanced visualization, increasing surgical precision and reducing the risk of complications. Robotic-assisted systems can help guide the surgeon's movements, ensuring more accurate placement of the artificial disc and minimizing the risk of nerve or spinal cord injury. Intraoperative navigation systems can also improve the surgeon's ability to navigate complex anatomy or perform revision surgeries, where scar tissue and altered anatomy can make the procedure more challenging. As these technologies continue to advance and become more widely available, it is expected that they will play a more significant role in cervical disc replacement procedures.

In conclusion, cervical disc replacement represents a promising surgical option for patients with persistent neck pain due to cervical spine pathologies that have not responded to conservative treatments. With ongoing research and advancements in technology, such as improved implant materials and designs, minimally invasive surgical techniques, patient-specific implants and 3D printing, and robotic-assisted surgery and navigation, the future of cervical disc replacement surgery holds great potential for further improving patient outcomes and expanding its indications for use.

Chapter 12

Cervical Fusion Surgery

Stabilizing the Spine to Alleviate Pain

Cervical fusion surgery, specifically anterior cervical discectomy and fusion (ACDF), is a widely used surgical procedure for treating various neck pain-causing conditions, such as cervical disc herniation, degenerative disc disease, and spinal instability. The primary goal of this surgery is threefold: to alleviate pain, stabilize the cervical spine, and restore the neck's normal function. This chapter delves into a comprehensive and scientifically accurate discussion of cervical fusion surgery, addressing its indications, techniques, potential risks, and post-operative care.

Cervical fusion surgery is typically performed when non-surgical treatments fail to provide sufficient relief from neck pain and associated symptoms. Conservative treatments such as physical therapy, medications, and injections are usually tried before considering surgery. However, when the patient's quality of life is significantly impacted or neurological symptoms become severe, surgical intervention may be warranted.

The cervical fusion surgery process involves the removal of the problematic intervertebral disc and fusing the adjacent vertebrae to stabilize the spine. In most cases, the procedure is carried out using the anterior approach, known as anterior cervical discectomy and fusion (ACDF). However, alternative approaches such as posterior cervical fusion and minimally invasive techniques are also available, depending on the patient's specific condition and the surgeon's preference.

During an ACDF procedure, the surgeon makes a small incision in the front of the neck to access the cervical spine. After the removal of the affected intervertebral disc, the adjacent vertebrae are prepared for fusion. A bone graft or an interbody cage filled with bone graft material is then placed in the disc space to promote bone growth and fusion. To provide additional stability, a metal plate and screws may be used during the fusion process.

The cervical fusion surgery aims to achieve long-term pain relief and improved function for patients suffering from neck pain due to degenerative conditions or spinal instability. However, the success of the surgery depends on several factors, including the patient's overall health, the severity of the condition being treated, and adherence to post-operative care and rehabilitation guidelines. Studies have reported success rates of approximately 80-95% for cervical fusion surgery in terms of pain relief and improved function.

Despite the high success rates, cervical fusion surgery, like any surgical intervention, carries some potential risks and complications. Some of the most common risks include infection, bleeding, nerve or spinal cord injury, nonunion or pseudarthrosis, adjacent segment degeneration, hardware failure, and general anesthesia complications. It is essential for patients to be well-informed of these risks before deciding to undergo the procedure.

Following cervical fusion surgery, patients require a period of recovery and rehabilitation to regain strength, mobility, and function. Post-operative care includes pain management, wound care, activity restrictions, physical therapy, the use of a cervical collar or brace, and regular follow-up visits with the surgeon. Adhering to the prescribed post-operative care plan and rehabilitation guidelines can significantly impact the fusion process and recovery.

Cervical fusion surgery is a proven and effective treatment option for individuals suffering from neck pain due to conditions such as cervical disc herniation, degenerative disc disease, and spinal instability. By stabilizing the spine and alleviating pressure on the spinal nerves, this procedure can significantly improve patients' quality of life. A thorough discussion with their healthcare provider is crucial for patients considering cervical fusion surgery to determine if this procedure is the right course of action for their specific situation.

Cervical fusion surgery is often considered when conservative treatments such as physical therapy, medications, and injections have been unsuccessful in providing adequate relief for neck pain and associated symptoms. There are several specific conditions that may necessitate cervical fusion surgery, and these are discussed in greater detail below.

Cervical disc herniation is a condition that arises when the soft, gel-like nucleus of an intervertebral disc protrudes through the tough outer layer, known as the annulus fibrosus. This herniation can potentially compress nearby nerves, leading to pain, numbness, and weakness in the neck, shoulders, arms, and hands. Cervical fusion surgery may be indicated for patients with cervical disc herniation who have not responded to conservative treatment measures and continue to experience significant discomfort or functional impairment.

Degenerative disc disease is another condition that may warrant cervical fusion surgery. With age-related wear and tear, the intervertebral discs can undergo degeneration, causing pain and reducing the disc's ability to act as a cushion between the vertebrae. When non-surgical treatments are ineffective, and the patient's quality of life is significantly affected, cervical fusion surgery may be considered to provide stability and relieve pain.

Cervical spondylosis, also known as cervical osteoarthritis, is a degenerative condition involving the spinal joints and ligaments. This degeneration can lead to neck pain and stiffness, affecting the individual's daily activities and overall well-being. If conservative treatments fail to provide relief, cervical fusion surgery may be recommended to address the underlying spinal instability and alleviate pain.

Cervical stenosis is a condition characterized by the narrowing of the spinal canal in the neck region, which can compress the spinal cord or nerve roots. This compression can result in pain, numbness, and weakness in the extremities. In cases where conservative treatments have not provided sufficient relief, and the patient's symptoms significantly impact their daily functioning, cervical fusion surgery may be considered as a treatment option.

Spinal instability can also necessitate cervical fusion surgery. Certain conditions, such as trauma, tumors, or infections, can lead to abnormal motion between the cervical vertebrae, causing pain and neurological symptoms. In these cases, cervical fusion surgery may be indicated to provide stability and alleviate the associated pain and neurological symptoms, particularly when non-surgical interventions have been unsuccessful.

Cervical fusion surgery techniques have evolved over time to provide patients with various options tailored to their specific needs. The most common technique is the anterior cervical discectomy and fusion (ACDF). Other alternatives include posterior cervical fusion and minimally invasive cervical fusion surgery, which are suitable for certain cases depending on the underlying condition and patient factors.

In the anterior cervical discectomy and fusion (ACDF) procedure, the surgeon makes a small incision in the front of the neck, usually on the left or right side, to access the cervical spine. This approach allows the surgeon to directly visualize the affected intervertebral disc and adjacent vertebrae while minimizing disruption to surrounding tissues. After making the incision, the surgeon gently retracts the muscles, trachea, and esophagus to expose the affected area of the spine.

The next step in the ACDF procedure is the removal of the damaged intervertebral disc. The surgeon carefully removes the disc material, taking care to avoid damaging the surrounding nerves and spinal cord. In some cases, additional bone spurs or thickened ligaments may also be removed to decompress the nerves and spinal cord further.

Once the disc has been removed, the adjacent vertebrae are prepared for fusion. The surgeon removes any remaining disc material and creates a rough surface on the endplates of the vertebrae to encourage bone growth. A bone graft or an interbody cage filled with bone graft material is then placed in the empty disc space. The bone graft, which can be harvested from the patient's hip or obtained from a bone bank, promotes new bone growth and ultimately leads to the fusion of the adjacent vertebrae.

To provide immediate stability and support during the fusion process, a metal plate and screws are often used to hold the vertebrae in the correct position. These implants, usually made of titanium, are secured to the vertebral bodies, ensuring proper alignment and immobilization. Over time, as the bone graft fuses the vertebrae together, the metal implants become less critical but usually remain in place unless they cause complications.

Posterior cervical fusion is an alternative technique that involves accessing the cervical spine through an incision in the back of the neck. This approach is primarily used when the source of instability or compression is located at the back of the spinal column, such as in cases of cervical stenosis with foraminal narrowing or cervical facet joint arthritis. In this procedure, the surgeon removes any compressive structures and fuses the vertebrae from the posterior side using bone grafts, rods, and screws. While posterior cervical fusion can effectively treat specific conditions, it may be associated with more extensive muscle dissection and a longer recovery period compared to ACDF.

Minimally invasive cervical fusion surgery is another option that aims to minimize tissue damage, reduce post-operative pain, and promote faster recovery. These procedures use smaller incisions and specialized instruments, such as tubular retractors and endoscopes, to perform the fusion while preserving the surrounding soft tissues. Minimally invasive techniques can be applied to both anterior and posterior approaches, depending on the patient's needs and the surgeon's expertise. Although minimally invasive cervical fusion surgery may offer some advantages, it is not suitable for all patients and conditions, and careful patient selection is crucial for optimal outcomes.

Posterior cervical fusion is a surgical technique that aims to stabilize the cervical spine by accessing it through an incision in the back of the neck. This approach is generally reserved for specific situations where the primary cause of instability or compression is located at the posterior

241

aspect of the spinal column. The following paragraphs will delve into the procedure, its indications, advantages, and potential complications.

Indications for Posterior Cervical Fusion: Posterior cervical fusion is particularly useful in cases of cervical stenosis with foraminal narrowing, cervical facet joint arthritis, and other conditions affecting the posterior elements of the spine. Foraminal narrowing, also known as foraminal stenosis, is a condition where the openings through which spinal nerves exit the spinal canal become constricted, leading to nerve compression and associated pain, numbness, and weakness in the upper extremities. Similarly, cervical facet joint arthritis is the degeneration of the small joints that connect adjacent vertebrae, causing pain, stiffness, and reduced range of motion in the neck.

Procedure Overview: During a posterior cervical fusion, the patient is positioned face-down on the operating table under general anesthesia. The surgeon makes an incision in the midline of the back of the neck, exposing the affected area of the cervical spine. Depending on the specific condition being treated, the surgeon may remove bone spurs, thickened ligaments, or degenerated facet joints to decompress the spinal nerves or spinal cord. Once the decompression is complete, the fusion process begins by placing bone graft material along the posterior aspect of the vertebrae, typically in the form of a bone graft, which may be harvested from the patient's hip or obtained from a bone bank. To enhance stability, the surgeon may also use metal rods, screws, or plates to hold the vertebrae in place while the bone graft fuses with the adjacent vertebrae.

Advantages of Posterior Cervical Fusion: One of the primary advantages of the posterior approach is the ability to directly address the pathology affecting the posterior elements of the cervical spine. By accessing the spine through the back of the neck, the surgeon can achieve optimal visualization and decompression of the affected spinal nerves or spinal cord. Additionally, the posterior approach allows for better stabilization of the spine in cases where multiple levels of fusion are required or when there is significant spinal instability.

Potential Complications: As with any surgical procedure, posterior cervical fusion carries some risks and complications. Some common complications associated with this procedure include infection, bleeding,

242

nerve injury, and hardware failure. Although rare, there is also a risk of nonunion or pseudarthrosis, which occurs when the vertebrae do not fuse properly, necessitating further surgical intervention. Patients should discuss these potential risks with their surgeon to make an informed decision about undergoing the procedure.

Posterior cervical fusion is a valuable surgical option for patients experiencing neck pain and neurological symptoms due to conditions affecting the posterior aspects of the cervical spine. By directly addressing the source of instability or compression, this procedure can provide significant relief and improved function for affected individuals.

Minimally invasive cervical fusion surgery is an alternative to traditional open surgery techniques that offers several potential benefits, including reduced tissue damage, decreased post-operative pain, and faster recovery times. This approach has been developed to minimize the invasiveness of the procedure while maintaining the same goals of spinal stabilization and pain relief.

One of the primary advantages of minimally invasive cervical fusion surgery is the utilization of smaller incisions. This results in less disruption to the surrounding muscles, ligaments, and other soft tissues, which may lead to a quicker recovery and reduced post-operative pain. Smaller incisions also lower the risk of infection and minimize scarring.

To perform minimally invasive cervical fusion surgery, specialized instruments and advanced imaging technology, such as intraoperative fluoroscopy or computer-assisted navigation, are used to guide the surgeon during the procedure. These tools allow for precise placement of the interbody device and screws while minimizing the risk of injury to the surrounding structures.

Anterior Cervical Discectomy and Fusion (ACDF) using minimally invasive techniques is an approach that involves the same basic principles as the traditional ACDF but employs smaller incisions and specialized retractors to minimize tissue disruption. The procedure is performed under fluoroscopic guidance to ensure accurate placement of the interbody device and hardware.

Minimally Invasive Posterior Cervical Fusion is a technique that involves accessing the cervical spine through small incisions in the back of the neck. The surgeon uses specialized instruments and retractors to minimize muscle dissection and damage while stabilizing the spine with rods and screws.

Cervical Disc Arthroplasty using minimally invasive techniques are used in some cases, when a patient may be a candidate for cervical disc replacement instead of fusion. This procedure involves the removal of the damaged disc and the insertion of an artificial disc device through a small incision in the front of the neck. Minimally invasive techniques can be applied to this procedure as well, resulting in reduced tissue damage and quicker recovery.

Lateral Mass Fusion using minimally invasive techniques is a procedure that is performed through small incisions in the back of the neck and involves the placement of screws into the lateral masses of the cervical vertebrae to stabilize the spine. This technique can be performed with minimally invasive retractors and instruments to minimize soft tissue disruption.

It is essential to note that not all patients may be suitable candidates for minimally invasive cervical fusion surgery. Factors such as the severity of the spinal condition, the patient's overall health, and the surgeon's experience and expertise in minimally invasive techniques must be considered when determining the appropriate surgical approach. In some cases, traditional open surgery may still be the best option to ensure the desired outcome.

Minimally invasive cervical fusion surgery represents a promising alternative to traditional open techniques, offering several potential benefits, including reduced tissue damage, decreased post-operative pain, and faster recovery times. By utilizing specialized instruments, advanced imaging technology, and meticulous surgical techniques, this approach aims to provide effective spinal stabilization and pain relief while minimizing the invasiveness of the procedure.

As with any surgical procedure, cervical fusion surgery carries some potential risks and complications. It is essential for patients to discuss these risks with their surgeon to make an informed decision about undergoing the procedure. One such risk is the possibility of infection. Although uncommon, surgical site infections can occur after cervical fusion surgery.

Infections after cervical fusion surgery are typically classified as superficial or deep. Superficial infections involve the skin and subcutaneous tissues around the surgical incision, while deep infections may involve the spinal column, bone grafts, or implanted hardware. Symptoms of infection may include redness, swelling, increased pain, fever, and discharge from the surgical site.

The risk of infection can be minimized through various preventive measures taken by the surgical team, such as proper sterilization techniques and the administration of prophylactic antibiotics before and during the procedure. Additionally, patients can lower their risk of infection by maintaining good hygiene and following the surgeon's post-operative care instructions.

When infections do occur, they are typically treated with antibiotics. The choice of antibiotic depends on the type of bacteria causing the infection, which can be determined through laboratory testing. In some cases, patients may require intravenous antibiotics for a more effective treatment.

In severe cases or when conservative treatments fail to resolve the infection, additional surgery may be required to clean the infected area. This may involve removing the infected tissue, bone graft, or implanted hardware. In cases where hardware removal is necessary, the surgeon may decide to perform a revision surgery to stabilize the spine once the infection has been successfully treated.

It is crucial to address infections promptly and effectively to prevent complications such as delayed bone fusion, hardware failure, or the spread of infection to other parts of the body. Patients experiencing symptoms of infection after cervical fusion surgery should contact their healthcare provider immediately for evaluation and appropriate treatment.

Bleeding during or after cervical fusion surgery is a potential concern that can lead to complications if not managed appropriately. Although some blood loss is expected during any surgical procedure, excessive bleeding can increase the risk of postoperative complications, prolong the recovery period, and, in rare cases, may even be life-threatening.

Surgeons take several precautions to minimize blood loss during cervical fusion surgery. These measures include the use of electrocautery devices, which use heat to seal blood vessels, and hemostatic agents, which promote clotting and help control bleeding. In addition, meticulous surgical techniques and careful dissection of tissues can help minimize blood loss during the procedure.

Despite these efforts, excessive bleeding can still occur in some cases. This may result from a patient's specific anatomy, the presence of underlying medical conditions, or the use of certain medications that interfere with blood clotting, such as anticoagulants or antiplatelet drugs. It is essential for patients to inform their surgeon of all medications they are taking before undergoing surgery, as some medications may need to be temporarily discontinued or adjusted to reduce the risk of excessive bleeding.

If excessive bleeding does occur during or after surgery, various interventions may be employed to manage the situation. This can include administering blood-clotting agents, the use of blood conservation techniques, or, in severe cases, performing a blood transfusion. Blood transfusions involve the administration of donated blood or blood products to replace the lost blood and maintain the patient's hemoglobin levels within a safe range. While blood transfusions can be lifesaving, they are not without risks, such as allergic reactions, infections, or transfusion reactions. As a result, transfusions are typically reserved for situations in which the benefits outweigh the potential risks.

While bleeding is a potential risk during cervical fusion surgery, surgeons take numerous precautions to minimize blood loss and manage any excessive bleeding that may occur. Patients should have a thorough discussion with their healthcare provider about the risks of bleeding and the potential need for blood transfusion before undergoing cervical fusion surgery. By understanding these risks and working closely with their healthcare team, patients can better prepare for their surgery and optimize their chances for a successful outcome.

During cervical fusion surgery, there is a small risk of nerve or spinal cord injury. Although rare, these injuries can occur due to multiple factors, such as inadvertent damage to the spinal cord or nerves, excessive bleeding causing compression, or misplacement of surgical hardware. The risk of nerve or spinal cord injury can be minimized by selecting an experienced surgeon and using advanced intraoperative monitoring techniques.

Nerve or spinal cord injuries that occur during cervical fusion surgery can manifest in various ways, depending on the severity and location of the injury. These injuries can lead to temporary or permanent neurological symptoms, which may include numbness, tingling, or burning sensations in the neck, shoulders, arms, or hands. In more severe cases, patients may experience weakness or paralysis of the affected muscles, loss of coordination, or difficulties with fine motor tasks.

Recovery from nerve or spinal cord injuries depends on the extent of the damage and the patient's overall health. In some cases, nerve injuries may resolve spontaneously over time as the nerves regenerate and heal. However, this process can be slow and may take several months or even years. In cases of severe or permanent nerve damage, patients may require additional treatments such as medications, physical therapy, occupational therapy, or assistive devices to help manage their symptoms and improve their quality of life.

In the event of a spinal cord injury during cervical fusion surgery, the consequences can be more severe and potentially life-altering. Patients may experience a loss of sensation, muscle strength, and reflexes below the level of the injury. In the most severe cases, complete paralysis of the upper or lower extremities may occur, necessitating long-term care and rehabilitation. Patients who suffer from spinal cord injuries during cervical fusion surgery may require a multidisciplinary approach to their care, involving various medical specialists such as neurologists, physiatrists, physical therapists, and occupational therapists.

To minimize the risk of nerve or spinal cord injuries during cervical fusion surgery, surgeons may employ intraoperative neuromonitoring techniques. These techniques involve the use of specialized equipment to monitor the electrical activity of the spinal cord and nerves during surgery, allowing the surgeon to identify and respond to any potential issues in real-time. Intraoperative neuromonitoring has been shown to reduce the risk of nerve or spinal cord injuries and improve the overall safety of cervical fusion procedures.

Despite the potential risks associated with nerve or spinal cord injuries during cervical fusion surgery, it is important to remember that these complications are relatively rare. By carefully selecting an experienced surgeon and discussing any concerns or questions with the surgical team, patients can feel more confident in their decision to undergo this procedure to alleviate their neck pain and improve their quality of life.

Nonunion, also known as pseudarthrosis, is a potential complication of cervical fusion surgery in which the vertebrae do not properly fuse together. This lack of fusion may result from various factors, such as poor bone quality, smoking, inadequate immobilization, infection, or issues related to surgical technique.

In the context of cervical fusion surgery, nonunion can lead to persistent neck pain, instability, and neurological symptoms. It is important to identify the underlying cause of nonunion to determine the appropriate course of action for addressing this complication.

Several risk factors may increase the likelihood of nonunion following cervical fusion surgery. Patient-related factors, such as age, obesity, diabetes, and osteoporosis, can negatively impact the fusion process by impairing bone healing and growth. Lifestyle factors, including smoking and excessive alcohol consumption, can also hinder the fusion process by reducing blood flow and oxygen supply to the bone graft site.

Surgical factors, such as inadequate bone graft material, poor graft positioning, or improper hardware placement, can contribute to nonunion as well. Infections occurring in the early post-operative period may disrupt the fusion process, leading to nonunion and necessitating additional treatment. Silicon nitride implants demonstrate considerable antibacterial behaviors that are probably multifactorial, and related to surface chemistry, texture, and electrical charge. The surface chemistry and natural nanostructure topography of the silicon nitride implant provides an optimal environment for stimulation of bone growth and fusion.

To diagnose nonunion, surgeons will typically assess the patient's symptoms, perform a physical examination, and use imaging studies such as X-rays, CT scans, or MRI scans to evaluate the fusion site. It is essential to distinguish between a delayed union, which may still progress to a successful fusion, and a true nonunion that requires intervention.

Treatment options for nonunion following cervical fusion surgery depend on the underlying cause and severity of the condition. Conservative treatments may include prolonged immobilization using a cervical collar or brace, activity modification, and pain management. Additionally, addressing modifiable risk factors such as smoking cessation, improving nutrition, and managing chronic health conditions may enhance the chances of successful fusion.

In cases where conservative treatments are unsuccessful or when the nonunion is causing significant pain, instability, or neurological symptoms, further surgical intervention may be necessary. Revision surgery may involve removing any hardware that has failed or is contributing to the nonunion, debriding the fusion site to promote new bone growth, and utilizing a new bone graft or additional bone graft material. Surgeons may also use bone morphogenetic proteins (BMPs), which are proteins that stimulate bone growth, or autologous platelet-rich plasma (PRP) to enhance the healing process.

Nonunion or pseudarthrosis is a potential complication of cervical fusion surgery that may require further intervention to achieve successful fusion. Identifying and addressing the underlying causes and risk factors for nonunion can significantly improve patient outcomes and overall quality of life.

Adjacent segment degeneration (ASD) is a potential long-term complication following cervical fusion surgery. The fusion of one or more spinal segments alters the biomechanics of the cervical spine, leading to increased stress and load on the adjacent, unfused segments. Over time, this increased stress can result in accelerated degeneration of the adjacent intervertebral discs, facet joints, and other spinal structures, leading to neck pain, stiffness, and in some cases, neurological symptoms.

The exact cause of ASD is not entirely understood, but several factors are thought to contribute to its development. One factor is the altered spinal biomechanics resulting from the immobilization of the fused segment. The loss of motion in the fused area causes the adjacent segments to compensate by increasing their range of motion, thus bearing additional stress. This biomechanical change may lead to increased wear and tear on the adjacent intervertebral discs and facet joints, ultimately causing degeneration.

In addition to biomechanical factors, patient-related factors such as age, overall health, and pre-existing spinal degeneration can also play a role in the development of ASD. Older patients and those with a history of degenerative spinal conditions may be at a higher risk for ASD following cervical fusion surgery. Moreover, lifestyle factors such as obesity, poor posture, and lack of physical activity can contribute to spinal degeneration and may exacerbate ASD.

The onset of ASD can vary greatly between individuals. Some patients may develop symptoms within a few years following cervical fusion surgery, while others may not experience any issues until several years or even decades later. The management of ASD typically begins with conservative treatments such as medications, physical therapy, and lifestyle modifications. However, if these conservative treatments fail to provide adequate relief or if the patient develops significant neurological symptoms, additional surgery may be required.

To address ASD, surgeons may consider various surgical options, including decompression procedures such as laminectomy or foraminotomy, or further spinal fusion to stabilize the degenerated adjacent segments. The choice of surgical intervention will depend on the specific location and severity of the degeneration and the patient's overall health and preferences.

To minimize the risk of ASD following cervical fusion surgery, it is crucial for patients to adhere to post-operative care and rehabilitation guidelines provided by their healthcare team. Maintaining a healthy lifestyle, practicing good posture, and engaging in regular physical activity can help preserve spinal health and may reduce the likelihood of developing ASD. Additionally, emerging surgical techniques and technologies, such as motion-preserving devices and minimally invasive procedures, are being developed and studied to address the potential negative consequences of spinal fusion surgery, including ASD.

Hardware failure is a potential complication that can occur following cervical fusion surgery. Although this complication is relatively uncommon, it is crucial to understand the factors that can contribute to hardware failure, its signs and symptoms, and the management strategies employed to address it.

During cervical fusion surgery, metal hardware such as plates, screws, and rods may be used to stabilize the spine and provide support while the fusion process occurs. These hardware components are typically made from materials such as titanium or stainless steel, which are biocompatible and resistant to corrosion. However, in some cases, the hardware can break or become loose, leading to complications.

There are several factors that can contribute to hardware failure. Excessive stress on the spinal hardware due to strenuous activities, incorrect surgical technique, poor bone quality, or noncompliance with post-operative activity restrictions may increase the risk of hardware failure. Furthermore, certain patient-related factors, such as obesity, smoking, and underlying health conditions like osteoporosis, can compromise the stability and strength of the hardware components.

Patients who experience hardware failure may exhibit signs and symptoms such as increased pain, swelling, or inflammation around the surgical site. In some cases, hardware failure can also cause neurological symptoms if the loose or broken components impinge on the spinal nerves or spinal cord. The presence of these symptoms warrants further investigation using imaging studies, such as X-rays or CT scans, to determine the cause and extent of the hardware failure.

Treatment for hardware failure depends on the severity and specific circumstances of the case. In some instances, conservative management with pain medications, activity modifications, and physical therapy may be sufficient to address the issue. However, in more severe cases or when conservative management is ineffective, revision surgery may be necessary. Revision surgery typically involves the removal or replacement of the failed

251

hardware components and, in some cases, additional procedures to ensure successful fusion and stabilization of the spine.

To minimize the risk of hardware failure, patients should follow their surgeon's post-operative guidelines, engage in appropriate rehabilitation programs, and maintain a healthy lifestyle to promote optimal bone health. Additionally, surgeons should employ meticulous surgical techniques and choose the most suitable hardware components for each patient, taking into consideration the patient's individual anatomy and risk factors. By working collaboratively, healthcare providers and patients can optimize the outcomes of cervical fusion surgery and reduce the likelihood of hardware-related complications.

General anesthesia is a medically induced state of unconsciousness that allows patients to undergo surgeries, such as cervical fusion, without experiencing pain or discomfort. While general anesthesia is considered safe and has been utilized in millions of procedures worldwide, it is essential to be aware of the potential complications associated with its use.

Allergic reactions to the anesthetic agents or adjunct medications used during general anesthesia are rare but can occur. These reactions can range from mild symptoms, such as rash or itching, to more severe manifestations, including difficulty breathing, low blood pressure, and, in extreme cases, anaphylaxis—a potentially life-threatening allergic reaction. Patients with a history of allergies to medications or those who have experienced adverse reactions to anesthesia in the past should inform their healthcare providers to reduce the risk of an allergic reaction during surgery.

Breathing difficulties can arise during general anesthesia due to various factors. The administration of anesthetic agents can depress the respiratory system, leading to decreased oxygen levels in the blood (hypoxia) or a buildup of carbon dioxide (hypercapnia). Additionally, the placement of an endotracheal tube—a flexible tube inserted into the trachea to maintain an open airway and facilitate mechanical ventilation—may cause complications, such as injury to the airway or difficulty placing the tube correctly. Anesthesiologists monitor patients closely during surgery to detect and manage any respiratory complications that may arise.

Adverse effects on the cardiovascular system are another potential complication of general anesthesia. The anesthetic agents can cause changes in blood pressure, heart rate, and cardiac output. While these effects are typically well-controlled, they can pose risks for patients with pre-existing cardiovascular conditions, such as heart disease, hypertension, or arrhythmias. In rare instances, general anesthesia can lead to more severe cardiovascular complications, including heart attack, stroke, or even cardiac arrest. To minimize these risks, a thorough pre-operative evaluation is conducted to identify patients with underlying heart conditions and develop an appropriate anesthetic plan.

It is also important to note that the risk of complications from general anesthesia is influenced by several factors, such as age, overall health, and the presence of chronic medical conditions. Elderly patients, those with obesity, and individuals with conditions like diabetes or obstructive sleep apnea may face an increased risk of complications during general anesthesia. In these cases, a comprehensive pre-operative assessment and careful monitoring during surgery are crucial to ensure patient safety.

While general anesthesia is a vital component of many surgical procedures, including cervical fusion surgery, it carries potential risks, such as allergic reactions, breathing difficulties, and adverse effects on the cardiovascular system. Patients should discuss their medical history and any concerns about anesthesia with their healthcare providers to ensure that all necessary precautions are taken for a safe and successful surgical experience.

Following cervical fusion surgery, patients embark on a recovery and rehabilitation journey to regain strength, mobility, and functionality in the neck. Proper post-operative care and adherence to prescribed guidelines are crucial in ensuring a successful recovery and optimal outcomes.

Pain management is a vital aspect of post-operative care, as patients typically experience some degree of discomfort after surgery. A combination of medications, including opioids, non-steroidal anti-inflammatory drugs (NSAIDs), and muscle relaxants, may be prescribed to alleviate pain. Over time, as the healing process progresses, patients can expect a gradual decrease in pain levels.

In addition to managing pain, wound care is essential in preventing infections and promoting proper healing. Surgeons provide specific instructions for keeping the surgical site clean and dry. This may involve timely removal of dressings, cleaning the incision area with appropriate antiseptic solutions, and monitoring for any signs of infection, such as redness, swelling, or discharge.

Activity restrictions play a significant role in preventing complications and promoting successful fusion. For several weeks after surgery, patients should avoid strenuous activities that strain the neck, such as heavy lifting, bending, or twisting. Surgeons will typically advise on when it is safe to resume normal activities and return to work, based on individual progress and recovery.

Physical therapy is a cornerstone of the rehabilitation process, helping patients regain strength, flexibility, and range of motion in the neck. A physical therapist will design a personalized program that may include exercises, stretching, and manual therapy techniques. Consistent participation in physical therapy is crucial for a successful recovery and minimizing the risk of long-term complications.

Some patients may need to wear a cervical collar or brace during the initial healing phase to provide support and limit neck motion. The surgeon will recommend the appropriate type of collar or brace and specify the duration of use. It is essential to follow these recommendations to ensure proper healing and spinal alignment.

Regular follow-up visits with the surgeon are necessary for monitoring the progress of fusion and healing. These appointments may involve imaging studies such as X-rays or CT scans to assess the success of the fusion process. Patients should also use these visits as an opportunity to discuss any concerns or questions they may have about their recovery.

Post-operative care and recovery following cervical fusion surgery involve a combination of pain management, wound care, activity restrictions, physical therapy, use of supportive devices, and regular follow-up visits. By adhering to these guidelines and working closely with healthcare professionals, patients can achieve a successful recovery and improve their overall quality of life.

Long-term outcomes and prognosis following cervical fusion surgery can vary among patients, but the procedure has been shown to provide significant pain relief and improved function for many individuals suffering from neck pain due to degenerative conditions or spinal instability. The long-term success of the surgery depends on several factors, including the patient's overall health, the severity of the condition being treated, and adherence to post-operative care and rehabilitation guidelines.

Success rates for cervical fusion surgery have been reported in the range of approximately 80-95% in terms of pain relief and improved function. However, certain factors can negatively impact the fusion process and overall success rate. For instance, smoking can hinder bone healing, while obesity can place additional strain on the spine and slow down the recovery process. Moreover, patients with poor bone quality, such as those with osteoporosis, may experience a higher risk of complications or unsuccessful fusion.

The timeframe for successful fusion can vary between patients, as it may take anywhere from 3 to 12 months, depending on factors like age, overall health, and the extent of the surgery. To positively impact the fusion process, it is essential for patients to adhere to post-operative care and rehabilitation guidelines provided by their healthcare team. This may include following prescribed medication regimens, engaging in physical therapy, and avoiding activities that place undue stress on the healing spine.

While cervical fusion surgery can offer lasting relief for many patients, some may require additional surgery in the future due to adjacent segment degeneration or hardware-related complications. Adjacent segment degeneration refers to the increased stress on the spinal levels adjacent to the fused segment, leading to accelerated degeneration and potential need for further surgical intervention. Hardware-related complications, such as broken or loose screws, may also necessitate revision surgery. The risk of needing additional surgery can be minimized by maintaining a healthy lifestyle, practicing good posture, and engaging in regular physical activity that strengthens the muscles supporting the spine.

Many patients who undergo cervical fusion surgery report an improvement in their overall quality of life. The pain relief and increased mobility that often follow the procedure can significantly enhance an individual's sense of well-being. The ability to return to work and daily activities without being hampered by chronic neck pain contributes to this improvement in quality of life. It is essential for patients to maintain realistic expectations regarding the potential outcomes of the surgery and to closely follow their healthcare team's recommendations to maximize their chances of a successful long-term outcome.

In conclusion, cervical fusion surgery has emerged as a reliable and effective treatment option for individuals experiencing neck pain due to various conditions, such as cervical disc herniation, degenerative disc disease, and spinal instability. This surgical procedure aims to stabilize the spine and alleviate pressure on spinal nerves, thereby significantly improving the patient's quality of life.

Before considering cervical fusion surgery, it is crucial to explore and exhaust all conservative treatment options. Surgery should only be pursued when conservative treatments have failed to provide adequate relief and when the patient's quality of life is severely impacted by their neck pain and associated symptoms. It is important to note that while the success rates of cervical fusion surgery are generally high, individual outcomes can vary, and no surgical procedure is without risks.

Understanding the potential risks and complications associated with cervical fusion surgery is essential for patients to make informed decisions. These risks may include infection, bleeding, nerve or spinal cord injury, nonunion or pseudarthrosis, adjacent segment degeneration, hardware failure, and complications related to general anesthesia. By discussing these risks and complications with their healthcare provider, patients can better assess the potential benefits and drawbacks of the procedure.

Post-operative care and rehabilitation play a vital role in ensuring the best possible outcomes following cervical fusion surgery. Adhering to a comprehensive rehabilitation program, including physical therapy, activity restrictions, and cervical collar or brace use, as prescribed by the healthcare provider, can significantly impact the fusion process and overall recovery. Patients must also be diligent about wound care, pain management, and follow-up visits to monitor their progress and address any potential issues that may arise during the healing process.

In addition to the surgical procedure itself, lifestyle modifications can contribute to long-term success and improved quality of life for patients who have undergone cervical fusion surgery. Maintaining a healthy weight, engaging in regular physical activity, practicing good posture, and seeking prompt treatment for any future neck or spine-related issues can help minimize the risk of complications and the need for additional surgery.

Ultimately, the decision to undergo cervical fusion surgery should be made through a thorough discussion between the patient and their healthcare provider, considering the patient's unique medical history, symptoms, and individual needs. By understanding the potential benefits, risks, and post-operative care requirements associated with cervical fusion surgery, patients can make well-informed decisions that support their long-term health and well-being.

Chapter 13

Post-Surgical Care and Recovery

Regaining Strength and Function after Neck Surgery

The post-surgical care and recovery process plays a critical role in determining the success of neck surgery. Appropriate care, rehabilitation, and adherence to the prescribed regimen can greatly improve the outcomes of the surgery and help patients regain strength and function. This chapter will provide a comprehensive overview of the post-surgical care and recovery process, including pain management, wound care, physical therapy, and rehabilitation. It will also discuss potential complications and strategies to prevent them, as well as provide guidance for resuming daily activities and achieving long-term success.

Pain management is a crucial aspect of post-surgical care, as it helps patients recover more comfortably and quickly while enabling them to participate more effectively in physical therapy. A variety of medications may be prescribed to manage acute postoperative pain following neck surgery. The choice and dosage of medications will depend on several factors, including the patient's medical history, the type of surgery performed, and the severity of the pain.

Opioids are a class of medications that act on the central nervous system to provide relief from moderate to severe pain. Commonly prescribed opioids after neck surgery may include morphine, oxycodone, or hydromorphone. While these medications can be highly effective in managing postoperative pain, they also carry the risk of side effects such as drowsiness, constipation, and respiratory depression. Furthermore, long-term use of opioids can lead to dependence or addiction. Therefore, opioids are typically prescribed for short-term use and are carefully monitored by the healthcare team.

Acetaminophen, also known as paracetamol, is a widely used analgesic and antipyretic medication that can help manage mild to moderate pain following neck surgery. It is often combined with other pain-relieving medications, such as opioids or NSAIDs, to provide more comprehensive pain management. Acetaminophen is generally well-tolerated and has a lower risk of side effects than opioids or NSAIDs. However, excessive use of acetaminophen can lead to liver damage, so it is essential to follow the prescribed dosage and not exceed the recommended daily limit.

Non-steroidal anti-inflammatory drugs (NSAIDs) are another class of medications that can help manage postoperative pain after neck surgery. These medications, such as ibuprofen, naproxen, or celecoxib, work by reducing inflammation and providing analgesic effects. NSAIDs are particularly useful for managing pain caused by inflammation, which is common following surgery. While generally effective and well-tolerated, NSAIDs can also cause side effects, particularly when used for prolonged periods. Potential side effects include gastrointestinal issues, such as ulcers or bleeding, and an increased risk of cardiovascular events. Patients with a history of gastrointestinal or cardiovascular issues should discuss the risks and benefits of NSAIDs with their healthcare provider.

In some cases, additional medications may be prescribed to enhance pain relief and address specific postoperative symptoms. For example, muscle relaxants such as cyclobenzaprine or baclofen may be used to help alleviate muscle spasms that can occur after surgery. Additionally, medications like gabapentin or pregabalin, which are typically used to treat nerve pain, may be prescribed for patients experiencing neuropathic pain following neck surgery.

Overall, the appropriate choice and combination of pain medications will be individualized based on the patient's needs and medical history. It is essential to follow the healthcare provider's recommendations and openly communicate any concerns or side effects related to pain management.

Ice therapy, also known as cryotherapy, is a widely used method to manage pain and inflammation following neck surgery. By applying cold temperatures to the affected area, ice therapy constricts blood vessels, which reduces blood flow and subsequently minimizes swelling and inflammation. Additionally, the cold temperature temporarily numbs the nerves in the area, providing pain relief and improving patient comfort during the early stages of recovery.

When utilizing ice therapy, it is crucial to take precautions to avoid frostbite or skin damage. Patients should always wrap the ice pack or cold compress in a thin cloth or towel to provide a barrier between the skin and the ice. Direct contact with the ice can cause skin irritation, burns, or even frostbite.

As the surgical site is often sensitive and tender, it is essential to follow the surgeon's recommendations on the appropriate frequency and duration of ice therapy. Typically, ice packs are applied for 20-30 minutes every 2-3 hours during the first 48-72 hours after surgery. Applying ice for longer periods or more frequently may lead to tissue damage or slow down the healing process. It is important to allow the skin to return to normal temperature between applications to avoid any adverse effects.

Patients should be aware of signs that ice therapy may be causing harm, such as persistent redness, blisters, or numbness that does not subside after removing the ice pack. If any of these symptoms occur, patients should discontinue ice therapy and consult their healthcare provider for further guidance.

261

While ice therapy is generally considered safe and effective for reducing postoperative pain and inflammation, it may not be suitable for all patients. Individuals with certain medical conditions, such as Raynaud's disease, peripheral artery disease, or peripheral neuropathy, should discuss the risks and benefits of ice therapy with their healthcare provider before implementing it into their post-surgical care routine.

Ice therapy can be a valuable tool for managing pain and inflammation following neck surgery when used correctly and under the guidance of a healthcare professional. By following the appropriate application techniques and paying close attention to any potential adverse effects, patients can safely and effectively incorporate ice therapy into their post-surgical care and recovery plan.

Proper wound care is vital to prevent infection and promote healing following neck surgery. The surgeon will typically provide detailed instructions on how to care for the incision site, and it is crucial for patients to adhere to these guidelines to ensure a smooth recovery process.

One of the key aspects of wound care is maintaining cleanliness and dryness at the incision site. Patients should be advised to clean the area gently with mild soap and water, taking care not to rub or scrub the wound. After cleaning, the incision should be patted dry using a clean, soft towel or sterile gauze. The surgeon may also provide specific instructions for showering or bathing, as submerging the incision site in water for prolonged periods can increase the risk of infection.

Changing dressings as instructed is another essential component of wound care. The surgeon will typically provide guidance on the frequency of dressing changes, which may vary depending on the type of surgery and the patient's individual healing progress. When changing the dressing, patients should wash their hands thoroughly with soap and water to minimize the risk of introducing bacteria to the wound. Wearing disposable gloves can provide an additional layer of protection.

It is important for patients to avoid touching the incision site with unwashed hands, as this can introduce harmful bacteria and increase the risk of infection. Additionally, patients should refrain from using any ointments or creams on the wound without the surgeon's consent, as these products may interfere with the healing process or cause irritation. In some cases, the surgeon may prescribe a topical antibiotic ointment to be applied to the incision site to help prevent infection.

Patients should also closely monitor the incision for signs of infection, such as increased redness, swelling, warmth, or discharge. Other symptoms that may indicate an infection include fever, chills, or increased pain at the incision site. If any of these signs are observed, it is essential for the patient to report their concerns to their healthcare provider promptly, as early intervention can help prevent more serious complications.

Proper wound care is an essential aspect of post-surgical care and recovery for neck surgery patients. By following the surgeon's recommendations for incision care, patients can minimize the risk of infection and promote efficient healing. This includes keeping the incision site clean and dry, changing dressings as instructed, and monitoring for signs of infection. Adherence to these guidelines can help ensure a successful recovery and optimize long-term outcomes.

Closing the incision after neck surgery is an essential step in the surgical process, as it helps promote healing and reduce the risk of complications such as infection or excessive scarring. Surgeons typically use sutures or staples to close the incision, depending on the type and location of the surgery, the surgeon's preference, and the patient's individual factors.

Sutures are strands of material, either absorbable or non-absorbable, that are threaded through the skin and underlying tissues to hold the wound edges together. Absorbable sutures are made from materials designed to break down and be absorbed by the body over time, typically within a few weeks to several months. These sutures do not require removal and are often used for deeper tissue layers or for patients who may have difficulty attending follow-up appointments for suture removal.

Non-absorbable sutures, on the other hand, are made from materials that are not broken down by the body. These sutures need to be removed by the surgeon or healthcare provider once the incision has healed sufficiently. The timing for suture removal varies depending on the type of surgery, the location of the incision, the patient's healing progress, and the surgeon's recommendations. Generally, non-absorbable sutures are removed 10-14 days after surgery.

Staples are small, metal clips that are used to close incisions, providing a secure and efficient method of wound closure. Similar to non-absorbable sutures, staples need to be removed once the wound has healed. The timeline for staple removal depends on the same factors as non-absorbable suture removal, including the type of surgery, the location of the incision, and the patient's healing progress.

During the removal process, whether for sutures or staples, the healthcare provider will carefully examine the incision to ensure that it is healing appropriately and that there are no signs of infection or other complications. If the incision is healing well, the sutures or staples will be removed using a sterile technique and specialized instruments designed to minimize discomfort and prevent damage to the surrounding tissues. Patients may experience mild discomfort during the removal process, but this is typically well-tolerated and short-lived.

After suture or staple removal, patients should continue to monitor the incision site for any signs of complications, such as increased redness, swelling, warmth, or discharge. If any of these signs are present, it is crucial to notify the healthcare provider promptly to address potential issues and ensure proper healing.

Early mobilization after neck surgery is a crucial aspect of post-surgical care, playing a key role in promoting recovery and preventing complications. By initiating movement and walking soon after surgery, patients can reduce the risk of complications such as deep vein thrombosis (DVT), pneumonia, and muscle atrophy. This section will delve into the benefits of early mobilization, the process of initiating movement, and the necessary precautions that should be taken.

The benefits of early mobilization are well-documented in scientific literature. Initiating movement shortly after surgery can improve blood circulation, which in turn helps prevent the formation of blood clots in the deep veins of the legs, known as DVT. Additionally, early mobilization encourages deeper breathing and the clearance of secretions in the lungs, reducing the risk of postoperative pneumonia. Furthermore, engaging in gentle movement can help prevent muscle atrophy and stiffness, which are common consequences of prolonged immobility after surgery.

To ensure a safe and effective early mobilization process, patients are typically encouraged to begin moving and walking as soon as it is medically approved, usually within the first 24 hours after surgery. The surgical team, including nurses, physical therapists, and physicians, will assess the patient's condition and provide guidance on when it is appropriate to start mobilizing. It is essential to follow the recommendations of the healthcare team, as they will consider factors such as the patient's medical history, the type of surgery, and the patient's overall stability before allowing them to move.

When initiating early mobilization, patients should start with small movements, such as gentle neck stretches, shifting positions in bed, and performing deep breathing exercises. Gradually, they can progress to more extensive activities, such as sitting up in bed, standing, and taking short walks with assistance. The surgical team will provide specific instructions on the appropriate level of activity and the precautions that should be taken to prevent injury or strain on the surgical site. For instance, patients may be advised to use a neck brace or collar to support the neck during the initial stages of mobilization, or they may be instructed to avoid certain movements that may exacerbate their condition.

Throughout the early mobilization process, it is crucial for patients to pay close attention to their bodies and communicate any pain, discomfort, or concerns to their healthcare team. The team can then make necessary adjustments to the patient's activity level or provide additional guidance to ensure a safe and effective recovery.

Early mobilization is a vital component of post-surgical care, offering numerous benefits for patients recovering from neck surgery. By initiating movement and walking shortly after surgery, patients can reduce the risk of complications such as DVT, pneumonia, and muscle atrophy. It is essential to follow the guidance of the surgical team and take necessary precautions to ensure a safe and effective early mobilization process.

Physical therapy is an essential component of post-surgical care for neck surgery patients, as it helps restore strength, flexibility, and function to the neck and surrounding muscles. Working with a skilled physical therapist can significantly improve the patient's recovery outcomes and overall quality of life.

The initial phase of physical therapy typically focuses on pain relief and reducing inflammation. The physical therapist may use various modalities, such as ice, heat, electrical stimulation, and ultrasound, to help alleviate pain and swelling. Gentle manual therapy techniques, like soft tissue mobilization and joint mobilization, can also be employed to decrease stiffness and improve range of motion in the neck.

As the patient progresses in their recovery, the physical therapist will design a customized rehabilitation program that addresses the patient's specific needs and recovery goals. This program may include a combination of manual therapy, stretching exercises, strengthening exercises, and functional training.

Manual therapy is a hands-on approach that involves various techniques to improve joint mobility, reduce muscle tightness, and alleviate pain. These techniques may include joint mobilizations, soft tissue mobilization, and myofascial release. Manual therapy can help restore normal movement patterns and facilitate the healing process.

Stretching exercises are crucial for maintaining and improving flexibility in the neck and surrounding muscles. The physical therapist will guide the patient through a series of gentle stretches that target specific muscle groups and help restore normal range of motion. These exercises should be performed regularly and within the patient's comfort zone to avoid overstretching or causing further injury.

Strengthening exercises are vital for rebuilding the strength and endurance of the neck muscles and supporting structures. Weak or imbalanced muscles can contribute to neck pain and increase the risk of reinjury. The physical therapist will prescribe a progressive strengthening program that targets the deep neck flexors, cervical extensors, and other key muscle groups. This program may include exercises using resistance bands, free weights, or the patient's body weight.

Functional training involves exercises and activities that mimic the patient's daily tasks and help improve their ability to perform these tasks without pain or discomfort. The physical therapist will work with the patient to identify any movement patterns or habits that may contribute to neck pain and provide guidance on how to modify these patterns to promote long-term recovery. This may include instruction on proper lifting techniques, workstation ergonomics, and sleep positioning.

Throughout the rehabilitation process, the physical therapist will also provide guidance on proper posture and body mechanics to prevent future neck pain and reduce the risk of injury. This may involve educating the patient on the importance of maintaining a neutral spine position, engaging in regular postural breaks, and using supportive devices, such as pillows or lumbar rolls, when necessary.

Physical therapy is a crucial aspect of post-surgical care for neck surgery patients, as it helps restore strength, flexibility, and function to the neck and surrounding muscles. By following a customized rehabilitation program that includes manual therapy, stretching exercises, strengthening exercises, and functional training, patients can significantly improve their recovery outcomes and reduce the risk of future neck pain and injury.

A home exercise program is a crucial component of the post-surgical rehabilitation process for patients recovering from neck surgery. This individualized program, developed by the physical therapist, is designed to complement supervised therapy sessions and facilitate continued progress toward regaining strength, flexibility, and function in the neck and surrounding muscles.

The home exercise program typically includes a combination of stretching exercises, strengthening exercises, and postural awareness activities. Stretching exercises aim to improve the flexibility and range of motion of the neck muscles and joints, which can help reduce stiffness and discomfort. Strengthening exercises focus on building and maintaining muscle strength in the neck, upper back, and shoulders, which is vital for providing adequate support to the cervical spine and preventing future neck pain. Postural awareness activities, on the other hand, help patients develop and maintain proper alignment and positioning of the head, neck, and shoulders during daily activities, thus reducing strain on the cervical spine.

267

To ensure the effectiveness and safety of the home exercise program, it is essential for patients to follow the instructions provided by their physical therapist. This includes adhering to the recommended frequency, duration, and intensity of the exercises. Overdoing exercises or performing them incorrectly can lead to increased pain or even injury, so patients should always consult their therapist if they are uncertain about the proper technique or if they experience pain while performing the exercises.

Regular communication between the patient and physical therapist is also important for monitoring progress and adjusting the home exercise program as needed. The physical therapist will periodically reassess the patient's recovery status, taking into consideration factors such as pain levels, range of motion, strength, and functional abilities. Based on this assessment, the therapist may modify the home exercise program to ensure that it remains challenging and effective for the patient's current level of recovery.

In addition to the prescribed exercises, patients should also be mindful of incorporating regular physical activity into their daily routines. This can include low-impact activities such as walking, swimming, or cycling, which can help improve overall fitness, promote circulation, and reduce the risk of complications associated with a sedentary lifestyle. However, it is essential for patients to consult their healthcare team before starting any new exercise or physical activity, especially during the early stages of recovery.

A well-designed home exercise program is an integral part of the post-surgical recovery process for patients who have undergone neck surgery. By consistently performing the prescribed exercises and maintaining open communication with their physical therapist, patients can improve their chances of achieving optimal recovery outcomes and preventing future neck pain.

Infection is a potential complication after neck surgery, and it is essential to take proactive steps to prevent it. One of the primary ways to minimize the risk of infection is through proper wound care, as discussed earlier in the chapter. Ensuring that the incision site remains clean and dry, and changing dressings as instructed by the surgeon, can help create an environment conducive to healing and reduce the chances of bacterial growth.

Maintaining good personal hygiene is another vital aspect of infection prevention. Patients should wash their hands frequently and thoroughly with soap and water, particularly before and after touching the surgical site or changing dressings. Hand sanitizer with at least 60% alcohol content can also be used if soap and water are not readily available. When bathing or showering, patients should avoid direct water pressure on the incision site and ensure that the area is gently patted dry afterward.

Avoiding contact with individuals who are sick or have infections is crucial during the recovery period, as patients may be more susceptible to infections while their immune system is focused on healing the surgical site. Additionally, patients should be cautious in public spaces and avoid touching surfaces that may harbor bacteria, such as door handles, elevator buttons, and handrails.

Surgeons may also prescribe prophylactic antibiotics to patients to further reduce the risk of infection, particularly in cases where the surgery involves implanted hardware, or the patient has a history of previous infections. The use of prophylactic antibiotics should be tailored to the patient's specific risk factors and the type of surgery performed, considering the potential benefits and risks associated with antibiotic use, such as the development of antibiotic-resistant bacteria.

In addition to these preventive measures, patients should monitor the incision site for signs of infection, such as increased redness, swelling, warmth, or discharge, as well as fever or chills. If any of these symptoms are present, it is important to notify the healthcare provider promptly so that appropriate interventions can be initiated. Early recognition and treatment of infection can help prevent more severe complications and promote a successful recovery.

Infection prevention after neck surgery involves a combination of proper wound care, good personal hygiene, avoidance of exposure to potential sources of infection, and, in some cases, the use of prophylactic antibiotics. By taking these precautions and closely monitoring the surgical site for signs of infection, patients can minimize their risk of complications and support a more successful recovery process.

Deep vein thrombosis (DVT) is a serious medical condition in which blood clots form in the deep veins, typically in the legs or pelvis. These clots can break loose and travel to the lungs, causing a life-threatening pulmonary embolism. Preventing DVT is an essential aspect of post-surgical care, particularly for patients who have undergone neck surgery, as their mobility may be temporarily limited. Several strategies can be employed to minimize the risk of DVT, including early mobilization, compression stockings, leg exercises, and blood-thinning medications.

As discussed earlier, mobilization plays a crucial role in DVT prevention. Encouraging patients to start moving and walking as soon as it is safe and medically approved helps increase blood flow and reduces the risk of clot formation. Gradually increasing the level of activity in the days and weeks following surgery can further promote circulation and minimize the risk of DVT.

Compression stockings, also known as graduated compression stockings, are another useful tool in DVT prevention. These specialized stockings apply gentle pressure to the legs, which helps improve blood flow and prevents blood from pooling in the veins. The pressure exerted by the stockings is strongest at the ankle and gradually decreases up the leg, encouraging blood flow back toward the heart. Compression stockings should be worn as directed by the surgeon or healthcare provider, and the appropriate level of compression should be determined based on the patient's individual risk factors and needs.

Leg exercises can also contribute to DVT prevention by promoting circulation and reducing blood stagnation in the veins. Patients can perform simple exercises, such as ankle pumps and foot circles, while seated or lying down. These exercises involve gently flexing and pointing the toes or rotating the feet in circles, which can stimulate blood flow in the calf muscles and prevent blood from pooling in the veins. It is essential to follow the healthcare provider's recommendations for the appropriate frequency and duration of these exercises to maximize their effectiveness.

In some cases, blood-thinning medications, also known as anticoagulants, may be prescribed to reduce the risk of DVT. These medications work by inhibiting the blood's clotting ability, making it less likely for clots to form in the deep veins. The decision to prescribe blood-thinning medications will depend on the patient's risk factors, the type of surgery, and the surgeon's recommendations. It is essential to closely follow the prescribed regimen and attend regular follow-up appointments to monitor the medication's effectiveness and ensure the patient's safety.

Preventing DVT after neck surgery involves a multifaceted approach that includes early mobilization, compression stockings, leg exercises, and, in some cases, blood-thinning medications. By following the surgeon's recommendations and adhering to these preventive measures, patients can significantly reduce their risk of developing DVT and its associated complications.

Returning to work after neck surgery is a crucial milestone in the recovery process, and it is essential to plan for this transition carefully to ensure a smooth and successful reintegration into the workplace. The timeline for resuming work activities depends on various factors, including the patient's occupation, the type of surgery, and their individual recovery progress.

For patients with sedentary jobs that primarily involve sitting and minimal physical activity, the return to work timeline may be shorter. Generally, these patients can expect to resume work within 2-4 weeks after surgery. However, it is important to note that patients may still need to make adjustments to their work environment to accommodate any lingering discomfort or mobility limitations. This may include using ergonomic office equipment, such as adjustable chairs, desks, and computer monitors, to maintain proper posture and reduce strain on the neck. It is also important for patients to take regular breaks to stand up, stretch, and change positions throughout the day to minimize the risk of developing additional neck pain or discomfort.

For patients with physically demanding jobs that involve heavy lifting, repetitive motions, or extended periods of standing or bending, the return-to-work timeline may be longer. In these cases, it is not uncommon for patients to require a recovery period of 6-12 weeks or more, depending on the complexity of the surgery and the patient's individual healing progress. The surgeon and physical therapist will provide guidance on when it is safe to resume specific work activities, and they may recommend a gradual return to work to ensure the patient does not overexert themselves or risk injury.

In addition to the physical aspects of returning to work, it is important to consider the psychological and emotional factors that may impact the patient's ability to resume their job duties. Anxiety, depression, and other mental health concerns can arise during the recovery process, and it is essential to address these issues to ensure a successful return to work. Patients may benefit from discussing their concerns with their healthcare team, who can provide support and resources to help manage these emotions.

When planning for the return-to-work, it is important for patients to communicate openly with their employer about their recovery progress and any accommodations they may need in the workplace. This may include temporary adjustments to their job responsibilities, modified work hours, or additional breaks for stretching and rest. Employers are often willing to make reasonable accommodations to support the employee's successful return to work, especially when these accommodations are supported by recommendations from the patient's healthcare team.

In conclusion, the timeline for returning to work after neck surgery is highly individualized and depends on various factors, including the patient's occupation, the type of surgery, and their recovery progress. By working closely with their healthcare team and employer, patients can develop a tailored plan for a safe and successful return to work that accommodates their specific needs and promotes long-term neck health.

The ability to safely resume driving and travel after neck surgery is an important consideration for patients, as it can significantly impact their daily lives and routines. The decision to return to driving and travel should be based on several factors, including the patient's overall recovery progress, neck mobility, and the specific type of surgery they have undergone.

Before resuming driving, patients must ensure they have sufficient neck mobility to safely check blind spots and maneuver their vehicle. The ability to move the neck comfortably and without pain is crucial for maintaining situational awareness and reacting to potential hazards on the road. Additionally, patients should no longer be taking narcotic pain medications, as these can impair cognitive function and reaction time, posing a risk to both the patient and other road users.

The specific timeline for resuming driving depends on the patient's individual recovery progress and the type of neck surgery they have undergone. For example, patients who have undergone minimally invasive procedures or those that require a shorter recovery period may be able to resume driving sooner than those who have had more extensive surgeries. In general, patients may be able to resume driving within 2-4 weeks after surgery, but it is essential to consult with the surgeon and follow their recommendations.

Regarding long-distance travel, especially air travel, patients should discuss their plans with their surgeon before booking a trip. The risk of developing deep vein thrombosis (DVT) and other complications may be heightened during long flights, as passengers are often seated for extended periods, and cabin pressure can affect blood circulation. To mitigate the risk of DVT, patients can take several precautions during long flights, such as wearing compression stockings, performing leg exercises, and staying well-hydrated. The surgeon may also provide additional recommendations based on the patient's individual risk factors.

When planning a trip, it is important for patients to consider their physical limitations and ensure that their destination can accommodate their needs. This may include researching accessible accommodations, transportation options, and activities that are suitable for their recovery stage. In some cases, the surgeon may advise postponing long-distance travel until the patient has made more progress in their recovery.

Resuming driving and travel after neck surgery should be done cautiously and under the guidance of the patient's healthcare team. By ensuring they have regained sufficient neck mobility, are no longer taking narcotic pain medications, and have taken appropriate precautions for long-distance travel, patients can safely reintegrate these activities into their lives as they continue to recover.

Resuming recreational activities and exercise after neck surgery is an important aspect of the recovery process, as it helps to improve overall physical fitness, support mental well-being, and reduce the risk of recurrence. However, it is essential to approach the reintroduction of physical activities with caution and under the guidance of a surgeon and physical therapist to avoid undue strain on the healing tissues and prevent complications.

In the initial weeks following surgery, patients should focus on low-impact activities that gently engage the neck and surrounding muscles without causing excessive strain. Walking is often the first form of exercise recommended, as it can help to improve circulation, maintain flexibility, and support cardiovascular health. Patients should start with short walks at a comfortable pace, gradually increasing the distance and intensity as tolerated.

Swimming is another low-impact activity that can be beneficial during the recovery process. The buoyancy of water helps to support the body, reducing the stress on the neck and spinal structures. Gentle swimming strokes, such as the breaststroke or sidestroke, are often preferred, as they involve minimal neck rotation and extension. Patients should consult with their healthcare team before resuming swimming to ensure it is safe and appropriate for their specific recovery timeline.

As patients progress in their recovery and regain strength and mobility in the neck, they can gradually incorporate more challenging exercises and recreational activities. Cycling, for example, can be a suitable activity for individuals recovering from neck surgery, provided they use proper posture and avoid excessive neck strain. Stationary bikes or recumbent bikes can be particularly helpful, as they allow for a more upright and supported position.

Strength training exercises, such as resistance band exercises or light weightlifting, can also be introduced as the patient's recovery progresses. It is essential to consult with a physical therapist to develop an appropriate strength training program tailored to the individual's needs and abilities.

The therapist will likely recommend starting with light weights and low resistance levels, focusing on proper form and technique to avoid injury.

When resuming more strenuous activities, such as running, high-intensity interval training, or contact sports, patients should proceed with caution and follow the guidance of their healthcare team. These activities often involve greater impact, rapid neck movements, or potential collisions, which could pose a risk to the healing tissues. It may be necessary to delay the resumption of these activities until the patient has achieved a sufficient level of strength, flexibility, and stability in the neck.

Throughout the recovery process, it is crucial for patients to listen to their bodies and avoid pushing through pain or discomfort. Pain can be an indicator of excessive strain on the healing tissues or a sign that the activity is too intense for the current stage of recovery. Patients should communicate any concerns or challenges related to their exercise regimen with their healthcare team, who can help to adjust the program as needed to ensure a safe and successful return to recreational activities and exercise.

Regular follow-up appointments with the surgeon and physical therapist are essential for closely monitoring the patient's recovery progress and ensuring the long-term success of the surgery. These appointments play a vital role in addressing any concerns, assessing the healing of the surgical site, and making necessary adjustments to the rehabilitation program.

The first follow-up appointment with the surgeon typically occurs within the first one to two weeks after surgery. During this visit, the surgeon will examine the incision site to ensure proper healing, evaluate the patient's overall progress, and address any potential complications or concerns. The surgeon may also provide updated guidance on activities, restrictions, and pain management strategies.

Additional follow-up appointments with the surgeon may be scheduled at regular intervals, such as at 6 weeks, 3 months, 6 months, and 1 year after surgery. The frequency and duration of these appointments may vary depending on the specific type of surgery and the patient's individual recovery progress. During these visits, the surgeon may assess the patient's range of motion, strength, and functional abilities. They may also order imaging studies, such as X-rays or MRIs, to evaluate the surgical site and surrounding structures for proper healing and alignment.

Physical therapy follow-up appointments are also a crucial component of the post-surgical recovery process. These appointments typically begin within the first few weeks after surgery and continue throughout the rehabilitation period. The frequency of physical therapy appointments may vary depending on the patient's needs and the therapist's recommendations. In general, patients may attend physical therapy sessions one to three times per week during the initial stages of recovery.

During physical therapy follow-up appointments, the therapist will assess the patient's progress, provide hands-on treatment, and guide them through a series of exercises designed to improve strength, flexibility, and function. The therapist will also monitor the patient's pain levels and make any necessary modifications to the rehabilitation program. As the patient progresses through their recovery, the physical therapist may adjust the frequency of appointments and update the home exercise program to ensure continued progress toward the patient's recovery goals.

Regular follow-up appointments with both the surgeon and physical therapist are crucial for monitoring the patient's recovery progress and ensuring the long-term success of the surgery. These appointments provide an opportunity to address any concerns, assess the healing of the surgical site, and make any necessary adjustments to the rehabilitation program. By actively engaging in the recovery process and maintaining open communication with the healthcare team, patients can maximize their chances of a successful outcome after neck surgery.

Adopting and maintaining a healthy lifestyle is crucial for preventing future neck pain and promoting overall well-being. Several components contribute to a healthier lifestyle, including maintaining a healthy weight, regular exercise, good posture, proper body mechanics, and ergonomic adjustments to workstations and sleeping environments.

Maintaining a healthy weight is essential, as excess weight can place undue stress on the neck and spine, leading to discomfort and potential injury. Patients can achieve a healthy weight through a balanced diet that includes a variety of fruits, vegetables, whole grains, lean proteins, and healthy fats. Additionally, engaging in regular physical activity can help with weight management and improve overall health. It is recommended that adults aim for at least 150 minutes of moderate-intensity aerobic activity or 75 minutes of vigorous-intensity aerobic activity per week, combined with muscle-strengthening activities on two or more days per week.

Regular exercise is not only beneficial for weight management but also for maintaining and improving neck strength and flexibility. Incorporating neck-specific exercises, as prescribed by a physical therapist or healthcare provider, can help strengthen the muscles supporting the neck and improve posture. Additionally, engaging in activities that promote overall flexibility, such as yoga or Pilates, can help prevent muscle imbalances that may contribute to neck pain.

Practicing good posture is vital for reducing strain on the neck and spine. Maintaining proper alignment of the head, neck, and shoulders can help minimize the risk of pain and injury. Patients should be mindful of their posture during daily activities, such as sitting at a desk, standing, and even using electronic devices. Healthcare providers or physical therapists can provide guidance on techniques to improve posture and reduce the risk of neck pain.

Using proper body mechanics during daily activities is another essential component of a healthy lifestyle. This includes lifting objects with the legs rather than the back and avoiding excessive twisting or bending of the neck. By being mindful of body mechanics, patients can minimize the risk of strain and injury to the neck and surrounding structures.

Ergonomic adjustments to workstations and sleeping environments can also play a significant role in reducing neck strain. For instance, adjusting the height of a computer monitor to eye level, using a supportive chair that promotes proper posture, and placing frequently used items within easy reach can help minimize strain on the neck during work hours. In addition, using a supportive pillow that maintains the natural curve of the neck and sleeping in a position that promotes proper spinal alignment can reduce the risk of neck pain during sleep.

Maintaining a healthy lifestyle that encompasses a balanced diet, regular exercise, good posture, proper body mechanics, and ergonomic adjustments can significantly contribute to the prevention of future neck pain and overall well-being. By incorporating these components into daily life, patients can minimize the risk of neck-related issues and enjoy a higher quality of life.

In some cases, patients may continue to experience residual pain after neck surgery. This can be due to various factors, such as nerve irritation, inflammation, or inadequate healing. It is essential to work closely with the healthcare team, including the surgeon, primary care physician, and physical therapist, to identify the cause of the pain and develop an appropriate pain management strategy tailored to the patient's specific needs.

Medications may play a role in ongoing pain management, depending on the source and severity of the pain. For mild to moderate pain, over-the-counter analgesics such as acetaminophen and non-steroidal anti-inflammatory drugs (NSAIDs) may be recommended. For more severe or persistent pain, prescription medications, such as opioids, muscle relaxants, or nerve pain medications like gabapentin, may be considered. It is crucial to follow the healthcare provider's guidance on the appropriate dosage and duration of these medications to minimize the risk of side effects and dependence.

Physical therapy is another essential component of ongoing pain management. Patients who continue to experience pain after surgery may benefit from modifications to their rehabilitation program, which may include adjustments to their exercise routine or the incorporation of additional therapeutic techniques. For example, manual therapy techniques such as joint mobilization or soft tissue manipulation can help alleviate pain by improving joint mobility and reducing muscle tension.

Complementary therapies can also play a role in managing residual pain after neck surgery. Acupuncture, for instance, has been shown to provide pain relief for some patients by stimulating the release of endorphins, the body's natural painkillers. Similarly, massage therapy can help alleviate pain by reducing muscle tension, improving circulation, and promoting relaxation. These therapies should be pursued in consultation with the healthcare team to ensure they are appropriate for the patient's specific situation and do not interfere with other aspects of their care.

In some instances, additional medical interventions may be necessary to address the underlying cause of ongoing pain. This may include further diagnostic tests, such as imaging studies or nerve conduction studies, to identify any structural or neurological issues that may be contributing to the pain. In rare cases, additional surgical procedures may be recommended to correct any identified issues or to revise the initial surgery if it is determined to be the cause of the persistent pain.

Ongoing pain management after neck surgery requires a multidisciplinary approach that considers the unique needs of each patient. By working closely with the healthcare team and exploring a combination of medical, physical, and complementary therapies, patients can develop an effective pain management strategy that helps them achieve optimal recovery and long-term pain relief.

Despite appropriate post-surgical care and recovery efforts, some patients may continue to experience pain or limited mobility after neck surgery. This can be due to various factors, including incomplete healing, nerve damage, scar tissue formation, or the development of new or unrelated issues.

In such cases, it is important to communicate these concerns to the healthcare team promptly. The team may perform a thorough physical examination and gather a detailed medical history to better understand the patient's symptoms. They may also recommend additional diagnostic tests, such as imaging studies (e.g., X-rays, MRI, or CT scans), nerve conduction studies, or electromyography, to identify any underlying structural or neurological issues contributing to the persistent pain or limited mobility.

Based on the findings of these tests, the healthcare team may suggest adjustments to the patient's rehabilitation program, including changes to the frequency or intensity of physical therapy sessions or the incorporation of additional modalities, such as manual therapy or aquatic therapy. These adjustments aim to improve the patient's symptoms and facilitate a more complete recovery.

In some cases, non-surgical interventions may be recommended to address the ongoing pain or mobility issues. These interventions can include pain-relieving medications, anti-inflammatory medications, nerve blocks, or radiofrequency ablation. Alternative therapies, such as acupuncture, massage, or chiropractic care, may also be considered, depending on the patient's preferences and the nature of their symptoms.

If non-surgical treatments are unsuccessful and the patient continues to experience significant pain or functional limitations, the healthcare team may discuss the possibility of revision surgery. This option is generally considered a last resort, as it carries its own set of risks and potential complications. The specific type of revision surgery will depend on the cause of the patient's ongoing symptoms and may involve procedures such as spinal fusion, disc replacement, or the removal of scar tissue or bone spurs. It is crucial for the patient to thoroughly discuss the potential risks and benefits of revision surgery with their healthcare team before making a decision.

Throughout the process of addressing persistent pain or limited mobility, maintaining open communication with the healthcare team is essential. By actively participating in their care and recovery, patients can improve their chances of achieving a successful outcome and regaining their quality of life after neck surgery.

Recovering from neck surgery can indeed be a challenging and emotional experience. The physical limitations and discomfort that patients may experience during the recovery process can contribute to feelings of frustration, anxiety, or depression. It is essential to acknowledge and address these emotions, as they can impact the overall success of the recovery and the patient's quality of life.

One of the first steps in addressing these emotional and psychological factors is for patients to develop realistic expectations about their recovery. Understanding the timeline and potential limitations can help minimize feelings of disappointment or frustration. Communication with the healthcare team is crucial, as they can provide guidance and reassurance throughout the recovery process.

Social support is another essential component in managing the emotional challenges that may arise during recovery. Connecting with friends and family members, sharing concerns and feelings, and seeking their assistance when needed can help alleviate feelings of isolation and stress. In addition, joining support groups or connecting with others who have undergone similar procedures can provide a sense of camaraderie and understanding.

In some cases, patients may benefit from professional mental health support. Psychotherapy, such as cognitive-behavioral therapy (CBT), can help patients develop coping strategies to manage their emotions and adjust to the changes in their physical abilities. CBT can also help patients identify and challenge negative thought patterns that may contribute to feelings of anxiety or depression. If necessary, a mental health professional may recommend medication to help manage these symptoms.

Mindfulness practices, such as meditation or deep breathing exercises, can also be beneficial in managing emotional and psychological factors during recovery. These practices can help patients develop a greater sense of self-awareness, allowing them to recognize and process their emotions more effectively. Mindfulness practices have been shown to reduce stress, anxiety, and depression, and can also improve overall well-being.

Engaging in enjoyable and relaxing activities can further help patients cope with the emotional challenges of recovery. These activities may include listening to music, reading, or engaging in hobbies that do not place strain on the neck. It is important to balance rest and activity to promote physical healing while also maintaining emotional well-being.

Addressing emotional and psychological factors during the recovery process is essential for a successful outcome after neck surgery. By acknowledging and managing these emotions, seeking support from friends, family, and mental health professionals, and engaging in self-care activities, patients can facilitate a more positive recovery experience and improve their overall quality of life.

In conclusion, post-surgical care and recovery serve as crucial elements in achieving optimal outcomes after neck surgery. Pain management, wound care, physical therapy, and rehabilitation are all essential components of a successful recovery, each playing a unique role in helping patients regain strength and function in their necks. By strictly adhering to the surgeon's recommendations and engaging in a comprehensive recovery plan, patients can maximize their chances of a successful outcome.

Patience and commitment to the recovery process are vital, as healing may take time and require dedication to prescribed therapies and exercises. It is important for patients to understand that their active participation in the recovery process can significantly impact the results of their surgery. A strong support system, including friends, family, and healthcare professionals, can help patients maintain motivation and a positive mindset throughout the recovery journey.

Open communication with the healthcare team is essential, as it allows patients to express their concerns, ask questions, and receive guidance tailored to their unique needs and circumstances. The healthcare team can assist in identifying potential challenges and developing strategies to overcome them, such as modifying the rehabilitation program or providing additional support resources.

Moreover, addressing the emotional and psychological aspects of recovery is crucial for overall well-being. Patients should not hesitate to seek help from mental health professionals or support groups if they experience feelings of frustration, anxiety, or depression during their recovery. These resources can provide valuable coping strategies and encouragement, facilitating a more positive recovery experience.

Lastly, long-term success after neck surgery depends on the patient's ability to maintain a healthy lifestyle and incorporate the lessons learned during recovery into their daily routines. This may include continued participation in physical therapy, maintaining good posture, and practicing proper body mechanics during activities to prevent future neck pain and complications.

With appropriate care, support, and commitment, most patients can successfully recover from neck surgery and enjoy an improved quality of life. The journey to recovery may be challenging, but the rewards of reduced pain and increased functionality make the effort worthwhile.

Chapter 14

Posture and Ergonomics

Aligning the Body to Reduce Neck Strain and Discomfort

The relationship between posture, ergonomics, and neck pain is well established in scientific literature. Poor posture and suboptimal ergonomics can lead to muscle imbalances, fatigue, and strain, contributing to the development or exacerbation of neck pain. Conversely, maintaining good posture and applying ergonomic principles can help alleviate existing neck pain, prevent its recurrence, and promote overall musculoskeletal health. This chapter will discuss the importance of posture and ergonomics in the context of neck pain, provide guidance on proper body alignment, and offer practical tips for optimizing ergonomics in various settings.

Good posture is essential for maintaining the proper alignment of the body's musculoskeletal system. This alignment allows for efficient movement and weight distribution while minimizing strain on muscles, ligaments, and joints. Good posture is particularly important when considering the prevention and management of neck pain. The cervical spine, which comprises the uppermost part of the vertebral column, supports the weight of the head and provides mobility and stability to the neck. When an individual's posture is poor, it can lead to a variety of issues that contribute to neck pain.

Poor posture can result in muscle imbalances, as some muscles may become overworked and tight, while others become weak and underutilized. These imbalances can place additional strain on the cervical spine and surrounding structures, increasing the likelihood of developing neck pain. For example, forward head posture, commonly observed in individuals who spend long hours working at a computer or using mobile devices, can cause tightening of the muscles at the back of the neck and weakness in the deep neck flexor muscles. This muscle imbalance contributes to increased stress on the cervical vertebrae, intervertebral discs, and ligaments, which may lead to pain and discomfort.

In addition to muscle imbalances, poor posture can place increased stress on the cervical spine itself. When the head is held in a forward or slouched position, the weight distribution on the cervical vertebrae shifts, increasing the compressive forces on the anterior portion of the intervertebral discs. Over time, this uneven weight distribution may lead to disc degeneration, herniation, or other spinal abnormalities that can cause neck pain. Furthermore, poor posture can exacerbate existing spinal conditions, such as cervical spondylosis or osteoarthritis, by placing additional stress on the affected joints and surrounding tissues.

By practicing good posture, individuals can help reduce neck strain, prevent the onset of neck pain, and improve their overall musculoskeletal health. Maintaining proper alignment of the head, neck, and shoulders promotes balanced muscle activation, reduces stress on the cervical spine, and facilitates optimal biomechanics during movement. In addition, good posture can enhance breathing efficiency, circulation, and nervous system function, further contributing to overall well-being.

It is important to recognize that good posture is not a static position, but rather a dynamic state that involves maintaining proper body alignment during various activities, such as sitting, standing, walking, and even sleeping. Cultivating good posture requires consistent practice, awareness, and attention to the body's positioning and movement patterns.

Incorporating exercises that target postural muscles, such as the deep neck flexors, upper back muscles, and core, can help improve postural stability and promote a more balanced musculoskeletal system. In combination with ergonomic adjustments and lifestyle modifications, maintaining good posture can play a crucial role in the prevention and management of neck pain.

Posture is influenced by various factors, both intrinsic and extrinsic, that can have a significant impact on an individual's overall musculoskeletal health and their susceptibility to neck pain. Understanding these factors and addressing any issues that may contribute to poor posture is essential for the effective prevention and management of neck pain.

Muscle strength and flexibility play a crucial role in maintaining proper body alignment. When muscles are weak or imbalanced, they may not provide adequate support for the spine and other structures, leading to poor posture and, ultimately, neck pain. For example, weak core muscles can result in an exaggerated lumbar curve, causing compensatory changes in the thoracic and cervical regions. Likewise, tight or inflexible muscles in the chest, shoulders, and neck can pull the head and shoulders forward, leading to a slouched posture that places increased strain on the cervical spine.

Joint mobility also has a significant impact on posture. Reduced range of motion in the spine, shoulders, or hips can limit an individual's ability to maintain proper alignment, potentially contributing to poor posture and neck pain. In some cases, joint mobility issues may stem from underlying conditions such as arthritis or previous injuries, necessitating targeted interventions to address the root cause of the problem.

Body weight is another factor that influences posture. Excess body weight, particularly in the abdominal area, can shift the body's center of gravity forward, placing additional strain on the spine and promoting poor posture. Furthermore, carrying excess weight can exacerbate muscle imbalances and joint mobility issues, compounding the negative effects on posture and neck pain.

Habitual movement patterns, developed over time through repetitive activities or prolonged postures, can also contribute to poor posture. These patterns may include crossing the legs while sitting, cradling a phone between the ear and shoulder, or leaning to one side when standing. Over time, these habits can lead to muscle imbalances and postural changes that increase the risk of neck pain.

External factors such as poorly designed furniture or equipment can have a substantial impact on posture. Chairs that do not provide adequate lumbar support or encourage slouching, desks that are too high or low, and computer monitors that force users to crane their necks can all contribute to poor posture and neck strain. In these cases, addressing the underlying ergonomic issues is essential for improving posture and preventing neck pain.

Finally, sedentary lifestyles and excessive sitting can negatively impact posture. Prolonged sitting can lead to muscle imbalances, decreased joint mobility, and reduced core strength, all of which contribute to poor posture and increased neck pain. Incorporating regular movement and exercise into daily routines can help counteract the negative effects of sedentary behavior and promote better posture.

Various factors influence posture, including muscle strength and flexibility, joint mobility, body weight, habitual movement patterns, poorly designed furniture or equipment, and sedentary lifestyles. Addressing these factors is crucial for maintaining proper body alignment, preventing neck pain, and promoting overall musculoskeletal health.

Ergonomics is a multidisciplinary field that combines knowledge from various disciplines, including biomechanics, physiology, psychology, and engineering, to study the interactions between humans and their environment. The primary goal of ergonomics is to optimize human well-being and performance by designing and arranging workspaces, systems, and products that minimize strain, discomfort, and the risk of injury. In the context of neck pain, ergonomics emphasizes the importance of proper body mechanics, posture, and equipment design to alleviate existing discomfort and prevent the development of musculoskeletal disorders.

A key aspect of ergonomics is the assessment and modification of workplace and home environments to support natural body alignment and encourage healthy movement patterns. This involves the consideration of various factors, such as chair design, desk height, monitor positioning, and the arrangement of frequently used items, to create an environment that promotes comfort, efficiency, and overall health. In addition to physical factors, ergonomic principles also address cognitive and organizational aspects of work, such as task design, workload, and job rotation, to reduce the risk of repetitive strain injuries and the development of chronic pain conditions.

When addressing neck pain, ergonomic interventions aim to minimize the load on the cervical spine and surrounding muscles by encouraging proper head and neck alignment and reducing awkward or repetitive movements. This can be achieved through a combination of equipment adjustments, education on proper body mechanics, and the implementation of regular breaks and stretching routines to prevent muscle fatigue and promote flexibility.

In recent years, the widespread use of electronic devices, such as smartphones, tablets, and laptops, has introduced new ergonomic challenges. Prolonged use of these devices, often in non-ergonomic positions, can contribute to increased neck strain and the development of "tech neck." Ergonomic principles can be applied to the use of electronic devices by promoting proper device posture, incorporating voice-activated features, and implementing regular breaks and stretching routines to mitigate the risk of neck pain and other musculoskeletal issues.

Overall, the principles of ergonomics play a crucial role in the prevention and management of neck pain by addressing the underlying causes of strain and discomfort. By incorporating ergonomic principles into daily life, individuals can not only reduce the risk of developing neck pain but also enhance their overall musculoskeletal health and quality of life.

Achieving good posture is a vital aspect of preventing and alleviating neck pain. Good posture involves maintaining the natural curves of the spine and positioning the head, shoulders, and pelvis in a balanced alignment. This proper alignment can be achieved by focusing on several key areas of the body.

Firstly, when standing or sitting, it is essential to keep the head centered over the shoulders. This involves maintaining the chin parallel to the floor and avoiding forward head posture, which is commonly observed when using electronic devices or working at a desk. Forward head posture can lead to increased strain on the neck muscles and contribute to neck pain and discomfort.

Next, the shoulders should be drawn back and down, engaging the shoulder blades and opening the chest. This position promotes optimal alignment of the upper body and prevents the development of rounded shoulders, which can exacerbate neck pain. By maintaining this open chest position, individuals can alleviate tension in the neck and upper back muscles and improve overall posture.

To maintain a neutral spine, individuals should engage their core muscles, which helps preserve the natural curves of the cervical, thoracic, and lumbar regions. Engaging the core muscles not only contributes to proper spinal alignment but also provides essential support for the entire body, promoting balance and stability. A strong core is a critical component of good posture and plays a significant role in preventing and alleviating neck pain.

In addition to focusing on the upper body, proper posture involves positioning the pelvis so that the hips are level and the lower back is supported. This alignment can be achieved by tilting the pelvis slightly forward or backward until a comfortable, neutral position is found. The pelvis serves as the base for the spine, and maintaining a level and supported position can help reduce strain on the neck and promote overall spinal health.

Lastly, when standing or sitting, it is important to distribute body weight evenly across both feet or across the sit bones, respectively. Uneven weight distribution can lead to imbalances in the body and contribute to poor posture and musculoskeletal discomfort. By ensuring that body weight is evenly distributed, individuals can promote optimal alignment and reduce the risk of developing neck pain.

Good posture is a multifaceted concept that involves attention to various areas of the body. By focusing on proper alignment of the head, shoulders, spine, and pelvis, and ensuring even weight distribution, individuals can achieve good posture and reduce the risk of neck pain and discomfort.

Maintaining good posture throughout the day is essential for preventing and managing neck pain. One effective strategy for ensuring proper alignment is to perform regular posture checks. Individuals can do this by standing against a wall, making sure that their head, shoulders, and hips are touching the wall while maintaining a small gap between the wall and their lower back. This position helps to encourage a neutral spine and proper alignment of the head, shoulders, and hips, reducing strain on the neck and other musculoskeletal structures.

In addition to posture checks, strengthening the core, upper back, and neck muscles is crucial for supporting good posture. Engaging in targeted exercises, such as planks for core stability, rows for upper back strength, and various neck stretches to improve flexibility, can help to correct muscle imbalances and reduce the risk of neck pain. A well-rounded exercise program that includes both strengthening and flexibility exercises can provide the necessary support for proper body alignment and reduce the strain on the cervical spine.

Another helpful tip for maintaining good posture, particularly when sitting, is to use lumbar rolls or cushions to support the lower back. By providing additional support to the lumbar region, these aids can help to maintain the natural curve of the spine and prevent excessive slouching or rounding of the back, which can contribute to neck strain. Placing a lumbar roll or cushion between the chair and the small of the back can encourage proper spinal alignment and minimize discomfort associated with poor sitting posture.

Finally, practicing mindfulness and body awareness is essential for maintaining good posture throughout the day. By paying close attention to the body's alignment and making adjustments as needed, individuals can develop a greater understanding of their habitual movement patterns and identify areas that require improvement. Incorporating mindfulness practices, such as meditation or yoga, can help to cultivate greater body awareness and encourage the adoption of healthier postural habits. This heightened sense of body awareness can be invaluable in preventing neck pain and promoting overall musculoskeletal health.

The workplace is a significant contributor to the development and exacerbation of neck pain, given the considerable amount of time individuals spend in office environments. Office ergonomics plays a critical role in preventing and managing neck pain, as it emphasizes the importance of creating a comfortable and efficient workspace that minimizes strain on the cervical spine and surrounding musculature. Inadequately designed workstations, extended periods of sitting, and repetitive movements can lead to neck strain, discomfort, and the development of musculoskeletal disorders. By incorporating ergonomic principles into the office setting, employees can decrease the likelihood of neck pain, enhance productivity, and improve overall well-being.

Poorly designed workstations often fail to provide the necessary support and alignment required for maintaining good posture. For instance, chairs lacking appropriate lumbar support or adjustability may force individuals into awkward positions that place undue stress on the neck and shoulders. Likewise, improperly positioned monitors can lead to excessive neck flexion or extension, contributing to muscle strain and discomfort. Addressing these issues through the implementation of ergonomic principles can significantly impact neck pain prevention and management.

Prolonged sitting is another factor that can contribute to neck pain in office environments. Sitting for extended periods places increased pressure on the discs and joints of the cervical spine, while also contributing to muscle imbalances and fatigue. To counteract the negative effects of prolonged sitting, employees should adopt strategies such as taking regular breaks, incorporating movement and stretching into their daily routines, and considering the use of sit-stand workstations. These practices can help alleviate muscle fatigue, promote circulation, and maintain spinal health.

Repetitive movements, often required by specific job tasks, can also contribute to neck pain. Activities such as prolonged typing, mouse usage, or continuous phone handling can lead to muscle strain and the development of repetitive stress injuries. Office ergonomics aims to mitigate these risks by encouraging the use of ergonomic equipment, such as keyboards with wrist rests and hands-free phone headsets, as well as promoting proper body mechanics and postural awareness.

Implementing ergonomic principles in the office environment not only helps to prevent and manage neck pain but also has a positive impact on overall health and well-being. A comfortable and efficient workspace can lead to reduced physical strain, improved mental focus, and increased job satisfaction. By emphasizing the importance of office ergonomics, employers can create a healthier and more productive work environment for their employees, which, in turn, can lead to reduced healthcare costs and increased productivity.

Office ergonomics is a vital component in the prevention and management of neck pain. By addressing issues related to workstation design, prolonged sitting, and repetitive movements, employees can minimize the risk of developing neck pain, enhance their productivity, and improve their overall well-being. Implementing ergonomic principles in the workplace is not only beneficial for neck pain relief but also contributes to a healthier and more efficient work environment.

Optimizing the office workstation is essential in creating an ergonomically sound environment that minimizes neck strain and promotes overall well-being. One of the key aspects of a well-designed workstation is selecting an adjustable chair that provides adequate lumbar support and encourages a neutral spine. The chair's seat height should be adjusted so that the feet rest flat on the floor, with the knees aligned with or slightly lower than the hips. This positioning ensures proper weight distribution and reduces stress on the lower back and cervical spine.

In addition to chair adjustments, proper monitor placement is crucial for minimizing neck strain. The computer monitor should be positioned at eye level and approximately an arm's length away, allowing the user to maintain a neutral head position while working. When using multiple monitors, it's essential to position them close together and at the same height to reduce excessive head movement, which can lead to neck discomfort and fatigue.

The arrangement of the keyboard and mouse also plays a significant role in promoting a comfortable and ergonomically sound workstation. The keyboard and mouse should be positioned at a height and distance that allow the forearms to remain parallel to the floor and the elbows to be bent at approximately a 90-degree angle. This positioning minimizes strain on the wrists and forearms and encourages proper upper body alignment. The use of a wrist rest can further alleviate strain on the wrists and help maintain a neutral wrist position while typing.

Organizing frequently used items, such as phones and office supplies, within easy reach is another important aspect of an ergonomically optimized workstation. This organization minimizes unnecessary movement and strain on the neck, shoulders, and upper back. Ensuring that frequently accessed items are within close proximity allows for more efficient and comfortable movement throughout the workday.

Lastly, using a document holder when referring to printed materials can significantly reduce neck strain caused by frequent head movements. The document holder should be placed at the same height and distance as the computer monitor, allowing for easy reference without requiring the user to continually shift their gaze and head position. This alignment helps maintain a neutral head posture, reducing the risk of developing neck pain and discomfort.

By implementing these strategies to optimize the office workstation, individuals can create an ergonomically sound environment that promotes proper body mechanics, minimizes neck strain, and enhances overall comfort and productivity.

Sedentary behavior and prolonged sitting can contribute to neck pain and other musculoskeletal issues. One way to counteract the effects of sitting is for employees to take regular breaks throughout the day. Standing up and moving around for a few minutes every 30 to 60 minutes can help reduce muscle fatigue, promote circulation, and alleviate stiffness in the neck and shoulders. Incorporating short walking breaks or engaging in light physical activity during these breaks can further enhance the benefits of movement, reducing the risk of developing musculoskeletal problems related to a sedentary lifestyle.

In addition to taking regular breaks, it is essential for employees to stretch throughout the day to alleviate tension and maintain flexibility in the neck and shoulders. Gentle neck and shoulder stretches can be performed at the workstation or during breaks, helping to relieve muscle tightness, improve range of motion, and prevent muscle imbalances that contribute to neck pain. Examples of effective stretches include neck tilts, rotations, and shoulder rolls. When performing these stretches, individuals should move slowly and smoothly, holding each stretch for 15 to 30 seconds and repeating as necessary.

Finally, employees should consider using a sit-stand workstation as a means of reducing the strain on the cervical spine and promoting better posture. A sit-stand workstation allows individuals to alternate between sitting and standing positions throughout the day, helping to decrease the pressure on the spine, engage different muscle groups, and encourage proper body mechanics. Research has shown that using a sit-stand workstation can help reduce the risk of developing neck pain and improve overall musculoskeletal health. To optimize the benefits of a sit-stand workstation, employees should aim to maintain proper posture and body alignment while standing, ensuring that the monitor, keyboard, and other workstation components are adjusted appropriately for each position.

By incorporating movement and stretching into the workday, employees can minimize the negative effects of sedentary behavior and reduce the risk of developing neck pain. These practices not only contribute to better musculoskeletal health but also enhance overall well-being, productivity, and quality of life.

The home environment plays a crucial role in maintaining proper posture and preventing neck pain. Applying ergonomic principles in domestic settings can help individuals maintain good posture, promote spinal alignment, and minimize strain on the neck and other musculoskeletal structures.

One essential aspect of home ergonomics is investing in supportive furniture. Selecting chairs and sofas that provide adequate lumbar support and encourage a neutral spine can greatly impact an individual's posture and comfort. It is important to avoid furniture that forces the body into slouched or awkward positions, as this can lead to muscle imbalances and strain on the cervical spine. When choosing furniture, consider the design, adjustability, and materials to ensure they provide the necessary support and promote proper body alignment.

Another critical component of home ergonomics is optimizing sleep ergonomics. Sleep is essential for overall health and well-being, and the way

293

individuals sleep can significantly impact their neck and spinal health. To create an ergonomically sound sleep environment, it is crucial to use a supportive pillow that maintains the natural curve of the neck. There are various types of pillows available, including memory foam, latex, and feather pillows, designed to provide optimal support for different sleeping positions. Individuals should choose a pillow that suits their preferred sleeping position and offers the appropriate level of firmness to support the cervical spine.

In addition to selecting the right pillow, it is vital to choose a mattress that provides proper spinal support. A mattress that is too soft or too firm can lead to improper spinal alignment and exacerbate neck pain. Individuals should consider their body type, weight, and sleep preferences when selecting a mattress, and should look for one that offers a balance of comfort and support.

Sleeping position also plays a significant role in maintaining spinal alignment and preventing neck pain. Sleeping on the back or side with a pillow between the knees can help promote spinal alignment and minimize strain on the neck. Stomach sleeping should be avoided, as it often forces the neck into an unnatural position, increasing the risk of pain and discomfort.

Lastly, practicing proper lifting techniques can help prevent neck pain and other musculoskeletal injuries at home. When lifting heavy objects, it is essential to engage the legs and core muscles, keep the object close to the body, and avoid twisting the spine. By using proper body mechanics and maintaining a neutral spine during lifting, individuals can minimize strain on the neck and other vulnerable areas of the body.

Incorporating ergonomics into the home environment is an essential step in preventing and managing neck pain. By investing in supportive furniture, optimizing sleep ergonomics, and practicing proper lifting techniques, individuals can help maintain proper posture, reduce strain on the neck, and promote overall musculoskeletal health.

The increasing use of electronic devices, such as smartphones, tablets, and laptops, has led to the emergence of "tech neck" – a term used to describe neck pain and strain resulting from prolonged device use. The issue arises when individuals frequently bend their necks forward to view their devices, which can place excessive strain on the cervical spine and supporting muscles. This section will delve into strategies to minimize the risk of developing tech neck, including maintaining proper device posture, taking frequent breaks, and implementing voice-activated features.

Maintaining proper device posture is crucial in preventing tech neck. Holding devices at eye level or using a stand can help avoid excessive neck flexion, reducing the stress placed on the cervical spine. When using a device, it is essential to keep the shoulders relaxed and the elbows close to the body. This position minimizes muscle tension in the neck, shoulders, and upper back. Additionally, if using a laptop, consider investing in a laptop stand and external keyboard and mouse to create a more ergonomically friendly setup that encourages better posture.

Taking frequent breaks from device use is another important strategy in combating tech neck. Prolonged device use can cause muscle fatigue and strain, which can exacerbate neck pain. Limiting continuous device use and taking breaks to stretch and reposition the body can help alleviate this strain. During these breaks, individuals can perform gentle neck and shoulder stretches and engage in activities that promote better posture, such as standing or walking. It is also beneficial to practice the 20-20-20 rule: every 20 minutes, take a 20-second break to look at something 20 feet away. This can help reduce eye strain and encourage a change in posture.

Implementing voice-activated features can further help minimize the risk of developing tech neck. By utilizing voice recognition or dictation software, individuals can reduce the need for constant typing and screen interaction. This can lead to less time spent looking down at devices and more time spent maintaining proper posture. Many smartphones, tablets, and laptops come equipped with built-in voice-activated features, making it easy to incorporate this technology into daily device use.

Ergonomic practices surrounding electronic devices are crucial in preventing and managing tech neck. By maintaining proper device posture, taking frequent breaks, and utilizing voice-activated features, individuals can reduce neck strain and discomfort associated with prolonged device use. Implementing these strategies not only contributes to neck pain relief but also promotes overall musculoskeletal health and well-being.

In conclusion, posture and ergonomics are essential factors in the prevention and management of neck pain. The importance of maintaining proper body alignment cannot be overstated, as it significantly reduces strain on the cervical spine and supporting structures. By paying close attention to body mechanics and making conscious efforts to preserve the natural curves of the spine, individuals can alleviate discomfort and prevent the onset of neck pain. Furthermore, adopting a mindful approach to posture can also lead to improvements in balance, mobility, and overall musculoskeletal health.

Optimizing both workplace and home environments is another crucial component in addressing neck pain. By creating ergonomic spaces that support proper alignment, individuals can minimize strain on the cervical spine and prevent the development of musculoskeletal disorders. This includes selecting appropriate furniture and equipment, adjusting workstations to accommodate individual needs, and incorporating regular breaks and movement into daily routines. These adjustments not only contribute to neck pain relief but also promote a more comfortable and productive environment.

Practicing healthy habits when using electronic devices is also essential in managing neck pain. The widespread use of smartphones, tablets, and other devices has led to an increase in neck strain and discomfort, resulting from prolonged and repetitive use. By being mindful of device posture, taking frequent breaks, and utilizing voice-activated features, individuals can mitigate the negative effects of device use on their necks and overall health.

Implementing these posture and ergonomic principles offers benefits beyond neck pain relief. Improved posture and ergonomics can lead to enhanced overall well-being, increased productivity, and a better quality of life. By making a conscious effort to prioritize posture and ergonomics in daily life, individuals can not only protect their necks but also foster an environment that supports long-term health and wellness.

Chapter 15

Exercise and Neck Pain

Maintaining Mobility and Preventing Recurrence

Neck pain is a common ailment, affecting millions of people worldwide. It can arise from various causes, such as poor posture, muscle strain, degenerative disc disease, and more. Maintaining mobility and preventing the recurrence of neck pain is crucial for overall well-being. Exercise has been shown to be an effective tool in managing and preventing neck pain by strengthening the muscles, improving flexibility, and promoting better posture. This chapter will discuss the scientifically accurate information regarding the role of exercise in managing neck pain, the types of exercises recommended, and the precautions to be taken when incorporating exercise into a neck pain management plan.

The importance of muscle strengthening for neck pain management cannot be understated. Weak or imbalanced neck muscles can contribute to neck pain by placing additional stress on the cervical spine and surrounding structures. By performing targeted exercises, individuals can strengthen these muscles, helping to support the head and spine more effectively. Strong neck muscles can decrease the risk of pain and injury, as well as improve overall function and mobility.

Muscle strengthening exercises for the neck focus on the various muscle groups that provide support and stability to the cervical spine. These groups include the deep neck flexors, extensors, lateral flexors, and rotators. Strengthening these muscles can help restore balance and stability to the cervical spine, alleviating pain and reducing the likelihood of future issues.

The deep neck flexors, specifically the longus colli and longus capitis, are crucial for maintaining proper cervical alignment and posture. Weakness in these muscles can lead to an imbalance in the neck's muscle system, causing increased stress on other muscles and spinal structures. Strengthening the deep neck flexors can help improve cervical alignment and reduce the strain on other muscles, contributing to decreased neck pain.

The neck extensors, which include the splenius capitis, splenius cervicis, semispinalis capitis, and upper trapezius muscles, are essential for providing stability to the back of the neck and head. Weakness in these muscles can result in poor posture, muscle imbalances, and increased strain on the cervical spine. By strengthening the neck extensors, individuals can improve overall neck stability, reducing the likelihood of pain and injury.

The lateral flexors, consisting of the scalene muscles, sternocleidomastoid, and levator scapulae, are responsible for side-to-side neck movements. Imbalances in these muscles can cause increased tension and strain on the neck and surrounding structures. Strengthening the lateral flexors can help to restore balance to the neck muscles and promote proper cervical alignment, reducing the likelihood of neck pain.

The neck rotators, such as the obliquus capitis superior and inferior, are responsible for rotating the head and neck. Strengthening these muscles can help to maintain proper cervical alignment and reduce strain on the surrounding structures, contributing to a decrease in neck pain.

It is important to note that muscle strengthening exercises should be performed with proper technique and under the guidance of a healthcare professional, such as a physical therapist or physician. This ensures that the exercises are done safely and effectively, minimizing the risk of injury or exacerbating existing pain. Gradual progression and consistency are key to achieving the desired results from a neck muscle strengthening program.

Muscle strengthening is a vital component of neck pain management. By targeting the various muscle groups responsible for neck stability and function, individuals can improve overall neck health and reduce the risk of pain and injury. It is essential to perform these exercises with proper technique and under professional guidance to ensure safety and effectiveness.

Improving flexibility is an essential aspect of managing and preventing neck pain, as muscle stiffness and limited range of motion can exacerbate the condition. When muscles in the neck, shoulders, and upper back are tight or inflexible, they can place additional strain on the cervical spine, potentially causing pain and discomfort. By regularly stretching these muscles, individuals can improve their flexibility and reduce the likelihood of experiencing neck pain.

Stretching exercises can be performed either dynamically or statically, depending on the individual's needs and preferences. Dynamic stretches involve moving the body through a range of motion, which can help to warm up the muscles and prepare them for activity. Static stretches, on the other hand, involve holding a stretched position for an extended period, typically between 15 and 60 seconds. Both types of stretches can be effective in improving flexibility and alleviating muscle tension in the neck, shoulders, and upper back.

There are several specific stretches that can be beneficial for improving flexibility in the neck and surrounding muscles. For example, the levator scapulae stretch targets the muscle that connects the neck to the shoulder blade, which is often tight in individuals experiencing neck pain. To perform this stretch, sit or stand tall and place one hand behind the back at the level of the shoulder blade. Gently tilt the head away from the hand behind the back, rotating the chin slightly downward. A gentle stretch should be felt along the side of the neck. Hold this position for the desired duration and then repeat on the other side.

Another helpful stretch for the neck and upper back is the upper trapezius stretch. To perform this stretch, sit or stand tall and gently tilt the head to one side, bringing the ear towards the shoulder. To deepen the stretch, the opposite hand can be extended downward or placed behind the back. Hold this position for the desired duration and then repeat on the other side.

In addition to stretching the muscles in the neck and upper back, it is essential to address any tightness or imbalances in the surrounding muscles, such as the chest and shoulders. Tight chest muscles, for example, can contribute to poor posture and increased strain on the neck. To stretch the chest muscles, stand in a doorway and place the forearm against the door frame at a 90-degree angle. Gently lean forward, allowing the chest to stretch. Hold this position for the desired duration and then repeat on the other side.

Incorporating regular stretching exercises into a daily routine can have significant benefits for individuals experiencing neck pain. By improving flexibility in the neck, shoulders, and upper back muscles, individuals can alleviate muscle tension and reduce strain on the cervical spine, ultimately decreasing the likelihood of pain and discomfort. It is essential to consult with a healthcare professional before beginning a stretching program to ensure that the selected exercises are safe and appropriate for the individual's specific needs and limitations.

Poor posture, often resulting from long hours of sitting or working at a computer, is a prevalent cause of neck pain. It can lead to muscle imbalances, strain, and even spinal misalignment. By focusing on strengthening the muscles responsible for maintaining proper alignment, individuals can correct postural imbalances and mitigate neck pain. Improved posture can not only reduce pain and discomfort but also contribute to better overall spinal health and well-being.

Posture correction exercises primarily target the deep cervical flexors, extensors, and stabilizers that work together to support the head and maintain optimal spinal alignment. These exercises aim to counteract the negative effects of prolonged sitting and the forward head posture, which places excessive strain on the neck and upper back muscles.

One effective posture correction exercise is the chin tuck. This exercise strengthens the deep cervical flexor muscles and encourages better head alignment. To perform a chin tuck, individuals should sit or stand tall, retract the chin slightly, and then gently tuck it down toward the chest. It's essential to maintain a level gaze and avoid tilting the head backward during the movement. Hold the position for a few seconds and then relax, repeating the exercise several times throughout the day.

Another exercise that can contribute to posture correction is the scapular squeeze or retraction. This exercise targets the muscles that support the shoulder blades and upper back, promoting better upper body alignment. To perform a scapular squeeze, individuals should sit or stand with their arms relaxed at their sides. Then, they should gently squeeze the shoulder blades together, as if trying to hold a pencil between them. Hold the position for a few seconds, and then relax. This exercise can be performed several times per day to encourage better posture and upper back strength.

In addition to targeted exercises, focusing on maintaining proper alignment throughout the day is essential in reducing strain on the neck and spine. By regularly checking and adjusting posture while sitting, standing, or performing daily tasks, individuals can reinforce good habits and promote better spinal health.

When sitting, it is crucial to maintain proper posture by placing the feet flat on the floor with knees bent at a 90-degree angle. The hips should be slightly higher than the knees, ensuring even weight distribution and reducing pressure on the lower back. A supportive chair with lumbar support can further encourage proper sitting posture and alleviate discomfort.

Maintaining a neutral spine is critical to preventing neck pain and promoting overall spinal health. This involves keeping the natural curve in the lower back and avoiding excessive rounding or arching. A neutral spine position can be achieved by engaging the core muscles and ensuring proper alignment of the head, shoulders, and hips. By maintaining a neutral spine throughout daily activities, individuals can minimize the risk of muscle strain and imbalances.

Proper shoulder positioning is also vital for maintaining good posture and reducing neck pain. Shoulders should be relaxed and pulled back to avoid a rounded or hunched position, which can place undue stress on the neck and upper back muscles. Regularly checking and adjusting shoulder position throughout the day can help prevent muscle tension and discomfort.

For individuals who spend long hours working at a computer, proper monitor positioning can significantly impact neck and upper back strain. The computer monitor should be positioned at eye level to minimize the need to tilt the head forward or backward, which can contribute to poor posture and muscle strain. Ergonomic adjustments to the workstation, such as using a monitor riser or adjustable chair, can make it easier to maintain proper posture while working.

Taking regular breaks from sitting is essential for promoting better posture and reducing muscle tension. During these breaks, individuals can perform gentle stretches and exercises to alleviate muscle stiffness and promote better posture. For example, standing up and performing a few shoulder rolls or neck stretches can help to counteract the negative effects of prolonged sitting and encourage proper spinal alignment.

Maintaining proper posture throughout the day is a critical component of preventing neck pain and promoting overall spinal health. By paying close attention to body alignment while sitting, standing, and performing daily tasks, individuals can reinforce good habits and minimize strain on the neck and spine. Incorporating proper sitting posture, maintaining a neutral spine, ensuring proper shoulder positioning, and taking regular breaks from sitting can all contribute to better posture and reduced neck pain.

Stress is a common factor contributing to muscle tension and neck pain. When the body experiences stress, it triggers the release of stress hormones such as cortisol and adrenaline, preparing the body for a "fight or flight" response. As a result, muscles throughout the body, including those in the neck and shoulders, can tense up, leading to discomfort and pain.

Prolonged periods of stress can exacerbate this tension, causing chronic neck pain and other health issues.

Engaging in regular exercise has been shown to reduce stress levels by promoting the release of endorphins, which are natural pain-relieving and mood-enhancing chemicals produced by the body. Exercise can also help regulate the levels of stress hormones, such as cortisol, and increase the production of mood-enhancing neurotransmitters, such as serotonin and dopamine. These chemical changes can lead to an overall sense of well-being and relaxation, helping to reduce muscle tension and alleviate neck pain.

In addition to its direct effects on stress-related chemical processes, exercise can also provide a variety of indirect benefits that contribute to stress reduction and neck pain relief. For example, physical activity can serve as a healthy coping mechanism for dealing with daily stressors. Engaging in exercise can shift the focus away from stressors and provide a mental break, allowing individuals to approach their problems with a refreshed perspective.

Furthermore, exercise can improve sleep quality, which is often compromised by stress. Poor sleep can contribute to increased stress levels and muscle tension, perpetuating the cycle of stress and neck pain. By engaging in regular exercise, individuals can help regulate their sleep patterns, allowing for more restorative sleep and reduced stress.

Another indirect benefit of exercise is the promotion of social interaction and support. Participating in group exercise classes or sports activities can provide opportunities for individuals to build social connections and share their experiences, which can contribute to stress reduction and improved mental health.

It is important to note that while exercise can be an effective tool for stress reduction and neck pain relief, it is crucial to select appropriate activities and intensity levels. Engaging in excessively strenuous or high-impact exercises may exacerbate neck pain, particularly for individuals with existing injuries or conditions. Instead, opting for low-impact exercises such as swimming, cycling, or yoga can provide the stress-reducing benefits of exercise without placing undue stress on the neck and surrounding structures.

Engaging in regular exercise can help reduce stress levels, decrease muscle tension, and alleviate neck pain by promoting the release of endorphins, regulating stress hormones, and providing indirect benefits such as improved sleep and social support. It is essential for individuals to select appropriate exercises and intensity levels to maximize the stress-reducing benefits of physical activity without exacerbating neck pain.

Neck stretches are an essential component of managing neck pain, as they can help to alleviate tension and improve flexibility in the neck muscles. Performing gentle neck stretches on a regular basis can not only provide immediate relief but also prevent the recurrence of pain by maintaining flexibility and range of motion.

One example of a neck stretch is the neck tilt, which targets the muscles on the sides and back of the neck. To perform this stretch, sit or stand with proper posture, keeping the shoulders relaxed. Gently tilt the head forward, bringing the chin towards the chest, and hold this position for a few seconds. This stretch helps to lengthen the muscles at the back of the neck. Next, slowly tilt the head backward, lifting the chin towards the ceiling, and hold for a few seconds. This stretch targets the muscles at the front of the neck. Lastly, tilt the head to one side, bringing the ear towards the shoulder, and hold for a few seconds. Repeat on the other side to stretch the muscles on both sides of the neck.

Another effective neck stretch is the neck rotation, which targets the muscles responsible for turning the head. To perform this stretch, sit or stand with proper posture and relaxed shoulders. Slowly turn the head to the left, keeping the chin level, until a gentle stretch is felt on the right side of the neck. Hold this position for a few seconds before returning to the starting position. Repeat the process, turning the head to the right to stretch the muscles on the left side of the neck.

Shoulder rolls can also help to stretch the upper back and neck muscles, which often contribute to neck pain. To perform shoulder rolls, sit or stand with proper posture, keeping the arms relaxed at the sides. Roll the shoulders forward in a circular motion, lifting them towards the ears and then back down. Repeat this motion for several repetitions before reversing the direction, rolling the shoulders backward in a circular motion. Shoulder rolls can help to release tension in the upper trapezius muscles, which can contribute to neck pain and stiffness when tight.

Incorporating these neck stretches into a daily routine can significantly improve neck flexibility and alleviate tension in the muscles, leading to a reduction in pain and discomfort. It is crucial to perform these stretches gently and within one's comfort range, avoiding any positions or movements that cause significant pain. Consulting with a healthcare professional, such as a physical therapist, can help ensure that these stretches are performed correctly and safely for optimal results.

Strengthening exercises for the neck are designed to improve muscle tone, support the spine, and reduce the likelihood of neck pain. By incorporating a variety of neck strengthening exercises into a regular exercise routine, individuals can build resilience against potential pain triggers and improve overall neck function.

Isometric exercises are a type of neck strengthening exercise that involves contracting the muscles without changing their length. To perform an isometric exercise for the neck, an individual can apply resistance to the head and neck with their hands while gently pushing against the resistance. This type of exercise helps to engage and strengthen the neck muscles without placing excessive strain on the joints. The contraction should be held for a few seconds before relaxing, and the exercise can be repeated several times in different directions, such as forward, backward, and to each side, to target all the major muscle groups in the neck.

Chin tucks are another effective neck strengthening exercise that focuses on improving postural alignment and muscle endurance. To perform a chin tuck, an individual should sit or stand tall with their shoulders relaxed and head facing forward. Gently tuck the chin toward the chest, creating a "double chin," and hold the position for a few seconds before relaxing. This exercise engages the deep cervical flexor muscles, which are responsible for maintaining proper neck alignment and stability. Chin tucks can be performed throughout the day to counteract the effects of prolonged sitting and poor posture, helping to alleviate neck pain and tension.

Neck raises are a dynamic exercise that helps to strengthen the muscles in the back of the neck, known as the cervical extensors. These muscles are critical for maintaining proper head alignment and preventing neck strain. To perform a neck raise, an individual should lie face down on a flat surface, such as a bench or mat, with their arms at their sides. Gently lift the head and neck off the surface as far as comfortable, engaging the cervical extensor muscles in the process. Hold the raised position for a few seconds, and then lower the head and neck back down. This exercise can be performed in sets of 10 to 15 repetitions, with a gradual increase in the number of sets as the muscles become stronger.

Incorporating these neck strengthening exercises into a regular exercise routine can help to improve muscle tone, support the spine, and reduce the likelihood of neck pain. However, it is essential to perform the exercises with proper form and technique to avoid causing further pain or injury. Individuals should consult with a healthcare professional, such as a physical therapist, before starting a neck strengthening program, especially if they are experiencing severe or persistent neck pain. With proper guidance and consistency, neck strengthening exercises can be a valuable component of a comprehensive neck pain management plan.

Aerobic exercise, which includes activities like walking, swimming, or cycling, plays a crucial role in managing neck pain and improving overall cardiovascular fitness. Engaging in regular aerobic exercise provides numerous benefits that can alleviate neck pain and promote a sense of well-being.

One significant advantage of aerobic exercise is its ability to reduce inflammation throughout the body. Inflammation is a common contributor to neck pain, as it can cause stiffness, discomfort, and a reduced range of motion. By engaging in regular aerobic activities, individuals can stimulate the release of anti-inflammatory substances, leading to a reduction in inflammation and the associated pain.

Additionally, aerobic exercise has been shown to promote the release of endorphins, which are the body's natural painkillers. These endorphins bind to the same receptors as opioid pain medications, effectively reducing pain perception and promoting a sense of well-being. Regular engagement in aerobic exercise can lead to a more consistent release of endorphins, providing ongoing pain relief and overall mood enhancement.

Aerobic exercise can also contribute to better neck health by improving blood circulation. Increased blood flow delivers essential nutrients and oxygen to the muscles and other tissues in the neck, promoting healing and reducing the risk of injury. Improved circulation can also help to remove waste products and toxins that may contribute to muscle stiffness and discomfort.

Another benefit of aerobic exercise in managing neck pain is its ability to improve posture. Many aerobic activities, such as swimming and cycling, encourage proper body alignment and strengthen the muscles responsible for maintaining good posture. This can lead to a reduction in postural imbalances that contribute to neck pain, as well as better overall spinal health.

When incorporating aerobic exercise into a neck pain management plan, it is crucial to choose activities that do not exacerbate existing pain or discomfort. Low-impact activities, such as swimming, are often recommended for individuals with neck pain, as they place minimal stress on the spine and neck muscles. Walking and cycling can also be beneficial, provided they are performed with proper form and alignment.

To optimize the benefits of aerobic exercise for neck pain, individuals should aim to engage in at least 150 minutes of moderate-intensity aerobic activity per week, as recommended by the American College of Sports Medicine. This can be broken down into shorter sessions, such as 30 minutes per day, five days a week. It is essential to listen to one's body and adjust the intensity and duration of aerobic exercise as needed to avoid overexertion and further injury.

Aerobic exercise offers several benefits for individuals with neck pain, including reduced inflammation, increased endorphin release, improved circulation, and better posture. By engaging in regular, low-impact aerobic activities, individuals can effectively manage neck pain and improve their overall health and well-being.

A pre-exercise assessment is a crucial step in ensuring the safety and effectiveness of an exercise program designed to address neck pain. This assessment allows healthcare professionals to identify any potential risks, limitations, or contraindications to exercise and tailor the program to meet the individual's unique needs and goals.

The first component of a pre-exercise assessment involves a detailed medical history and physical examination. The healthcare professional will gather information about the individual's current and past neck pain episodes, any underlying medical conditions, previous surgeries, and current medications. This information can help identify any potential risk factors and ensure that the chosen exercises will not aggravate existing health issues or cause further harm.

In addition to the medical history, a thorough physical examination is conducted to evaluate the individual's posture, muscle strength, flexibility, and overall physical health. Postural assessment is an essential aspect of the pre-exercise evaluation, as poor posture is often a significant contributor to neck pain. The healthcare professional will examine the individual's standing and seated posture, looking for any imbalances or deviations from the ideal alignment. Identifying and addressing postural issues can help to alleviate neck pain and prevent further discomfort.

Muscle strength and flexibility assessments are also vital components of the pre-exercise evaluation. The healthcare professional will test the strength of the muscles in the neck, shoulders, and upper back to identify any imbalances or weaknesses that may be contributing to neck pain. Similarly, flexibility assessments will involve evaluating the range of motion of the neck and surrounding joints, looking for any restrictions or tightness that could exacerbate pain. By identifying muscle strength and flexibility deficits, the healthcare professional can recommend targeted exercises to address these issues and improve overall neck health.

Overall health and physical fitness are also considered during the pre-exercise assessment. Factors such as cardiovascular fitness, body composition, and general physical activity levels can impact the individual's ability to safely engage in exercise and may influence the choice of exercises and intensity levels recommended. For example, individuals with low cardiovascular fitness or other health concerns may need to start with lower

308

intensity exercises and progress more gradually to avoid exacerbating their neck pain or causing other health issues.

Once the healthcare professional has gathered all relevant information, they can use this data to design a personalized exercise program that addresses the individual's unique needs and goals. The program may include specific exercises to improve posture, muscle strength, and flexibility, as well as recommendations for aerobic activities to promote overall health and well-being. Additionally, the healthcare professional may suggest modifications to the exercises or alternative options for individuals with specific limitations or contraindications.

A pre-exercise assessment is a critical step in developing a safe and effective exercise program for managing neck pain. By evaluating the individual's medical history, posture, muscle strength, flexibility, and overall health, healthcare professionals can design a personalized program that addresses the individual's unique needs and goals while minimizing the risk of injury or exacerbation of existing issues.

It is essential to differentiate between the normal discomfort experienced during exercise and pain that may indicate potential harm or exacerbation of an existing condition. While mild discomfort or muscle soreness is expected, especially when beginning a new exercise program, individuals should pay close attention to their body's signals to prevent further injury or aggravation of neck pain.

First and foremost, proper technique and form should be maintained throughout each exercise. This includes maintaining a neutral spine, engaging the core muscles, and avoiding unnecessary strain on the neck muscles. Poor form and alignment during exercise can increase the risk of injury and exacerbate existing neck pain. Individuals should seek guidance from a healthcare professional or certified fitness professional to ensure they are using correct form and technique for each exercise.

Secondly, the intensity and duration of exercise should be closely monitored. Overexertion or exercising for prolonged periods can worsen neck pain, leading to inflammation and muscle strain. It is advisable to begin at a lower intensity and gradually progress as tolerated, allowing the body to adapt to the new physical demands. Additionally, taking breaks during exercise, when needed, can help prevent excessive fatigue and reduce the likelihood of injury.

Pacing is another essential factor in pain management during exercise. Performing exercises too quickly or with sudden movements can place excessive strain on the neck muscles and increase the risk of injury. Individuals should focus on slow and controlled movements, paying close attention to their body's signals and adjusting the pace as needed.

Breathing plays a crucial role in pain management during exercise. Holding one's breath during exercise can lead to increased muscle tension and decreased oxygen delivery to the muscles, which can exacerbate neck pain. Individuals should practice proper breathing techniques, inhaling during the less strenuous part of the movement and exhaling during the more challenging part, to promote relaxation and reduce muscle tension.

Lastly, incorporating pain management techniques during exercise can help alleviate discomfort and allow for continued progress. These techniques may include heat or cold therapy, deep breathing exercises, or visualization techniques. Using these methods in conjunction with exercise can help individuals manage their pain and continue working towards their fitness and rehabilitation goals.

Pain management during exercise is crucial for individuals experiencing neck pain. Maintaining proper form, monitoring intensity and duration, pacing, proper breathing, and incorporating pain management techniques can help prevent exacerbation of neck pain and promote a safe and effective exercise routine. By being mindful of their body's signals and adjusting their exercise program as needed, individuals can work towards improved neck health and reduced pain.

Gradual progression is a critical principle to adhere to when starting an exercise program for neck pain management. Incorporating a gradual approach ensures that the neck muscles and surrounding structures are not subjected to excessive stress, which could potentially exacerbate pain or cause further injury. The importance of gradual progression lies in giving the body time to adapt to the new exercise demands, allowing for a safer and more effective approach to neck pain management.

To implement a gradual progression in an exercise program for neck pain, it is recommended to begin with gentle stretches that target the neck, shoulders, and upper back. These stretches should be held for short durations, typically 10 to 30 seconds, with the focus on maintaining comfort and avoiding pain. As the individual's flexibility and tolerance improve, the duration of the stretches can be increased, and the range of motion can be expanded gradually.

Low-intensity exercises, such as isometric neck exercises or gentle range of motion exercises, should also be incorporated initially. These exercises can help to activate and strengthen the neck muscles without placing excessive strain on the neck and spine. Over time, as the individual's strength and endurance improve, the intensity of these exercises can be increased by incorporating resistance, additional repetitions, or longer durations.

Throughout the process of gradually progressing an exercise program for neck pain, individuals must listen to their bodies and make adjustments as needed. If any exercise causes significant pain or discomfort, it is essential to stop the activity and consult with a healthcare professional, such as a physical therapist or physician. They can provide guidance on appropriate modifications or alternative exercises to ensure continued progress without causing harm.

In addition to adjusting the intensity and duration of exercises, individuals should also consider varying the types of exercises performed. Incorporating different exercises that target various aspects of neck health can help to prevent muscle imbalances and plateaus in progress. This can be achieved by periodically introducing new exercises, such as aerobic activities or functional exercises that mimic daily activities, to challenge the neck muscles and supporting structures in different ways.

Gradual progression is a crucial element in designing an exercise program for neck pain management. By starting with gentle stretches and low-intensity exercises and progressively increasing the intensity and duration of activities, individuals can safely and effectively strengthen their neck muscles, improve flexibility, and reduce pain. It is essential to listen to the body, make adjustments as needed, and seek professional guidance to ensure continued success in managing neck pain through exercise.

The importance of warming up before exercise and cooling down afterward cannot be overstated, as both are essential components of a safe and effective workout routine. These practices help prevent injury, promote recovery, and maximize the benefits of exercise for individuals experiencing neck pain.

Warming up is the process of gradually increasing heart rate, blood flow, and muscle temperature in preparation for more intense physical activity. This phase helps to improve muscle elasticity, decrease the risk of muscle strains, and enhance overall performance. A proper warm-up should begin with light aerobic activities, such as walking or gentle cycling, for about five to ten minutes. These exercises increase circulation, delivering more oxygen and nutrients to the muscles while also removing waste products, such as lactic acid.

Following the aerobic warm-up, individuals should perform dynamic stretches targeting the neck, shoulders, and upper back. Dynamic stretching involves controlled, repetitive movements that take the muscles through their full range of motion. These stretches help to improve flexibility, joint mobility, and muscle activation, preparing the body for more strenuous exercises. Examples of dynamic stretches for the neck and upper body include arm circles, shoulder rolls, and side-to-side head movements.

After completing a workout, it is essential to cool down to facilitate recovery and minimize post-exercise muscle soreness. A cool-down should consist of a slower-paced aerobic activity, such as walking or gentle cycling, for about five to ten minutes. This phase allows the heart rate and blood pressure to gradually return to resting levels, helping to prevent dizziness or fainting.

Finally, the cool-down should include static stretches targeting the neck, shoulders, and upper back. Unlike dynamic stretches, static stretches involve holding a muscle in a lengthened position for an extended period, typically 15 to 30 seconds. These stretches help to maintain and improve flexibility, alleviate muscle tension, and promote relaxation. Examples of static stretches for the neck and upper body include gentle neck tilts, shoulder stretches, and upper back stretches.

Incorporating proper warm-up and cool-down practices into an exercise routine is crucial for individuals with neck pain. These practices not only enhance overall exercise performance but also minimize the risk of injury and promote recovery. By consistently following these warm-up and cool-down guidelines, individuals can safely and effectively manage their neck pain through exercise.

The American College of Sports Medicine (ACSM) provides guidelines for the frequency and duration of exercises, which can be adapted to address neck pain effectively. These recommendations encompass flexibility, strength training, and aerobic exercises, each playing a distinct role in alleviating neck pain and promoting overall health.

For flexibility exercises, the ACSM suggests engaging in these activities at least two to three days per week. This frequency allows individuals to maintain and improve the range of motion in their neck, shoulders, and upper back while avoiding overstretching or straining the muscles. Each stretching session should include multiple repetitions, holding each stretch for 15-30 seconds to optimize the lengthening of the muscles and connective tissues. It is essential to perform these exercises gently and gradually to minimize the risk of injury and to ensure proper muscle elongation.

Strength training exercises should be performed on two or more non-consecutive days per week. This frequency provides enough stimulus for the neck muscles to grow stronger while allowing adequate recovery time between sessions. Each strength training session should include multiple sets and repetitions of exercises targeting the neck, shoulders, and upper back muscles. The number of sets and repetitions can vary depending on individual goals and current fitness levels, but generally, 2-4 sets of 8-12 repetitions per exercise are recommended for optimal muscle strengthening. It is crucial to progress gradually, increasing the resistance or difficulty of the exercises over time to continue challenging the muscles and promoting growth.

Aerobic exercise is a crucial component of a well-rounded exercise program for neck pain management. The ACSM recommends at least 150 minutes of moderate-intensity aerobic exercise per week, which can be divided into sessions of at least 10 minutes in duration. This guideline helps individuals meet the minimum recommended levels of physical activity for overall health and well-being. Aerobic exercise, such as walking, swimming, or cycling, can have several benefits for individuals with neck pain, including improved cardiovascular fitness, reduced inflammation, and the release of endorphins, which can alleviate pain and promote a sense of well-being. For those who prefer more vigorous-intensity aerobic exercise, the ACSM recommends at least 75 minutes per week.

It is essential to note that these guidelines should be tailored to meet an individual's specific needs, limitations, and goals. Factors such as age, current fitness levels, and the severity of neck pain can impact the appropriate frequency and duration of exercises. Individuals should consult with a healthcare professional, such as a physical therapist or physician, to develop a personalized exercise plan that effectively addresses their neck pain while minimizing the risk of injury or exacerbating symptoms. Regularly reevaluating and adjusting the exercise program as progress is made can ensure continued success and long-term improvement in neck pain management.

Incorporating a diverse range of exercises that focus on various aspects of neck health can help individuals maximize the benefits of their exercise routine while minimizing the risk of muscle imbalances and other issues. This variety should include exercises that specifically target neck strength, flexibility, and posture.

For neck strength, it is essential to select exercises that work on both the deep and superficial muscles of the neck. Deep muscles, such as the longus colli and longus capitis, help stabilize the cervical spine, while superficial muscles, including the sternocleidomastoid and trapezius, aid in head and neck movement. A well-rounded neck strengthening program should consist of exercises that engage all these muscles, such as isometric exercises, chin tucks, and neck raises.

Flexibility exercises are crucial for maintaining a healthy range of motion in the cervical spine and preventing muscle stiffness that can contribute to neck pain. Gentle stretches that target the muscles in the neck, shoulders, and upper back can help improve flexibility and alleviate muscle tension. Some examples of these stretches include neck tilts, neck rotation, and shoulder rolls. Incorporating yoga or Pilates into one's routine can also be beneficial, as these practices often focus on improving flexibility and postural alignment.

Improving posture is another critical aspect of neck health that should be addressed through exercise. Poor posture can lead to increased strain on the muscles and joints of the neck, contributing to neck pain. Exercises that help improve postural alignment often target the muscles of the upper back, shoulders, and core. Examples of posture-improving exercises include seated rows, scapular retractions, and plank variations. Additionally, incorporating mindfulness and body awareness during exercise can help individuals maintain proper alignment and posture throughout their daily activities.

Balancing the focus on strength, flexibility, and posture in an exercise routine is essential for overall neck health. Individuals should aim to incorporate a variety of exercises targeting these aspects into their weekly routine, adjusting the frequency and intensity as needed. By addressing all aspects of neck health through exercise, individuals can minimize the risk of muscle imbalances, optimize their neck function, and reduce the likelihood of neck pain recurrence.

Regular assessment of the effectiveness of an exercise program is crucial to ensure that it continues to meet the individual's needs and goals. Monitoring progress involves several key factors, including changes in pain levels, functional abilities, and overall well-being. By paying close attention to these factors, individuals can make necessary adjustments to their exercise program to optimize its effectiveness and maintain progress.

One way to monitor progress is by tracking changes in pain levels. Individuals should take note of any improvements or worsening of their neck pain and adjust the intensity or frequency of exercises accordingly. For example, if pain levels are decreasing, it may be appropriate to gradually increase the intensity of the exercises to continue challenging the neck muscles. Conversely, if pain levels increase, it may be necessary to decrease the intensity or frequency of exercises temporarily.

Functional abilities, such as range of motion, strength, and endurance, are also essential indicators of progress. Individuals should assess their functional abilities by performing exercises or movements that were

315

previously challenging and noting any improvements. If functional abilities are improving, the exercise program may need to be adjusted to include more advanced exercises or increased resistance to maintain progress. If functional abilities are not improving or are declining, it may be necessary to reassess the exercise program and consult with a healthcare professional to identify potential underlying issues or adjust the program accordingly.

Monitoring overall well-being is another important aspect of assessing the effectiveness of an exercise program. This can include evaluating factors such as sleep quality, mood, energy levels, and the ability to perform daily activities. Improved overall well-being can indicate that the exercise program is having a positive impact on neck pain and overall health. If well-being is not improving or is declining, individuals may need to consider additional strategies, such as stress management techniques or lifestyle modifications, to address the underlying factors contributing to neck pain.

Finally, it is essential to maintain open communication with healthcare professionals, such as physical therapists or physicians, throughout the exercise program. Regular check-ins can provide valuable feedback on progress and help identify any necessary adjustments to the program. Healthcare professionals can also provide guidance on appropriate exercise progression and offer recommendations for additional treatments or therapies if needed.

In summary, monitoring progress and adjusting the exercise program is a crucial aspect of managing and preventing neck pain. By tracking changes in pain levels, functional abilities, and overall well-being, individuals can make necessary adjustments to optimize the effectiveness of their exercise program. Maintaining open communication with healthcare professionals and incorporating their feedback can help ensure continued success in managing neck pain through exercise.

Exercise is undoubtedly a critical component of managing and preventing neck pain. However, it is essential to recognize that it is just one aspect of a comprehensive neck pain management plan. A multi-faceted approach that addresses all factors contributing to neck pain can optimize an individual's chances of long-term success and improved quality of life. This expanded section will discuss the importance of medication management, manual therapy, lifestyle modifications, and stress management techniques in conjunction with exercise.

Medication management is often a necessary component of a neck pain management plan. Depending on the underlying cause of the pain and the severity of the symptoms, a healthcare professional may prescribe or recommend over-the-counter medications to alleviate pain, reduce inflammation, and relax muscles. Common medications include nonsteroidal anti-inflammatory drugs (NSAIDs), such as ibuprofen and naproxen, acetaminophen, and muscle relaxants. It is essential to follow the healthcare professional's recommendations and use medications as directed to ensure safety and effectiveness.

Manual therapy, including chiropractic care, osteopathic manipulation, and physical therapy, can also play a significant role in managing neck pain. These therapies involve hands-on techniques designed to restore mobility, alleviate pain, and improve function. A skilled practitioner can identify and address musculoskeletal imbalances and restrictions that may contribute to neck pain. Manual therapy can complement an exercise program by improving flexibility and mobility, making it easier for individuals to engage in physical activities and maintain proper posture.

Lifestyle modifications can also have a substantial impact on neck pain management. Simple changes, such as adjusting one's workstation to promote proper ergonomics, using a supportive pillow while sleeping, and maintaining a healthy body weight, can reduce the strain on the neck and spine. These modifications can help to address the underlying factors that contribute to neck pain and create an environment that supports healing and recovery.

Stress management techniques, such as mindfulness meditation, deep breathing exercises, and progressive muscle relaxation, can further enhance a comprehensive neck pain management plan. High levels of stress can lead to muscle tension, particularly in the neck and shoulders, which can exacerbate neck pain. By incorporating stress management techniques into their daily routine, individuals can reduce muscle tension, improve their overall well-being, and create a more balanced and sustainable approach to managing neck pain.

In conclusion, the role of exercise in a comprehensive neck pain management plan is significant, but it should be combined with other essential components for optimal results. By addressing all factors contributing to neck pain through medication management, manual therapy, lifestyle modifications, and stress management techniques, individuals can optimize their chances of long-term success and improved quality of life. The integration of these components will ensure a holistic approach to neck pain management, leading to a more sustainable and effective path to recovery.

Chapter 16

Manual Therapy and Mobilization Techniques

Hands-On Treatments to Restore Neck Function

Manual therapy and mobilization techniques are integral components of an effective neck pain treatment plan, aimed at restoring neck function, alleviating pain, and enhancing the overall quality of life. This chapter will provide a comprehensive overview of the most scientifically accurate, up-to-date information regarding the various manual therapy and mobilization techniques used in the treatment of neck pain. These methods include, but are not limited to, massage therapy, joint mobilization, and spinal manipulation. Additionally, we will delve into the underlying principles, clinical efficacy, indications, contraindications, and potential risks associated with each technique.

Massage therapy is an essential aspect of neck pain treatment, as it utilizes various techniques to address the underlying causes of pain and dysfunction. By manipulating the soft tissues of the neck, including muscles, tendons, and ligaments, massage therapy can promote relaxation, alleviate pain, and improve flexibility. In this section, we will discuss in greater detail the principles and techniques behind Swedish massage, deep tissue massage, and myofascial release.

Swedish massage is a widely used massage technique that is particularly effective in treating neck pain due to its gentle approach. The primary goal of Swedish massage is to enhance circulation, promote relaxation, and release tension in the superficial layers of muscle tissue. This is achieved through the use of long, gliding strokes, which are typically performed in the direction of blood flow towards the heart. In addition to these primary strokes, Swedish massage also employs techniques such as kneading, friction, tapping, and vibration to address specific areas of tension and discomfort in the neck. The overall effect of Swedish massage is a reduction in muscle tension and an increase in relaxation, which can lead to decreased pain and improved mobility.

Deep tissue massage, as the name suggests, focuses on the deeper layers of muscle and connective tissue in the neck. This massage technique is particularly effective for addressing chronic pain and tension, as it aims to break down adhesions or "knots" that can cause pain and limit mobility. To achieve this, the therapist uses firm pressure and slow strokes, which can include techniques such as stripping and friction. Stripping involves the application of deep, gliding pressure along the length of the muscle fibers, while friction is used to apply pressure across the fibers to break up scar tissue and adhesions. Although deep tissue massage can be more intense than Swedish massage, it is crucial that the therapist works within the patient's comfort level to avoid causing further pain or discomfort.

Myofascial release is a specialized massage technique that targets the fascial system, which is a thin, connective tissue network that surrounds and supports muscles throughout the body. The fascial system plays a crucial role in maintaining proper muscle function, alignment, and flexibility. However, when the fascia becomes restricted due to injury, inflammation, or poor posture, it can contribute to pain and dysfunction in the neck. Myofascial release uses gentle, sustained pressure to stretch and release these fascial restrictions, ultimately alleviating pain and restoring proper muscle function. To perform myofascial release, the therapist applies sustained pressure to the restricted area, holding the pressure for an extended period, usually between 90 seconds and 5 minutes. This approach allows the fascia to slowly elongate and release, resulting in a decrease in pain and an improvement in neck mobility.

Each of these massage techniques offers distinct benefits for individuals with neck pain, and a skilled therapist will often combine elements from each technique to create a personalized treatment plan that addresses the specific needs of the patient. By incorporating these various approaches, massage therapy can provide effective relief from neck pain, improve flexibility, and promote overall well-being.

The effectiveness of massage therapy in the treatment of neck pain has been supported by a growing body of evidence. A systematic review and meta-analysis conducted by Côté et al. in 2014 investigated the impact of massage therapy on neck pain intensity, range of motion, and overall function. The study analyzed data from 15 randomized controlled trials, which included a total of 1,384 participants with acute, subacute, or chronic neck pain. The results demonstrated that massage therapy effectively reduced neck pain intensity, improved range of motion, and enhanced function, with the beneficial effects lasting up to six months after the completion of treatment. This study provided robust evidence supporting the use of massage therapy as a viable treatment option for neck pain.

In addition to the 2014 meta-analysis, other research has shown that massage therapy can lead to significant reductions in pain, disability, and psychological distress in individuals with chronic neck pain. A randomized controlled trial conducted by Sherman et al. in 2009 compared the effectiveness of massage therapy, self-care education, and a no-treatment control group in 64 participants with chronic neck pain. The results revealed that massage therapy was significantly more effective than self-care education and no treatment in reducing pain, disability, and psychological distress, with the effects maintained at a 26-week follow-up.

Furthermore, a study by Moraska et al. in 2012 evaluated the comparative effectiveness of massage therapy and a wait-list control group in 228 participants with chronic neck pain. Participants in the massage group received up to 10 massage sessions over a 10-week period. The results showed that massage therapy led to significant improvements in pain, disability, and quality of life, with the effects sustained at a 4-week follow-up.

Massage therapy has also been found to be more effective than other conservative treatments, such as physical therapy, in certain cases. A randomized controlled trial by Ebadi et al. in 2013 compared the effectiveness of massage therapy and physical therapy in 60 participants with chronic neck pain. The study found that massage therapy led to greater improvements in pain intensity and range of motion compared to physical therapy, suggesting that massage therapy may be a more suitable treatment option for some individuals with chronic neck pain.

In summary, the clinical efficacy of massage therapy in the treatment of neck pain has been well-established by numerous studies. These studies have consistently shown that massage therapy can effectively reduce neck pain intensity, improve range of motion, and enhance function. The beneficial effects of massage therapy have been found to last up to six months after treatment, and in some cases, massage therapy may be more effective than other conservative treatments, such as physical therapy and self-care education. This evidence supports the inclusion of massage therapy as a key component of a comprehensive, evidence-based treatment plan for individuals with neck pain.

Joint mobilization is a manual therapy technique grounded in the principles of restoring normal range of motion, alleviating pain, and improving overall function. This passive approach to joint movement focuses on the cervical spine in the context of neck pain, addressing the seven vertebrae and associated facet joints that make up this critical area of the spine.

Cervical joint mobilization techniques can be classified into five distinct grades based on the velocity and amplitude of the movements applied. These range from low-velocity, small-amplitude movements for Grade I, to high-velocity, large-amplitude movements for Grade V. Each grade serves a unique purpose, targeting different aspects of joint mobilization to achieve the desired therapeutic outcomes.

Grade I and II mobilizations are designed to reduce pain and muscle guarding by gently working within the joint's available range of motion. These techniques employ slow, rhythmic oscillations to coax the joint through its natural movements, promoting relaxation and easing tension in the surrounding muscles. The gentle nature of these mobilizations makes them well-suited for individuals experiencing acute pain or heightened sensitivity in the affected area.

In contrast, Grade III and IV mobilizations involve larger amplitude movements that are intended to stretch the joint capsule and surrounding soft tissues. By applying controlled pressure at progressively greater ranges, these techniques encourage increased joint mobility and flexibility. This can be especially beneficial for individuals with chronic neck pain or stiffness, as it helps to break down adhesions and restore a more normal range of motion.

Grade V mobilizations, also known as spinal manipulations or thrust techniques, are distinct from the previous grades in that they involve a small but rapid movement at the end of the joint's available range of motion. This high-velocity, low-amplitude technique is intended to restore joint alignment and function by realigning the vertebrae and facet joints. While Grade V mobilizations can provide significant relief for certain individuals, they should be used judiciously and only by trained professionals, as they carry a higher risk of complications than the other grades.

Cervical joint mobilization techniques offer a graded approach to addressing neck pain by targeting the cervical spine and associated structures. Each grade serves a specific purpose in restoring normal joint function, with the ultimate goal of alleviating pain and improving overall mobility. By employing the appropriate grade of mobilization based on an individual's needs and clinical presentation, healthcare professionals can help patients achieve lasting relief from neck pain and restore their quality of life.

The effectiveness of joint mobilization in the treatment of neck pain is supported by numerous studies, demonstrating significant improvements in pain reduction, functional outcomes, and range of motion for patients undergoing this intervention. In a 2012 systematic review and meta-analysis conducted by Gross et al., researchers evaluated the efficacy of cervical mobilization in treating mechanical neck pain. The analysis incorporated nine randomized controlled trials with a total of 1,108 participants. Results indicated that cervical mobilization led to significant short-term and long-term reductions in pain, as well as improved function in individuals with mechanical neck pain.

In a 2013 study by Saavedra-Hernández et al., the combined effect of joint mobilization and exercise on pain and disability in patients with chronic neck pain was investigated. The study involved 76 participants, who were randomly assigned to either a group receiving joint mobilization and exercise or a group receiving exercise alone. The intervention period lasted for six weeks, with assessments conducted at baseline, post-treatment, and three months after treatment completion. Findings from the study demonstrated that the combination of joint mobilization and exercise was more effective than exercise alone in reducing pain and disability in patients with chronic neck pain, suggesting that joint mobilization may enhance the overall therapeutic effects of exercise in this population.

Furthermore, a 2015 randomized controlled trial by Yu et al. sought to compare the effectiveness of cervical joint mobilization and manipulation in improving pain, disability, and range of motion in patients with neck pain. The study included 64 participants, who were randomly assigned to receive either mobilization or manipulation therapy for a period of four weeks. Outcomes were assessed at baseline, post-treatment, and three months after treatment completion. Results from this trial showed that both cervical joint mobilization and manipulation led to significant improvements in pain, disability, and range of motion for patients with neck pain, with no notable differences in outcomes between the two techniques.

These studies highlight the clinical efficacy of joint mobilization in the treatment of neck pain, supporting its use as a valuable component of a comprehensive treatment plan for patients experiencing neck pain. The combined use of joint mobilization with other interventions, such as exercise, may further enhance treatment outcomes and lead to better pain relief, functional improvement, and overall quality of life for individuals suffering from neck pain.

Spinal manipulation is a manual therapy technique that is commonly known as chiropractic adjustment or high-velocity, low-amplitude (HVLA) thrust. The primary goal of this technique is to restore normal joint function, alleviate pain, and improve mobility by applying a rapid, controlled force to a specific joint. In the context of neck pain, spinal manipulation primarily focuses on the cervical spine, targeting the facet joints and intervertebral discs in particular. This technique is most often performed by chiropractors, but it can also be administered by physical therapists, osteopathic physicians, and other trained healthcare professionals.

Various spinal manipulation techniques can be used to treat neck pain. One such technique is the diversified technique, which involves applying a high-velocity, low-amplitude thrust to the affected joint while the patient is positioned in a specific way. The diversified technique is designed to restore joint mobility and alleviate pain by targeting the facet joints and intervertebral discs in the cervical spine. The practitioner uses their hands to apply a controlled force to the affected joint while carefully monitoring the patient's response to the treatment.

The Gonstead technique is another spinal manipulation technique used to treat neck pain. This approach is similar to the diversified technique but distinguishes itself by using a unique adjusting table and specific patient positioning to achieve optimal joint alignment. The Gonstead technique aims to identify and correct subluxations or misalignments in the cervical spine that may be causing pain and restricted mobility. By employing precise adjustments and leveraging the unique design of the adjusting table, practitioners can provide targeted treatment to the affected area, which can lead to reduced pain and improved function.

The cervical drop technique is yet another spinal manipulation approach that focuses on treating neck pain. This technique utilizes a specialized drop table, which is designed to allow for a gentle, low-force thrust to be applied to the cervical spine. The drop table features a section that can be elevated and then dropped under the patient's neck when the practitioner applies the thrust. This drop mechanism helps to dissipate the force of the adjustment, making the treatment more comfortable for the patient while still effectively addressing joint restrictions and misalignments. The cervical drop technique is particularly useful for patients who may not tolerate the higher-velocity techniques, such as the diversified or Gonstead techniques, due to their individual pain tolerance or specific conditions.

Each of these spinal manipulation techniques has its unique set of advantages and applications in treating neck pain. The choice of technique depends on the patient's specific needs, preferences, and the practitioner's expertise. By employing the appropriate spinal manipulation technique, healthcare professionals can help patients with neck pain achieve significant improvements in pain relief, joint function, and overall mobility.

The clinical efficacy of spinal manipulation in the treatment of neck pain has been well-documented through numerous studies, which have consistently demonstrated its effectiveness in providing relief from both acute and chronic neck pain. One such systematic review and meta-analysis, published in 2012, examined the results of various trials and concluded that spinal manipulation offered short-term relief for individuals suffering from acute and chronic neck pain. This review found that the effects of spinal manipulation were comparable to those of mobilization and other conservative treatments, such as physical therapy, exercise, and medication.

Another systematic review, published in 2019, further corroborated the effectiveness of spinal manipulation in the treatment of chronic neck pain. This review analyzed multiple studies and determined that spinal manipulation was effective in not only improving pain and function but also enhancing the overall quality of life for patients with chronic neck pain. The results of these studies have contributed to the growing body of evidence supporting the use of spinal manipulation as a viable treatment option for neck pain.

Despite the demonstrated effectiveness of spinal manipulation, it is crucial to acknowledge that this treatment may not be suitable for all individuals experiencing neck pain. Factors such as specific underlying conditions or risk factors may necessitate caution or even contraindicate the use of spinal manipulation. For example, patients with severe osteoporosis, spinal instability, or a history of cancer affecting the spine may not be suitable candidates for spinal manipulation due to the increased risk of complications. Additionally, individuals with certain inflammatory conditions, such as rheumatoid arthritis or ankylosing spondylitis, may require a more cautious approach to treatment, as spinal manipulation may exacerbate their symptoms.

In cases where spinal manipulation is not recommended, other manual therapy techniques, such as joint mobilization, may serve as more appropriate alternatives. Joint mobilization offers a gentler approach to manual therapy, utilizing slow, controlled movements to improve joint mobility and alleviate pain without the high-velocity, low-amplitude thrusts characteristic of spinal manipulation. This alternative treatment method can be particularly beneficial for patients who may be at higher risk for complications or those who prefer a more conservative approach to manual therapy.

The clinical efficacy of spinal manipulation in the treatment of neck pain has been well-established through numerous studies, demonstrating its effectiveness in providing relief from pain, improving function, and enhancing the quality of life for patients with acute and chronic neck pain. However, it is essential for healthcare professionals to recognize that spinal manipulation may not be suitable for all individuals experiencing neck pain and to carefully assess each patient's unique circumstances and risk factors before initiating treatment. In cases where spinal manipulation may not be appropriate, other manual therapy techniques, such as joint mobilization, can offer effective alternatives for the treatment of neck pain.

Manual therapy and mobilization techniques are versatile interventions that can effectively address a wide range of neck pain conditions. They are generally indicated for the treatment of various types of neck pain, including mechanical neck pain, cervical radiculopathy, and whiplash-associated disorders. In the following paragraphs, we will delve deeper into the specific indications and benefits of manual therapy and mobilization techniques for these conditions.

Mechanical neck pain, one of the most common types of neck pain, arises from various structures within the cervical spine, including muscles, ligaments, facet joints, and intervertebral discs. This pain often results from muscle imbalances, joint stiffness, or postural dysfunction. Manual therapy and mobilization techniques can help alleviate mechanical neck pain by restoring normal joint mobility, releasing muscle tension, and improving overall neck function. These techniques can also facilitate the correction of postural imbalances and reduce the likelihood of pain recurrence.

Cervical radiculopathy is a condition in which a nerve root in the cervical spine becomes compressed or irritated, causing pain, numbness, tingling, or weakness in the neck, shoulders, arms, or hands. Manual therapy and mobilization techniques can help alleviate cervical radiculopathy by reducing nerve root compression and inflammation. This can be achieved through the mobilization of cervical joints, the release of tight soft tissues, and the improvement of spinal alignment. Additionally, these techniques can help address underlying factors, such as muscle imbalances or joint stiffness, which may contribute to the development of cervical radiculopathy.

Whiplash-associated disorders refer to a range of symptoms that can occur following a sudden acceleration-deceleration force to the neck, typically during motor vehicle accidents. Common symptoms include neck pain, stiffness, headaches, and dizziness. Manual therapy and mobilization techniques can help alleviate whiplash-associated symptoms by promoting tissue healing, reducing inflammation, and restoring normal joint mobility and muscle function. These techniques can also aid in the prevention of chronic pain and disability following a whiplash injury.

Manual therapy and mobilization techniques may be particularly beneficial for individuals with muscle tightness, joint stiffness, or limited range of motion, as they can directly target these issues and restore normal neck function. These techniques can also be used in conjunction with other conservative treatments, such as exercise, stretching, and postural education, to enhance overall treatment outcomes. By incorporating manual therapy and mobilization techniques into a comprehensive, multimodal treatment plan, healthcare providers can optimize pain relief and functional improvements for individuals with various types of neck pain.

While manual therapy and mobilization techniques can be highly effective for treating neck pain, certain conditions may contraindicate their use or necessitate a more cautious approach. In these cases, it is crucial to identify and consider the contraindications to ensure patient safety and optimal treatment outcomes. Contraindications can be categorized into two types: absolute contraindications, which completely prohibit the use of manual therapy, and relative contraindications, which require a more cautious approach or modification of the treatment.

Absolute contraindications for manual therapy include the presence of spinal instability, which can result from trauma, degenerative changes, or congenital abnormalities. This condition poses a significant risk of causing further damage or neurological complications if manual therapy is applied. Severe osteoporosis is another absolute contraindication, as the weakened bone structure increases the risk of fractures during manual therapy. Acute fractures and dislocations also preclude the use of manual therapy, as these injuries require medical stabilization or surgical intervention before any form of manual treatment can be considered.

Infections involving the spinal column, such as discitis or vertebral osteomyelitis, are also absolute contraindications for manual therapy. Applying manual force in the presence of an active infection can exacerbate the condition, leading to the potential spread of infection or increased tissue damage.

Relative contraindications, on the other hand, require a more cautious approach or modification of the treatment plan. Spinal stenosis, a narrowing of the spinal canal that can compress the spinal cord or nerve roots, is one such condition. While manual therapy may still be beneficial for patients with spinal stenosis, practitioners must exercise caution and utilize gentle, controlled techniques to avoid exacerbating nerve compression.

Spondylolisthesis, a condition in which one vertebra slips forward over the one below it, is another relative contraindication for manual therapy. In these cases, the practitioner must assess the degree of slippage and the stability of the affected segment before determining the appropriate treatment approach, which may involve modified techniques or alternative interventions.

Inflammatory arthritis, such as rheumatoid arthritis or ankylosing spondylitis, also warrants a cautious approach to manual therapy. While some patients with inflammatory arthritis may benefit from gentle mobilization techniques, care must be taken to avoid exacerbating joint inflammation or causing additional damage to the affected structures.

A history of spinal surgery, especially if it involves instrumentation or fusion, is another relative contraindication for manual therapy. In these cases, the practitioner must have a thorough understanding of the surgical procedure, any resulting biomechanical changes, and the patient's current level of stability and function. This information is crucial for determining the most appropriate treatment approach and ensuring patient safety.

While manual therapy and mobilization techniques can be highly effective for treating neck pain, it is essential to identify and consider any contraindications to ensure patient safety and optimal treatment outcomes. A thorough assessment by a qualified healthcare professional is necessary to determine the most appropriate treatment approach based on the patient's specific condition and needs.

As with any intervention, manual therapy and mobilization techniques are not without risks. Although rare, potential adverse effects may include transient soreness, increased pain, or neurological symptoms. It is crucial to acknowledge and understand these risks to ensure patients receive the most appropriate and safe treatment.

Transient soreness is a common and mild side effect of manual therapy and mobilization techniques. This soreness may occur due to the manipulation of soft tissues and joints, causing a temporary inflammatory response. Generally, this soreness resolves within a day or two and can be managed with over-the-counter pain relievers or ice packs. Patients should be informed of this potential side effect and encouraged to report any lingering or worsening discomfort to their healthcare provider.

Increased pain following manual therapy interventions may result from the aggravation of pre-existing conditions or the inappropriate application of techniques. In some cases, increased pain may signal the presence of an undiagnosed underlying issue that requires further evaluation and a modified treatment approach. To minimize the risk of increased pain, healthcare providers should carefully assess each patient's medical history, symptoms, and physical examination findings to determine the most appropriate treatment plan.

Neurological symptoms, such as tingling, numbness, or weakness, may occasionally arise following manual therapy and mobilization techniques. These symptoms may result from the temporary irritation or compression of nerves within the cervical spine. Although typically transient, neurological symptoms should be closely monitored, and any persistent or worsening symptoms should be promptly evaluated by a healthcare professional to rule out more serious complications.

More severe complications, such as vertebral artery dissection or spinal cord injury, have been reported in the context of cervical spinal manipulation but are extremely rare. Vertebral artery dissection refers to a tear in the inner lining of the vertebral artery, which can potentially result in stroke or other serious neurological complications. Spinal cord injury may result from excessive force or inappropriate technique during cervical spinal manipulation, leading to damage to the spinal cord and potentially severe neurological deficits. A systematic review published in 2007 estimated the risk of serious complications following cervical spinal manipulation to be approximately 1 in 2 million treatments.

To minimize the risk of adverse effects, it is essential for manual therapy and mobilization techniques to be performed by qualified, trained healthcare professionals who possess a thorough understanding of the anatomy, biomechanics, and clinical presentation of neck pain. Proper training and experience can help practitioners recognize and avoid potentially harmful techniques, as well as tailor treatment plans to each patient's unique needs and contraindications.

Additionally, a comprehensive patient assessment, including a detailed medical history and physical examination, should be conducted prior to initiating any manual therapy interventions to identify any potential contraindications or risk factors. This assessment may include imaging studies, such as X-rays or magnetic resonance imaging (MRI), to rule out more serious underlying conditions or identify specific anatomical factors that may influence treatment selection.

While manual therapy and mobilization techniques can be highly effective in the treatment of neck pain, it is crucial to consider the potential risks and take appropriate measures to ensure patient safety. By working with qualified healthcare professionals and carefully assessing each patient's unique needs and risk factors, the benefits of manual therapy can be maximized while minimizing potential adverse effects.

In conclusion, manual therapy and mobilization techniques offer a diverse range of evidence-based approaches for addressing neck pain, ultimately contributing to enhanced patient outcomes. Techniques such as massage therapy, joint mobilization, and spinal manipulation have consistently demonstrated their ability to relieve pain, restore function, and improve overall quality of life for individuals suffering from neck pain. By targeting various structures within the cervical spine—including muscles, tendons, ligaments, facet joints, and intervertebral discs—these hands-on treatments can be customized to address the specific needs and preferences of each patient, ensuring a tailored approach to care.

Importantly, the successful implementation of manual therapy and mobilization techniques relies on the expertise of healthcare professionals, who must be cognizant of the potential risks and contraindications associated with these interventions. By conducting a comprehensive patient assessment prior to initiating treatment, healthcare providers can identify any potential contraindications or risk factors, ensuring a safe and effective treatment experience.

In addition to their standalone benefits, manual therapy and mobilization techniques can also be seamlessly integrated into a comprehensive, individualized treatment plan, which may incorporate other evidence-based interventions such as exercise, stretching, and postural education. This multidisciplinary approach to care allows healthcare providers to address the complex and multifaceted nature of neck pain, optimizing treatment outcomes and fostering a holistic approach to patient well-being.

Furthermore, the integration of manual therapy and mobilization techniques into the broader healthcare landscape highlights the importance of collaboration and communication among healthcare professionals. By working together across disciplines, healthcare providers can ensure that patients receive the most effective, evidence-based care, ultimately leading to a more efficient and patient-centered healthcare system.

Finally, ongoing research and innovation in the field of manual therapy and mobilization techniques continue to shed light on new and emerging approaches to the treatment of neck pain. As our understanding of the underlying mechanisms, efficacy, and safety of these interventions continues to evolve, healthcare professionals must remain committed to staying up-to-date with the latest scientific developments, ensuring that patients receive the most accurate, evidence-based care available.

In summary, manual therapy and mobilization techniques represent a valuable and effective approach to the treatment of neck pain. By leveraging the expertise of healthcare professionals, conducting thorough patient assessments, and integrating these techniques into comprehensive, individualized treatment plans, patients with neck pain can achieve optimal outcomes, returning to their daily activities with reduced pain and improved function.

Chapter 17

Lifestyle Modifications and Stress Management

Addressing the Psychological Factors that Contribute to Neck Pain

Neck pain is a common condition affecting millions of people worldwide. It can range from a mild annoyance to a debilitating issue that significantly impacts an individual's quality of life. While there are numerous physical factors that can contribute to neck pain, such as poor posture, injury, and muscle strain, psychological factors also play a significant role. This chapter will explore the various psychological factors that contribute to neck pain and provide evidence-based recommendations for lifestyle modifications and stress management techniques to address these factors.

Stress is a complex and multifaceted phenomenon that can have profound effects on the body, including contributing to neck pain. It is important to understand the various types of stress and how they can impact the body in order to effectively address the stress-related factors that contribute to neck pain.

There are two primary types of stress: acute stress and chronic stress. Acute stress is a short-term response to a specific stressor or event, such as an argument, deadline, or accident. The body's reaction to acute stress is primarily adaptive, helping individuals respond to immediate challenges or threats. However, chronic stress, which is the result of ongoing, persistent stressors, can have detrimental effects on the body, including increasing the risk of neck pain.

Chronic stress leads to the prolonged release of stress hormones, such as cortisol and adrenaline. These hormones, when present in the body for extended periods, can result in a state of physiological hyperarousal, causing the body to remain in a constant state of tension and alertness. This heightened state can lead to increased muscle tension, particularly in the neck and shoulders, as the body's muscles remain contracted in preparation for potential threats. Over time, this sustained muscle tension can cause pain, stiffness, and reduced range of motion in the neck.

The relationship between stress and neck pain can also be influenced by individual factors, such as personality traits and coping mechanisms. For example, individuals who exhibit Type A personality traits, such as competitiveness, impatience, and a strong need for control, may be more prone to experiencing stress-related neck pain due to their heightened sensitivity to stressors and tendency to internalize stress. Similarly, individuals who rely on maladaptive coping mechanisms, such as denial, avoidance, or substance use, may also be at a higher risk for developing stress-related neck pain.

In addition to the direct effects of stress on muscle tension and neck pain, stress can also exacerbate neck pain through indirect pathways. For example, stress can negatively impact sleep quality, leading to a cycle of poor sleep and increased pain. Additionally, stress can lead to poor posture, particularly for those who work in high-stress environments, such as office settings. Hunching over a computer or constantly cradling a phone between the shoulder and ear can further contribute to neck pain and stiffness.

Understanding the complex relationship between stress and neck pain is essential for developing effective interventions and lifestyle modifications that address both the physical and psychological aspects of neck pain. By managing stress through various techniques, such as exercise, relaxation, and cognitive-behavioral strategies, individuals can reduce muscle tension and alleviate neck pain, improving their overall quality of life.

Anxiety and depression are common psychological factors associated with neck pain. Individuals with anxiety disorders or depression often experience muscle tension and pain as part of their symptoms. This heightened muscle tension, particularly in the neck and shoulder areas, can be a result of the body's physiological response to stress and emotional distress. When an individual experiences anxiety or depression, the body's nervous system activates the release of stress hormones, which can cause muscles to tense up as part of the fight-or-flight response.

This connection between anxiety, depression, and neck pain can lead to a vicious cycle, as neck pain can exacerbate anxiety and depression symptoms, which in turn can worsen neck pain. For example, individuals with anxiety may focus excessively on their neck pain and catastrophize the situation, believing that the pain is indicative of a more severe issue or that it will never improve. This negative thinking pattern can contribute to increased anxiety levels, which can further aggravate muscle tension and pain.

Similarly, individuals with depression may experience a decreased ability to cope with the pain, as well as a lowered motivation to engage in activities that could help alleviate neck pain, such as exercise or seeking treatment. This lack of motivation and perceived helplessness can lead to increased pain levels and further exacerbate depressive symptoms.

Research has demonstrated a strong association between anxiety, depression, and neck pain. In a study published in the journal Pain, researchers found that individuals with high levels of anxiety and depression were more likely to report neck pain than those with lower levels of these psychological factors. Additionally, a systematic review published in the European Journal of Pain found that depression was a significant predictor of chronic neck pain.

Addressing anxiety and depression in the context of neck pain management is crucial for breaking this vicious cycle and improving overall well-being. Treatment approaches that target both the physical and psychological aspects of neck pain, such as cognitive-behavioral therapy, mindfulness-based stress reduction, and exercise, can help individuals better manage their anxiety and depression symptoms while also reducing muscle tension and pain. By recognizing the interconnected nature of anxiety, depression, and neck pain, individuals and healthcare providers can develop more effective, comprehensive treatment plans to improve the quality of life for those suffering from these conditions.

Somatization is a complex psychological phenomenon in which individuals experience physical symptoms that cannot be attributed to any identifiable medical condition. These symptoms are not intentionally produced or feigned and can cause significant distress and functional impairment. Somatization can manifest in various forms, including headaches, fatigue, gastrointestinal issues, and musculoskeletal pain, such as neck pain.

The relationship between somatization and neck pain is multifaceted. Individuals with somatization disorders may have a heightened sensitivity to pain, known as hyperalgesia, which can contribute to increased neck pain. This heightened sensitivity is believed to be a result of altered pain processing in the central nervous system. When an individual experiences stress or anxiety, the nervous system can become more sensitized, leading to a lower pain threshold and an exaggerated perception of pain.

Another factor contributing to neck pain in individuals with somatization disorders is the tendency to focus on bodily sensations, known as somatosensory amplification. This increased awareness and attention to bodily sensations can cause individuals to perceive and interpret normal or mild sensations as painful, leading to an increased experience of neck pain. This heightened focus on bodily sensations can create a feedback loop, as the more an individual focuses on their pain, the more intense it may become.

Furthermore, individuals with somatization disorders may exhibit maladaptive coping strategies, such as catastrophizing and avoidance behaviors. Catastrophizing refers to the tendency to view pain as

338

unbearable, uncontrollable, or never-ending. This negative thinking pattern can exacerbate neck pain by increasing stress, anxiety, and muscle tension. Avoidance behaviors, on the other hand, involve limiting or avoiding activities out of fear that they will cause pain. This avoidance can lead to physical deconditioning and increased muscle tension, ultimately worsening neck pain.

It is essential to recognize that individuals with somatization disorders are genuinely experiencing pain, even if the cause is not entirely understood. A comprehensive approach to managing neck pain in individuals with somatization disorders should involve addressing both the physical and psychological aspects of the condition. This may include interventions such as cognitive-behavioral therapy, which focuses on modifying maladaptive thought patterns and behaviors, and mindfulness-based techniques that can help individuals develop a more adaptive relationship with their bodily sensations. Additionally, physical treatments, such as exercise and manual therapy, can help improve muscle strength and flexibility, further reducing neck pain. By addressing both the physical and psychological components of somatization, individuals can effectively manage their neck pain and improve their overall quality of life.

Regular exercise has numerous benefits for overall health and well-being, including stress management and reduction of neck pain. Exercise helps in reducing muscle tension by increasing blood flow to the muscles, promoting relaxation, and improving flexibility. The release of endorphins, the body's natural painkiller, during exercise can also help alleviate neck pain and provide a sense of relaxation and well-being.

Aerobic exercise, also known as cardio, is an essential component of any exercise routine. Activities such as walking, swimming, cycling, and jogging can improve cardiovascular health, increase endurance, and promote relaxation. Engaging in moderate-intensity aerobic exercise for at least 150 minutes per week, or vigorous-intensity aerobic exercise for at least 75 minutes per week, is recommended for adults to achieve health benefits. Regular aerobic exercise has been shown to reduce muscle tension and stiffness, which can contribute to neck pain relief.

Strength training exercises focus on building and maintaining muscle strength, which can be beneficial for individuals experiencing neck pain. By

339

targeting the muscles in the neck, shoulders, and upper back, strength training exercises can help improve posture, provide better support for the cervical spine, and reduce the likelihood of developing muscle imbalances that can contribute to neck pain. It is recommended to engage in strength training exercises for all major muscle groups at least twice a week, with at least 48 hours of rest between sessions to allow for muscle recovery.

Yoga is a mind-body practice that combines physical postures, breath control, and meditation to promote relaxation, flexibility, and overall well-being. Practicing yoga regularly can help improve posture, increase muscle strength and flexibility, and reduce muscle tension in the neck and shoulders. Specific yoga poses, such as neck stretches, gentle backbends, and shoulder openers, can be particularly helpful for individuals experiencing neck pain. Furthermore, the mindfulness aspect of yoga practice can help individuals become more aware of their body's tension patterns and learn to release muscle tension more effectively.

Tai chi, a traditional Chinese martial art, combines slow, flowing movements with deep breathing and relaxation techniques. Regular practice of tai chi has been shown to improve balance, flexibility, and muscle strength, as well as reduce stress and anxiety. The gentle, flowing movements of tai chi can help alleviate neck pain by promoting relaxation and reducing muscle tension in the neck and shoulders. In addition, tai chi practice can help individuals develop a greater awareness of their body and learn to recognize and release tension patterns that contribute to neck pain.

Incorporating regular exercise into daily routines, including aerobic exercise, strength training, yoga, and tai chi, can help manage stress, reduce muscle tension, and alleviate neck pain. By engaging in a variety of physical activities that promote relaxation, improve posture, and increase muscle strength and flexibility, individuals can address both the physical and psychological factors contributing to neck pain and promote overall well-being.

Poor sleep quality and sleep disturbances are significant factors that can exacerbate neck pain. Numerous studies have demonstrated the association between sleep problems and increased neck pain, emphasizing the importance of addressing sleep issues as part of a comprehensive pain management strategy.

Creating a consistent sleep schedule is a crucial step in improving sleep quality. Maintaining a regular sleep pattern, including going to bed and waking up at the same time every day, helps regulate the body's internal clock and promotes better sleep. It is essential to prioritize sleep and make adjustments to daily routines to ensure sufficient sleep duration. Experts recommend that adults aim for 7-9 hours of sleep per night to support optimal health and well-being.

Optimizing the sleep environment can also contribute to improved sleep quality and reduced neck pain. Ensuring that the mattress and pillow provide adequate support and comfort is essential. A medium-firm mattress is generally recommended for spinal alignment, while a pillow that supports the natural curve of the neck can help prevent muscle strain during sleep. Additionally, maintaining a dark, quiet, and cool environment can enhance sleep quality by reducing external disturbances and facilitating the body's natural sleep processes. Using blackout curtains or an eye mask to block out light and using earplugs or a white noise machine to minimize noise can help create a more conducive sleep environment.

Incorporating relaxation techniques before bedtime can also help improve sleep quality and reduce neck pain. Developing a pre-sleep routine that includes activities that promote relaxation, such as reading, taking a warm bath, or practicing gentle stretching, can signal to the body that it is time to wind down and prepare for sleep. Mindfulness practices, such as meditation or deep breathing exercises, can also be beneficial in reducing stress and anxiety, which are common contributors to sleep disturbances and neck pain.

Furthermore, limiting exposure to electronic devices before bedtime can help improve sleep quality. The blue light emitted by screens on smartphones, tablets, and computers can interfere with the production of melatonin, a hormone that regulates sleep-wake cycles. Reducing screen time at least an hour before bedtime and engaging in relaxing activities instead can help promote better sleep.

Addressing sleep issues is a vital component of managing neck pain. By creating a consistent sleep schedule, optimizing the sleep environment, and incorporating relaxation techniques before bedtime, individuals can improve their sleep quality, which can, in turn, contribute to reduced neck pain and overall better health.

Improving workplace ergonomics is a critical aspect of addressing neck pain, as it helps create a supportive and healthy work environment. Poor posture, awkward workstations, and prolonged static positions can exacerbate neck pain and lead to musculoskeletal disorders. By implementing ergonomic principles and making adjustments to one's workspace, individuals can reduce neck pain and improve overall well-being.

One important aspect of workplace ergonomics is the proper positioning of computer monitors. The ideal placement of a computer monitor is at eye level or slightly below, at a distance of approximately 20-40 inches (50-100 cm) from the user. This positioning helps prevent excessive neck flexion or extension, which can contribute to neck pain. If necessary, the use of monitor risers or adjustable arms can help achieve the optimal monitor height and distance.

The choice of chair is another vital component of workplace ergonomics. Ergonomic chairs with proper lumbar support and adjustable features, such as seat height, backrest angle, and armrest height, can help promote a neutral spine posture and reduce strain on the neck and shoulders. Additionally, the use of footrests can help ensure the user's feet are firmly on the ground, further promoting proper posture.

Taking regular breaks to stretch and move throughout the day is an essential practice for preventing neck pain and promoting overall health. Prolonged sitting has been linked to numerous health issues, including neck pain, and periodic movement can help alleviate muscle tension and improve circulation. Microbreaks, which are brief periods of rest or movement every 20-30 minutes, can be particularly helpful in reducing neck pain. These breaks can include standing up, walking around, or performing simple stretches and exercises, such as neck rolls, shoulder shrugs, and seated spinal twists.

In addition to these measures, other ergonomic considerations can help reduce neck pain. For instance, placing frequently used items, such as the phone, within easy reach can help minimize excessive reaching and twisting. The use of document holders or stands can also help maintain a neutral neck posture while reading or referencing documents. Furthermore, positioning the keyboard and mouse at a comfortable height and distance can prevent excessive wrist extension and shoulder abduction, which can contribute to neck pain.

Addressing workplace ergonomics is crucial for preventing and managing neck pain. By making adjustments to one's workspace, such as optimizing monitor placement, using ergonomic chairs, and taking regular breaks, individuals can create a more comfortable and supportive work environment. Implementing these ergonomic principles can help reduce neck pain and contribute to overall health and well-being.

Mindfulness-Based Stress Reduction (MBSR) is an evidence-based approach to stress reduction that was developed by Dr. Jon Kabat-Zinn at the University of Massachusetts Medical Center in the late 1970s. MBSR is an eight-week program that combines mindfulness meditation, gentle yoga, and group discussions to help participants develop greater self-awareness, self-compassion, and coping skills for managing stress.

The core principles of MBSR revolve around cultivating mindfulness, which is the practice of purposefully paying attention to the present moment in a non-judgmental manner. Mindfulness meditation techniques used in MBSR include body scan meditation, sitting meditation, and walking meditation. These practices encourage individuals to develop a greater awareness of their thoughts, emotions, and bodily sensations, allowing them to recognize and respond to stressors more effectively.

Gentle yoga is another integral component of MBSR. Yoga practice in MBSR focuses on gentle stretches and postures designed to help participants develop body awareness, improve flexibility, and release muscle tension. By incorporating yoga into the MBSR program, participants can learn to recognize areas of tension in their bodies, including the neck, and work on releasing that tension through gentle movement and mindful breathing.

Research has demonstrated the effectiveness of MBSR in reducing stress, anxiety, and depression, all of which can contribute to neck pain. Studies have shown that MBSR participants report significant reductions in psychological distress and improvements in mental well-being following the program. Furthermore, research has found that MBSR can lead to reductions in the production of pro-inflammatory cytokines, which have been linked to chronic pain conditions, including neck pain.

By learning to be present and non-judgmental through mindfulness meditation and gentle yoga, individuals can develop a greater awareness of their body and tension patterns. This heightened body awareness can help individuals identify areas of tension, such as in the neck and shoulders, and learn to release that tension through mindful movement and relaxation techniques. As a result, MBSR can lead to reduced muscle tension and neck pain, improving overall well-being and quality of life.

Mindfulness-Based Stress Reduction (MBSR) is an effective approach to stress management that can help individuals address the psychological factors contributing to neck pain. Through mindfulness meditation and gentle yoga, MBSR participants can develop greater self-awareness, self-compassion, and coping skills, leading to reduced stress, anxiety, and depression. By cultivating mindfulness and body awareness, individuals can recognize and release tension in the neck, resulting in decreased neck pain and improved overall well-being.

Cognitive Behavioral Therapy (CBT) is a well-established and evidence-based psychotherapeutic approach that targets unhelpful thought patterns and behaviors contributing to various mental health conditions, including chronic pain. In the context of neck pain, CBT addresses the psychological factors that may exacerbate the experience of pain and hinder recovery.

CBT for neck pain typically involves several components, including psychoeducation, cognitive restructuring, behavioral activation, and relaxation techniques. Psychoeducation helps individuals understand the biopsychosocial model of pain, which acknowledges that pain is a complex interplay of biological, psychological, and social factors. By understanding this model, individuals can develop a more comprehensive understanding of their neck pain and the various factors that contribute to it.

Cognitive restructuring is a core component of CBT that focuses on identifying and challenging maladaptive thoughts related to pain, such as catastrophizing, negative self-talk, and overgeneralization. Catastrophizing, for example, involves magnifying the negative aspects of pain and feeling helpless in coping with it. Negative self-talk may involve thoughts such as "I can't handle this pain" or "I'll never get better." By examining the evidence supporting these thoughts and considering alternative, more balanced perspectives, individuals can reduce the emotional distress associated with their pain and develop a more adaptive mindset.

Behavioral activation is another key element of CBT for neck pain, which involves gradually reintroducing activities that have been avoided due to pain. Fear of movement and activity avoidance can perpetuate pain and disability, leading to a cycle of worsening pain and diminished quality of life. CBT helps individuals set realistic and achievable goals to gradually increase their level of activity and overcome their fear of movement. This process, known as graded exposure, allows individuals to regain their function and decrease the impact of pain on their daily lives.

Relaxation techniques, such as deep breathing, progressive muscle relaxation, and guided imagery, are also commonly integrated into CBT for neck pain. These techniques help individuals manage stress and anxiety, which can contribute to increased muscle tension and pain. Regular practice of relaxation techniques can promote a sense of calm and improve overall well-being, which can, in turn, alleviate neck pain.

CBT for neck pain is typically delivered in individual or group therapy sessions, with the duration and frequency of treatment varying based on individual needs. Research has consistently shown that CBT is effective in reducing pain, improving function, and enhancing the quality of life for individuals with chronic pain, including neck pain. By addressing the psychological factors that contribute to neck pain and providing individuals with the tools to develop more adaptive coping strategies, CBT can be a valuable component of a comprehensive neck pain management plan.

Progressive Muscle Relaxation (PMR) is a relaxation technique developed by American physician Edmund Jacobson in the early 20th century. The technique is based on the premise that physical relaxation can lead to mental relaxation, helping to reduce stress, anxiety, and pain. PMR has been extensively studied and found to be effective in managing various forms of pain, including neck pain, by decreasing muscle tension and promoting overall relaxation.

The PMR technique involves a step-by-step process of tensing and relaxing different muscle groups throughout the body. The individual starts by focusing on a specific muscle group, such as the muscles in the feet, and deliberately tenses the muscles for a few seconds, usually around five to ten seconds. The individual then relaxes the muscles for a longer period, typically 15 to 20 seconds, before moving on to the next muscle group. This process is repeated for each major muscle group in the body, working progressively from the feet to the head.

The regular practice of PMR can help individuals develop a greater awareness of their muscle tension patterns and learn how to release this tension effectively. As muscle tension is a common contributor to neck pain, the consistent practice of PMR can lead to a reduction in neck pain over time. Additionally, the relaxation response induced by PMR can help to counteract the stress response, further alleviating neck pain by reducing the stress-related muscle tension.

PMR has been shown to have numerous benefits beyond reducing muscle tension and neck pain. Studies have found that PMR can help improve sleep quality, reduce symptoms of anxiety and depression, and enhance overall well-being. These mental health benefits can further contribute to the reduction of neck pain, as improved mental health can lead to decreased muscle tension and a heightened ability to cope with pain.

To maximize the benefits of PMR, it is essential to practice the technique consistently and correctly. Individuals should aim to practice PMR daily or at least several times a week for optimal results. It is also important to find a quiet, comfortable environment for practicing PMR, free from distractions. Finally, focusing on deep, slow breathing during the PMR process can enhance relaxation and further reduce muscle tension.

Progressive Muscle Relaxation is an evidence-based relaxation technique that can effectively reduce muscle tension, anxiety, and pain, including neck pain. By regularly practicing PMR, individuals can become more aware of their muscle tension patterns and learn to release this tension, leading to a reduction in neck pain. Furthermore, the mental health benefits associated with PMR can contribute to a more comprehensive approach to managing neck pain, addressing both physical and psychological factors.

Biofeedback is a non-invasive technique that uses electronic devices to monitor and display an individual's physiological processes in real-time, such as muscle tension, heart rate, skin temperature, and brainwave activity. The goal of biofeedback is to help individuals gain greater awareness and control over these processes, allowing them to better manage stress, reduce muscle tension, and alleviate pain, including neck pain.

There are several types of biofeedback techniques, each targeting specific physiological processes. For addressing neck pain, electromyographic (EMG) biofeedback is particularly relevant. EMG biofeedback focuses on monitoring muscle tension by measuring electrical activity in the muscles. By observing the visual or auditory feedback provided by the biofeedback device, individuals can learn to recognize when their muscles are tense and develop strategies to relax them, ultimately reducing muscle tension and neck pain.

One of the key principles behind biofeedback is self-regulation. By gaining awareness of their physiological responses, individuals can learn to recognize their body's signals related to stress and tension. This awareness empowers them to take control of their body's reactions and modify their behaviors or thought patterns to reduce stress and muscle tension. As a result, biofeedback can help individuals develop better coping strategies for managing stress and alleviating neck pain in the long term.

Several studies have shown that biofeedback can be effective in reducing neck pain, especially when combined with other stress management techniques and interventions, such as cognitive-behavioral therapy, relaxation techniques, and exercise. For instance, a study conducted by Flor and Turk (1989) found that individuals who received EMG biofeedback, in conjunction with relaxation training and cognitive-behavioral therapy, experienced significant reductions in neck pain and improvements in daily functioning.

Biofeedback has several advantages as a treatment for neck pain. It is non-invasive, has no known side effects, and can be tailored to the specific needs of the individual. Additionally, the skills learned through biofeedback can be applied in various situations, allowing individuals to manage their stress and tension independently and proactively.

However, it is important to note that biofeedback may not be effective for everyone, and the success of the treatment depends on the individual's commitment and willingness to engage in the process. Furthermore, while biofeedback can be an effective tool for managing neck pain, it is not a cure-all solution. For optimal results, biofeedback should be incorporated into a comprehensive treatment plan that includes other evidence-based interventions, such as exercise, ergonomic adjustments, and psychological therapies.

Biofeedback is a promising technique for addressing the psychological factors that contribute to neck pain. By providing real-time feedback on muscle tension and other physiological processes, biofeedback helps individuals develop greater awareness and control over their body's responses to stress. This increased self-regulation can lead to reduced muscle tension and, ultimately, decreased neck pain. When combined with other stress management techniques and interventions, biofeedback can be an effective component of a comprehensive neck pain management plan.

Breathing techniques have long been recognized as an effective method for reducing stress, anxiety, and muscle tension. By deliberately controlling one's breath, individuals can encourage relaxation and alleviate the tension that contributes to neck pain. Two well-known deep breathing exercises that can be easily incorporated into daily routines are diaphragmatic breathing and paced breathing.

Diaphragmatic breathing, also known as belly breathing, involves engaging the diaphragm – the primary muscle responsible for respiration – to breathe more deeply and efficiently. This technique helps to reduce the activation of the sympathetic nervous system (the "fight or flight" response) and increase the activation of the parasympathetic nervous system (the "rest and digest" response), promoting relaxation and stress reduction. To practice diaphragmatic breathing, individuals can follow these steps in a comfortable position, either sitting or lying down:

First, place one hand on the chest and the other on the abdomen, just below the ribcage. Slowly inhale through the nose, allowing the abdomen to rise while keeping the chest relatively still. Exhale slowly through pursed lips, allowing the abdomen to fall back towards the spine. Continue this pattern of deep, slow breaths for several minutes, focusing on the sensation of the breath entering and leaving the body.

Paced breathing, also known as controlled breathing or slow breathing, involves consciously slowing down the breath to a specific rate, usually between four and six breaths per minute. This slower pace has been shown to stimulate the vagus nerve, which plays a crucial role in activating the parasympathetic nervous system and promoting relaxation. Paced breathing can be practiced using the following steps in a comfortable position, either sitting or lying down:

Begin by inhaling slowly through the nose for a count of four. Hold the breath for a count of four. Then exhale slowly through the mouth for a count of six. Pause for a count of two before inhaling again. Repeat this pattern for several minutes, focusing on maintaining a consistent rhythm and pace.

In addition to diaphragmatic and paced breathing, other breathing techniques, such as alternate nostril breathing, 4-7-8 breathing, and box breathing, have been shown to be effective in reducing stress, anxiety, and muscle tension. Regular practice of these techniques can help individuals develop greater self-awareness and self-regulation skills, enabling them to better manage stress and reduce the impact of psychological factors on neck pain.

Alternate nostril breathing is a technique that involves breathing in through one nostril while closing the other, then exhaling through the opposite nostril while closing the first one. This practice is thought to balance the two hemispheres of the brain and promote relaxation. The 4-7-8 breathing technique consists of inhaling for four counts, holding the breath for seven counts, and exhaling for eight counts, which is believed to help reduce anxiety and promote a sense of calm. Box breathing, also known as square breathing or four-square breathing, is a technique where inhalations, exhalations, and breath-holding are all done for an equal number of counts, typically four. This practice is often used by military personnel and athletes to manage stress and maintain focus.

Incorporating breathing exercises into daily routines can be a simple yet effective way to manage stress and neck pain. By dedicating just a few minutes each day to practicing these techniques, individuals can develop a greater sense of control over their stress levels and promote relaxation, ultimately reducing the tension that contributes to neck pain and improving overall well-being.

Acupuncture, originating from traditional Chinese medicine, has been practiced for thousands of years as a method to treat various ailments and maintain overall health. The technique entails inserting thin, sterile needles into specific points, known as acupuncture points or acupoints, on the body. These points correspond to meridians, which are channels through which energy, or "qi," is believed to flow. By stimulating these acupoints, acupuncture aims to restore balance in the flow of qi and promote the body's natural healing processes.

In recent years, scientific research has increasingly supported the efficacy of acupuncture in treating neck pain. Studies have shown that acupuncture can provide both short-term and long-term relief for individuals experiencing neck pain, as well as improve their overall functioning and quality of life. Moreover, evidence suggests that acupuncture can be a valuable adjunct therapy when combined with other treatments, such as exercise and stress management techniques.

The exact mechanisms through which acupuncture provides pain relief are not yet fully understood. However, several theories have been proposed to explain its effectiveness in reducing pain and muscle tension. One widely accepted theory is that acupuncture stimulates the release of endorphins, the body's natural painkillers. Endorphins are neurotransmitters that interact with the brain's opiate receptors to produce analgesic effects, reducing the perception of pain and promoting a sense of well-being.

Another theory suggests that acupuncture influences the nervous system by modulating pain signals sent to the brain. This modulation occurs through the activation of nerve fibers that transmit non-painful sensory information, ultimately inhibiting the transmission of pain signals. Additionally, acupuncture is believed to have anti-inflammatory effects, which can contribute to reduced pain and muscle tension. By decreasing local inflammation, acupuncture may promote the healing of injured tissues and reduce pain associated with musculoskeletal conditions like neck pain.

It is essential to note that the effectiveness of acupuncture may vary depending on the skill of the practitioner, the severity of the neck pain, and the individual's response to treatment. Therefore, it is crucial to seek care from a licensed and experienced acupuncturist who can develop a personalized treatment plan based on the individual's specific needs and condition. Furthermore, acupuncture is generally considered safe when performed by a qualified professional. However, some individuals may experience mild side effects, such as temporary soreness, bruising, or bleeding at the needle insertion sites.

Acupuncture is a promising treatment option for individuals experiencing neck pain. By stimulating specific points on the body, acupuncture can promote the release of endorphins, modulate pain signals, and reduce inflammation, resulting in decreased pain and muscle tension. When used in conjunction with other treatments, such as exercise and stress management techniques, acupuncture can be an effective component of a comprehensive neck pain management plan.

Massage therapy is a widely accepted non-invasive treatment that involves the manipulation of soft tissues, including muscles, tendons, and ligaments. It has been shown to provide numerous benefits for individuals experiencing neck pain by addressing both physical and psychological factors.

There are various types of massage techniques that can be employed to alleviate neck pain, each with its unique approach and benefits. Swedish massage, for example, utilizes long, flowing strokes and kneading techniques to relieve muscle tension, increase circulation, and promote relaxation. Deep tissue massage, on the other hand, focuses on the deeper layers of muscle and connective tissue, using slow, firm pressure to release chronic tension and knots. Myofascial release is another technique that targets the fascia, a connective tissue that surrounds muscles, to improve flexibility and reduce pain.

One of the primary benefits of massage therapy is its ability to reduce muscle tension, a common contributing factor to neck pain. By applying pressure and manipulating the soft tissues, massage therapists can help relax tight muscles, release trigger points, and improve overall muscle

351

function. The reduction in muscle tension not only alleviates pain but also improves range of motion and flexibility in the neck.

Massage therapy can also improve circulation, promoting the delivery of essential nutrients and oxygen to the muscles and facilitating the removal of metabolic waste products. This increased circulation can help reduce inflammation and promote healing in the affected tissues, leading to a decrease in neck pain and an improvement in overall function.

In addition to its physical benefits, massage therapy has been shown to have a significant impact on psychological well-being. Massage has been found to stimulate the release of endorphins, the body's natural painkillers, and other neurotransmitters, such as serotonin and dopamine, which can help improve mood and reduce anxiety. The relaxation response triggered by massage can also help lower cortisol levels, a stress hormone known to contribute to muscle tension and neck pain.

Furthermore, massage therapy can enhance the effectiveness of other treatments and interventions for neck pain. For example, massage can help improve the outcomes of physical therapy exercises by increasing flexibility and reducing pain, allowing for more effective stretching and strengthening of the affected muscles. Similarly, massage can complement chiropractic care by addressing soft tissue imbalances and promoting relaxation, thereby facilitating spinal adjustments and improving overall function.

It is essential to work with a qualified and experienced massage therapist who understands the specific needs of individuals with neck pain. The therapist should be able to tailor the massage techniques to address the individual's unique symptoms and preferences, ensuring a safe and effective treatment. While massage therapy can provide significant benefits for those experiencing neck pain, it is crucial to remember that it should be part of a comprehensive treatment plan that addresses both the physical and psychological factors contributing to neck pain.

Massage therapy can be a valuable addition to a neck pain management plan, offering numerous physical and psychological benefits. By reducing muscle tension, improving circulation, and promoting relaxation, massage can help alleviate neck pain and improve overall well-being. Integrating massage therapy with other treatments and interventions, such as exercise, stress management techniques, and chiropractic care, can provide a holistic approach to addressing the complex interplay of physical and psychological factors that contribute to neck pain.

Chiropractic care is a healthcare profession that focuses on the diagnosis, treatment, and prevention of musculoskeletal disorders, particularly those involving the spine and other joints. The primary objective of chiropractic care is to restore proper joint function and alleviate pain through the use of manual techniques, such as spinal manipulation and mobilization. Chiropractic treatment has been shown to be effective in reducing neck pain and improving function for some individuals.

Spinal manipulation, also known as chiropractic adjustment, involves the application of controlled force to specific joints in the spine. This technique is designed to improve joint mobility, relieve muscle tension, and promote proper alignment. Spinal manipulation has been found to provide short-term pain relief and functional improvements for individuals with acute and subacute neck pain. However, the evidence regarding the effectiveness of spinal manipulation for chronic neck pain is less conclusive, and further research is needed to determine its long-term benefits.

Mobilization is another manual technique used by chiropractors that involves the gentle, passive movement of joints within their normal range of motion. This technique aims to improve joint function and reduce muscle tension, which can help alleviate neck pain. Mobilization may be particularly beneficial for individuals with neck pain who are unable or unwilling to undergo spinal manipulation due to contraindications or personal preference.

In addition to manual techniques, chiropractors may also incorporate other therapies into their treatment plans, such as soft tissue techniques, therapeutic exercises, and postural advice. These adjunctive therapies can help address underlying muscle imbalances, poor posture, and other factors that may contribute to neck pain. By addressing these issues, chiropractic care can help improve overall musculoskeletal function and reduce the likelihood of recurring neck pain.

While chiropractic care may not directly address the psychological factors contributing to neck pain, it can help alleviate physical symptoms and improve overall well-being, which can, in turn, improve mental health. Research has shown that individuals who experience improvements in their physical pain levels often report corresponding improvements in their psychological well-being, including reduced stress, anxiety, and depression. By reducing physical discomfort and improving function, chiropractic care can indirectly contribute to better mental health for individuals with neck pain.

It is important to note that chiropractic care may not be appropriate for everyone, and certain conditions may contraindicate its use, such as severe osteoporosis, spinal instability, or active infections. Furthermore, while rare, there are potential risks associated with spinal manipulation, including temporary discomfort, disc herniation, or nerve injury. It is crucial for individuals considering chiropractic care for neck pain to consult with a qualified healthcare professional to discuss their specific needs and determine the most appropriate course of treatment.

Chiropractic care can be an effective component of a comprehensive neck pain management plan for some individuals. By addressing physical factors, such as joint dysfunction and muscle tension, chiropractic care can help alleviate neck pain and improve overall well-being, which can indirectly improve mental health. It is essential for individuals with neck pain to work closely with their healthcare providers to develop a personalized treatment plan that addresses both the physical and psychological aspects of their pain.

In conclusion, addressing the psychological factors that contribute to neck pain is essential for effective pain management. A comprehensive approach to neck pain management should consider both physical and psychological aspects, as they often interact and exacerbate each other.

Lifestyle modifications can significantly impact neck pain by addressing both physical and psychological contributors. Regular exercise not only helps in maintaining good physical health but also serves as a powerful tool for stress reduction. Exercise releases endorphins, the body's natural painkillers, which can help alleviate neck pain and enhance mood.

Moreover, engaging in regular physical activity can improve sleep quality, which plays a vital role in pain management and overall well-being.

Proper sleep is essential for both physical and mental health. Ensuring a consistent sleep schedule, creating a conducive sleep environment, and employing relaxation techniques before bedtime can improve sleep quality, thus reducing the likelihood of neck pain. Improved sleep can also enhance an individual's ability to cope with stress, further contributing to a reduction in neck pain.

Ergonomic improvements, particularly in the workplace, can help reduce neck pain by promoting proper posture and minimizing muscle strain. Implementing ergonomic measures such as adjustable chairs, monitor stands, and ergonomic keyboards can significantly reduce the risk of developing neck pain due to poor posture or repetitive strain.

Stress management techniques, including mindfulness-based stress reduction (MBSR), cognitive-behavioral therapy (CBT), progressive muscle relaxation (PMR), biofeedback, and breathing exercises, can help individuals better manage their stress and reduce muscle tension contributing to neck pain. These techniques equip individuals with the skills to recognize and address negative thought patterns and behaviors, promoting better coping strategies for stress and pain.

Integrative approaches, such as acupuncture, massage therapy, and chiropractic care, can also play a crucial role in a comprehensive neck pain management plan. Acupuncture has been shown to stimulate the body's natural healing processes and promote the release of endorphins, which can help reduce pain and muscle tension. Massage therapy can provide immediate relief from muscle tension, improve circulation, and promote relaxation. Chiropractic care, through spinal manipulation and other joint adjustments, can help alleviate physical symptoms and improve overall well-being, which can, in turn, improve mental health.

By considering both the physical and psychological aspects of neck pain, individuals can take a holistic approach to pain management and improve their overall quality of life. Adopting a multifaceted approach to address the complex interplay between physical and psychological factors can lead to more effective and lasting pain relief. Additionally, fostering an awareness

355

of the psychological factors contributing to neck pain can empower individuals to seek the appropriate interventions and take control of their pain management journey. Ultimately, addressing the psychological factors associated with neck pain can lead to a better understanding of the intricacies of pain management and promote a more comprehensive and effective approach to mitigating neck pain and its impact on daily life.

Chapter 18

Nutritional Support and Supplements

Essential Nutrients for Optimal Neck Health

Nutrition plays a vital role in maintaining overall health, including neck health. Adequate intake of essential nutrients can support muscle and joint function, reduce inflammation, and promote healing. This chapter will discuss the essential nutrients for optimal neck health and provide evidence-based recommendations for incorporating these nutrients through diet and supplementation.

Protein is an essential macronutrient that plays a crucial role in maintaining healthy muscles, tendons, and ligaments. It is a critical component in the structure, function, and regulation of the body's tissues and organs, including those that support the neck. The importance of adequate protein intake cannot be overstated, especially for individuals experiencing neck pain due to muscle strains or injuries. Consuming sufficient protein ensures that the body has the necessary building blocks to repair and maintain the tissues that support the neck, helping to alleviate pain and promote recovery.

There are various sources of protein, and incorporating a diverse range of these foods into one's diet can help ensure that all essential amino acids are obtained. Lean meats such as chicken, turkey, and lean cuts of beef and pork provide high-quality protein, as well as essential vitamins and minerals. Poultry and fish, including salmon, tuna, and other cold-water fish, are excellent sources of protein that also offer additional health benefits, such as omega-3 fatty acids, which can help reduce inflammation and support neck health.

For those who follow a vegetarian or vegan diet, legumes such as beans, lentils, and chickpeas are rich sources of plant-based protein. Nuts, including almonds, walnuts, and pistachios, and seeds, like chia, flax, and hemp seeds, provide not only protein but also healthy fats and other essential nutrients. Dairy products, including milk, yogurt, and cheese, are also high in protein, with the added benefit of being rich in calcium, which is essential for bone health.

Individual protein requirements may vary based on factors such as age, sex, and activity level. Generally, the recommended daily allowance (RDA) for protein is 0.8 grams per kilogram of body weight. However, this guideline may not be sufficient for all individuals, particularly those with increased protein needs due to factors such as injury, illness, or intense physical activity. In these cases, a higher protein intake may be necessary to support optimal recovery and overall health.

It is essential to consider not only the quantity of protein consumed but also the quality. Consuming complete proteins, which contain all essential amino acids, is critical for the body's ability to synthesize new proteins effectively. Most animal-based proteins are considered complete, while plant-based proteins often have one or more limiting amino acids. To ensure the intake of all essential amino acids, individuals following a plant-based diet should consume a variety of protein sources throughout the day.

Protein is a vital component of a healthy diet that supports optimal neck health. By consuming a diverse range of protein sources and ensuring adequate intake based on individual needs, individuals can support the repair and maintenance of the muscles, tendons, and ligaments that make up the neck and help alleviate pain and promote recovery.

Carbohydrates, as the body's primary source of energy, play a significant role in maintaining optimal neck health. When muscles and other tissues in the neck receive sufficient energy from carbohydrates, they can function efficiently, promoting overall neck health and reducing the risk of pain and injury. Carbohydrates can be categorized into two main types: simple carbohydrates and complex carbohydrates.

Simple carbohydrates, such as those found in sugar, candy, and processed foods, are quickly broken down by the body and can cause rapid spikes in blood sugar levels. While these simple carbohydrates provide energy, they do not offer substantial nutritional benefits and can contribute to weight gain and other health issues when consumed in excess.

In contrast, complex carbohydrates are composed of longer chains of sugar molecules, which take longer to break down and provide a more stable and prolonged source of energy. These complex carbohydrates can be found in whole grains, fruits, and vegetables, and they offer additional benefits beyond energy provision.

One significant advantage of complex carbohydrates is their fiber content. Fiber, an indigestible carbohydrate, plays a critical role in maintaining digestive health, regulating blood sugar levels, and promoting satiety. A diet rich in fiber can help prevent constipation, reduce the risk of developing chronic diseases such as heart disease and diabetes, and support weight management, which is essential for reducing the strain on neck muscles and joints.

In addition to fiber, complex carbohydrates are also rich in essential vitamins and minerals, such as B vitamins, vitamin C, potassium, and magnesium. These nutrients play vital roles in various bodily functions, including the maintenance of healthy muscles, nerves, and bones, which are crucial for optimal neck health.

The consumption of complex carbohydrates in place of simple carbohydrates can help to ensure a steady supply of energy for neck muscles and tissues, along with the added benefits of fiber, vitamins, and minerals. To support neck health, it is essential to consume carbohydrates within the recommended daily intake range of 45-65% of total daily caloric intake, focusing on complex carbohydrate sources. This range may vary depending on factors such as age, sex, activity level, and overall health. By prioritizing complex carbohydrates in the diet, individuals can support their neck health and overall well-being.

Fats play a crucial role in maintaining overall health, including the health of the neck and surrounding structures. As an essential component of nerve function, hormone production, and absorption of fat-soluble vitamins, healthy fats can contribute to a well-functioning neck by reducing inflammation and promoting tissue repair.

Unsaturated fats, which can be further divided into monounsaturated and polyunsaturated fats, are considered healthier than saturated and trans fats. Monounsaturated fats can help lower bad cholesterol levels and reduce inflammation, which may alleviate neck pain. They can be found in avocados, nuts like almonds, cashews, and peanuts, as well as seeds such as pumpkin and sesame seeds. Additionally, monounsaturated fats can be found in plant-based oils, such as olive oil, canola oil, and peanut oil.

Polyunsaturated fats are essential fats, meaning the body cannot produce them, and they must be obtained through diet. These fats include omega-3 and omega-6 fatty acids, which have numerous health benefits, including reducing inflammation and supporting brain and heart health. Omega-3 fatty acids are especially beneficial for neck health, as they have been shown to help alleviate pain and inflammation in joints and muscles. Sources of omega-3 fatty acids include fatty fish like salmon, mackerel, and sardines, as well as flaxseeds, chia seeds, and walnuts. Omega-6 fatty acids can be found in vegetable oils such as soybean, corn, and sunflower oil, and are also present in nuts and seeds.

Saturated fats, found in animal products like red meat, butter, and full-fat dairy, as well as some plant-based oils like coconut and palm oil, should be consumed in moderation. While they are not inherently unhealthy, excessive consumption of saturated fats has been linked to increased levels of bad cholesterol and an elevated risk of heart disease.

Trans fats, also known as partially hydrogenated oils, are artificially produced fats that have been associated with various health problems, including inflammation, increased bad cholesterol levels, and a higher risk of heart disease. Trans fats can be found in some processed foods, baked goods, and fried foods. It is recommended to avoid or limit trans fat consumption as much as possible to support overall health, including neck health.

Maintaining a balance of healthy fats in one's diet can contribute to better neck health by reducing inflammation and supporting proper nerve function, hormone production, and tissue repair. By focusing on consuming unsaturated fats from sources like avocados, nuts, seeds, olive oil, and fatty fish, while limiting the intake of saturated and trans fats, individuals can promote optimal neck health and overall well-being.

Vitamin D, often referred to as the "sunshine vitamin," is a fat-soluble vitamin that is essential for maintaining bone health and plays a crucial role in calcium absorption. It helps the body maintain adequate levels of calcium and phosphate in the blood, which are necessary for normal bone mineralization, muscle function, and overall health. Inadequate vitamin D levels can lead to weakened bones and an increased risk of fractures, which can contribute to neck pain.

The human body can produce vitamin D through exposure to sunlight. Ultraviolet B (UVB) radiation from the sun converts a precursor molecule in the skin, called 7-dehydrocholesterol, into vitamin D3, also known as cholecalciferol. The liver and kidneys then convert vitamin D3 into its active form, calcitriol, which the body uses to regulate calcium and phosphate metabolism.

Vitamin D can also be obtained through dietary sources and supplements. Fatty fish, such as salmon, mackerel, and sardines, are natural sources of vitamin D. Fortified foods, such as milk, orange juice, yogurt, and breakfast cereals, provide additional dietary sources of vitamin D. Vitamin D supplements are available in two forms: vitamin D2 (ergocalciferol) and vitamin D3 (cholecalciferol). Research suggests that vitamin D3 may be more effective in raising and maintaining adequate blood levels of vitamin D compared to vitamin D2.

The recommended daily intake of vitamin D varies based on factors such as age, sex, and life stage. For most adults aged 19-70, the Recommended Dietary Allowance (RDA) is 600 International Units (IU) per day, while adults aged 71 and older require 800 IU per day. However, some experts argue that higher daily intakes may be necessary for optimal health, particularly for those with limited sun exposure or increased risk factors for vitamin D deficiency.

Vitamin D deficiency can result from inadequate sun exposure, limited dietary intake, or impaired absorption due to gastrointestinal disorders. Symptoms of deficiency may include muscle weakness, bone pain, and an increased risk of fractures. Severe vitamin D deficiency in children can lead to rickets, a condition characterized by soft, weak bones, while adults may develop osteomalacia, a similar condition marked by bone pain and muscle weakness.

It is essential to maintain adequate vitamin D levels to support neck health and overall well-being. However, it is also important not to exceed the Tolerable Upper Intake Level (UL) of vitamin D, which is set at 4,000 IU per day for adults. Excessive vitamin D intake can lead to toxicity, causing symptoms such as nausea, vomiting, constipation, and in severe cases, kidney damage and the formation of calcium deposits in soft tissues. To ensure optimal vitamin D status, individuals should aim to strike a balance between sun exposure, dietary intake, and supplementation as needed, under the guidance of a healthcare professional.

Calcium is a crucial mineral for maintaining strong bones and teeth, as it is the primary component of bone mineral. Adequate calcium intake is essential for preventing conditions such as osteoporosis, which can lead to an increased risk of fractures and neck pain. Osteoporosis is a condition characterized by a decrease in bone mass and density, leading to fragile bones and an increased risk of fractures. As the neck is composed of various bones and joints, maintaining optimal calcium levels can help support neck health and reduce the risk of injuries and pain.

Good sources of calcium include dairy products such as milk, yogurt, and cheese, which are considered some of the most bioavailable sources of calcium. For individuals who are lactose intolerant or prefer non-dairy options, leafy green vegetables like kale, bok choy, and broccoli are excellent alternatives. These vegetables also provide other essential nutrients, such as vitamins and minerals, which can further support overall health. Fortified cereals and plant-based milk alternatives, like almond milk and soy milk, can also be valuable sources of calcium for those who have dietary restrictions or preferences. Additionally, calcium-rich foods like sardines and salmon with bones, almonds, and tofu made with calcium sulfate can contribute to meeting daily calcium requirements.

Calcium supplements can be beneficial for individuals who have difficulty meeting their daily calcium requirements through diet alone. There are several types of calcium supplements available, with the most common being calcium carbonate and calcium citrate. Calcium carbonate is typically more cost-effective and has a higher percentage of elemental calcium, but it should be taken with food for optimal absorption. Calcium citrate, on the other hand, is absorbed more easily and can be taken with or without food. It is important to consult with a healthcare professional before starting a calcium supplement regimen to determine the appropriate type and dosage based on individual needs.

The recommended daily intake of calcium for adults ranges from 1000-1300 mg, depending on age and sex. Women aged 19-50 and men aged 19-70 should aim for 1000 mg of calcium daily, while women over 50 and men over 70 should increase their intake to 1200 mg daily. It is essential to note that consuming excessive amounts of calcium through supplements can lead to adverse effects, such as constipation, kidney stones, and impaired absorption of other minerals like iron and zinc. Therefore, it is crucial to balance calcium intake from both dietary sources and supplements while considering individual needs and tolerances.

Calcium is a vital mineral for maintaining strong bones and teeth, and adequate calcium intake is essential for preventing conditions like osteoporosis that can contribute to neck pain. Consuming a balanced diet rich in calcium sources such as dairy products, leafy green vegetables, fortified cereals, and supplements, if necessary, can help support optimal neck health and reduce the risk of fractures and pain.

Magnesium is a crucial mineral that is involved in over 300 biochemical reactions in the body, including those related to muscle and nerve function, energy production, and bone health. It plays a particularly important role in maintaining the proper balance of calcium and potassium, which are essential for healthy muscle contractions and nerve transmission. As such, adequate magnesium intake is vital for optimal neck health, as it can help prevent muscle cramps, spasms, and stiffness that may contribute to neck pain.

There are several factors that can lead to magnesium deficiency, including poor dietary intake, reduced absorption due to gastrointestinal disorders, and increased excretion due to certain medications or medical conditions. Symptoms of magnesium deficiency can include muscle cramps, spasms, and weakness, as well as fatigue, anxiety, and insomnia, all of which can exacerbate neck pain. Therefore, ensuring adequate magnesium intake is essential for individuals experiencing neck pain, as well as for overall health and well-being.

Magnesium can be obtained from a variety of dietary sources. Nuts, such as almonds, cashews, and peanuts, are particularly rich in magnesium, as are seeds like pumpkin seeds, sunflower seeds, and chia seeds. Legumes, including beans, lentils, and chickpeas, are also good sources of magnesium, providing not only the essential mineral but also fiber, protein, and other nutrients. Whole grains, such as quinoa, brown rice, and whole wheat, contain higher levels of magnesium compared to their refined counterparts, making them a healthier option for those looking to increase their magnesium intake. Additionally, leafy green vegetables, like spinach, kale, and Swiss chard, are rich in magnesium and provide a host of other vitamins and minerals, further supporting overall health.

The bioavailability of magnesium from different food sources can vary, with plant-based sources often containing compounds like phytic acid or oxalates, which can inhibit magnesium absorption. However, consuming a varied diet that includes a range of magnesium-rich foods can help ensure adequate intake and absorption of the mineral. It's worth noting that some factors, such as excessive alcohol consumption, high intake of caffeine or salt, and chronic stress, can interfere with magnesium absorption or increase its excretion, potentially leading to suboptimal levels of the mineral.

For individuals who may not be able to meet their magnesium needs through diet alone, supplementation can be an option. Magnesium supplements come in various forms, including magnesium citrate, magnesium oxide, and magnesium glycinate, with varying degrees of bioavailability and side effects. Magnesium citrate and magnesium glycinate are generally well-absorbed and well-tolerated, while magnesium oxide tends to have lower bioavailability and may cause gastrointestinal side effects in some individuals. It is essential to consult with a healthcare professional before starting any magnesium supplement to determine the appropriate form and dosage based on individual needs and health status.

Magnesium plays a critical role in muscle and nerve function, energy production, and bone health, making it an essential nutrient for optimal neck health. Ensuring adequate magnesium intake through a varied diet rich in nuts, seeds, legumes, whole grains, and leafy green vegetables can help prevent muscle cramps, spasms, and stiffness that may contribute to neck pain. In some cases, supplementation may be necessary to meet individual magnesium needs and should be done under the guidance of a healthcare professional.

Omega-3 fatty acids, particularly eicosapentaenoic acid (EPA) and docosahexaenoic acid (DHA), are essential for reducing inflammation and promoting overall health. These polyunsaturated fatty acids play a crucial role in maintaining cell membrane integrity, supporting brain function, and modulating immune system responses. They have been shown to have numerous health benefits, including supporting joint health, improving cardiovascular health, and reducing the risk of chronic diseases such as diabetes and Alzheimer's disease.

For individuals with neck pain, omega-3 fatty acids may help alleviate pain and inflammation by reducing the production of pro-inflammatory compounds known as cytokines and prostaglandins. Research has shown that omega-3 supplementation can lead to a significant reduction in pain and stiffness in individuals with various musculoskeletal conditions, including neck pain.

Good sources of omega-3 fatty acids include fatty fish such as salmon, mackerel, and sardines, which are particularly rich in EPA and DHA. Plant-based sources of omega-3 fatty acids, such as flaxseeds, chia seeds, and walnuts, primarily contain alpha-linolenic acid (ALA), which the body can convert into EPA and DHA, albeit with limited efficiency. To ensure adequate intake of EPA and DHA, it is recommended to consume a combination of both animal and plant-based sources of omega-3 fatty acids.

The American Heart Association recommends consuming at least two servings of fatty fish per week, equivalent to approximately 500 mg of EPA and DHA per day, to support cardiovascular health. For individuals with neck pain or other inflammatory conditions, higher doses of omega-3 fatty acids may be necessary to achieve optimal benefits. Some studies have suggested that doses of 1000-3000 mg of EPA and DHA per day can provide significant anti-inflammatory and pain-relieving effects.

When considering omega-3 supplementation, it is essential to choose high-quality products that have been third-party tested for purity and potency. Fish oil supplements are a common source of EPA and DHA, but it is crucial to select products that have been purified to remove potential contaminants such as heavy metals and environmental pollutants. Algae-based supplements are an alternative source of EPA and DHA for individuals who prefer a plant-based option or have concerns about fish-derived products.

Omega-3 fatty acids play a vital role in reducing inflammation and promoting overall health, making them a crucial component of a comprehensive approach to neck pain management. Ensuring adequate intake of omega-3 fatty acids through diet or supplementation can help alleviate pain and inflammation associated with neck pain, as well as support overall health and well-being.

Antioxidants are compounds that help neutralize free radicals, which are unstable molecules that can cause oxidative stress, leading to inflammation and tissue damage. Free radicals are produced naturally in the body as a byproduct of normal metabolic processes, but their production can also be increased by external factors such as pollution, smoking, and exposure to radiation. When the production of free radicals exceeds the body's ability to neutralize them, oxidative stress occurs, which can contribute to a variety of health issues, including neck pain and inflammation.

Consuming a diet rich in antioxidant-containing foods can support neck health by reducing inflammation, promoting tissue repair, and protecting against oxidative stress-induced damage. Antioxidants work by donating electrons to free radicals, thereby stabilizing them and preventing them from causing further damage. There are numerous types of antioxidants, each with unique properties and functions in the body.

Vitamin C, also known as ascorbic acid, is a water-soluble antioxidant that plays a crucial role in collagen synthesis, which is essential for maintaining healthy connective tissues in the neck. Good sources of vitamin C include citrus fruits, strawberries, kiwi, bell peppers, and broccoli. The recommended daily intake of vitamin C for adults ranges from 75-90 mg, depending on age and sex.

Vitamin E is a fat-soluble antioxidant that helps protect cell membranes from oxidative damage. It also plays a role in maintaining healthy immune function and reducing inflammation. Good sources of vitamin E include nuts, seeds, vegetable oils, and leafy green vegetables. The recommended daily intake of vitamin E for adults is 15 mg.

Polyphenols are a large group of antioxidants found in plant-based foods, such as fruits, vegetables, and whole grains. These compounds have been shown to possess anti-inflammatory, anti-cancer, and heart-protective properties. Examples of polyphenol-rich foods include berries, cherries, dark chocolate, green tea, and red wine. Although there is no specific recommended daily intake for polyphenols, consuming a diverse array of plant-based foods can help ensure adequate polyphenol intake.

Carotenoids, such as beta-carotene, lycopene, and lutein, are antioxidants found in colorful fruits and vegetables. These compounds have been shown to support eye health, reduce the risk of certain cancers, and protect against oxidative damage. Good sources of carotenoids include carrots, sweet potatoes, tomatoes, spinach, and kale. There is no specific recommended daily intake for carotenoids, but consuming a variety of colorful fruits and vegetables can help ensure adequate intake.

Antioxidants play a critical role in protecting the body from oxidative stress and reducing inflammation, which can contribute to neck pain and other health issues. Consuming a diet rich in antioxidant-containing foods, such as fruits, vegetables, nuts, seeds, and whole grains, can support neck health and promote overall well-being. Additionally, supplementing with specific antioxidants, such as vitamin C and E, may be beneficial for individuals who have difficulty obtaining adequate amounts through diet alone. As always, it is essential to consult with a healthcare professional before starting any supplement regimen.

Curcumin, a bioactive compound found in turmeric, has gained increasing attention for its anti-inflammatory and pain-relieving properties. Derived from the rhizomes of the Curcuma longa plant, turmeric has been used in traditional medicine for centuries, and recent scientific research supports its potential benefits for individuals experiencing neck pain.

The anti-inflammatory effects of curcumin can be attributed to its ability to inhibit key inflammatory pathways in the body, such as nuclear factor-kappa B (NF-$\varkappa$B) and cyclooxygenase-2 (COX-2). By suppressing these inflammatory mediators, curcumin can effectively reduce inflammation and promote healing in the neck tissues. This may be particularly beneficial for individuals with neck pain resulting from conditions such as cervical spondylosis, muscle strains, or soft tissue injuries.

In addition to its anti-inflammatory effects, curcumin has been shown to possess analgesic properties, which can help alleviate pain. Curcumin acts on multiple pain pathways, including the modulation of serotonin and dopamine levels in the brain, which are neurotransmitters involved in the perception of pain. This pain-relieving effect of curcumin can contribute to improved neck function and overall quality of life for individuals experiencing neck pain.

To reap the benefits of curcumin, it can be incorporated into the diet through the consumption of turmeric, which can be added to dishes such as curries, soups, and rice. However, the bioavailability of curcumin from dietary sources is relatively low due to its poor absorption and rapid metabolism. To overcome this limitation, curcumin can also be taken as a dietary supplement, which often contains higher concentrations of the active compound.

When supplementing with curcumin, it is essential to choose a product that includes black pepper extract, or specifically, piperine. Piperine is an alkaloid found in black pepper that has been shown to significantly enhance the absorption of curcumin by inhibiting its metabolism in the liver and increasing its bioavailability. Some curcumin supplements incorporate patented formulations that combine curcumin with piperine or other bioavailability-enhancing agents, such as phospholipids, to further improve the absorption of the active compound.

The optimal dosage of curcumin for neck pain relief has not been definitively established, as research studies have used varying doses and formulations. However, a general guideline is to take between 500-1500 mg of curcumin per day, divided into multiple doses. It is crucial to consult with a healthcare professional before starting a curcumin supplement regimen to determine the appropriate dosage based on individual needs and to monitor for potential interactions with medications or adverse effects.

Curcumin has shown promise as a natural anti-inflammatory and pain-relieving compound, with potential benefits for individuals experiencing neck pain. Incorporating curcumin into the diet through turmeric or supplementation can contribute to reduced inflammation and pain, promoting healing and improved neck function. Selecting a high-quality curcumin supplement with enhanced bioavailability and consulting with a healthcare professional for personalized recommendations is essential for maximizing the potential benefits of this powerful compound.

Bromelain is a proteolytic enzyme derived from the stem, fruit, and juice of the pineapple plant (Ananas comosus). It has gained attention in recent years for its anti-inflammatory and analgesic properties, which can potentially benefit individuals with neck pain.

The anti-inflammatory effects of bromelain are attributed to its ability to modulate the production of pro-inflammatory mediators such as prostaglandins and leukotrienes. By inhibiting these mediators, bromelain can help reduce inflammation and swelling, which can contribute to neck pain. Additionally, bromelain has been shown to improve blood circulation, which can promote healing and reduce pain in injured tissues.

Bromelain's analgesic properties stem from its ability to block the activity of specific pain-inducing molecules, such as bradykinin, which can contribute to the sensation of pain. By reducing the levels of these molecules, bromelain may help alleviate pain in individuals with neck discomfort.

Numerous studies have been conducted to evaluate the efficacy of bromelain in managing pain and inflammation. Some research has shown that bromelain may be as effective as non-steroidal anti-inflammatory drugs (NSAIDs) in reducing pain and inflammation, with fewer side effects. However, more research is needed to confirm these findings and establish optimal dosing guidelines.

Incorporating bromelain into the diet can be achieved through consuming pineapple, particularly the core, which contains the highest concentration of the enzyme. However, the amount of bromelain in dietary sources may not be sufficient to provide significant therapeutic benefits. Bromelain supplements are available in various forms, including capsules, tablets, and powders, and can provide a more concentrated source of the enzyme.

The typical dosage for bromelain supplements ranges from 500-1000 mg per day, divided into multiple doses. It is recommended to take bromelain supplements on an empty stomach to maximize absorption and effectiveness. While bromelain is generally considered safe, it may cause mild side effects such as gastrointestinal discomfort or allergic reactions in some individuals. It is also essential to note that bromelain can interact with certain medications, such as blood thinners, and should be used with caution in individuals taking these medications.

Bromelain is a promising natural supplement that may help reduce inflammation and pain in individuals with neck discomfort. While further research is needed to confirm its efficacy and establish optimal dosing guidelines, incorporating bromelain through dietary sources or supplementation may provide additional support for neck pain management. As always, it is essential to consult with a healthcare professional before starting any new supplement regimen, especially if taking medications or managing a medical condition.

Individual needs for nutritional supplements can vary widely due to several factors, making it essential to tailor supplement regimens to each person's unique circumstances. One crucial factor to consider is age, as nutritional requirements change throughout the lifespan. For example, older adults may have different needs for certain nutrients, such as vitamin D and calcium, to support bone health and prevent age-related bone loss. Similarly, younger individuals may require additional nutrients to support growth and development.

Sex is another factor to consider when determining individual needs for nutritional supplements. Men and women have different nutritional requirements, which can influence the types and amounts of supplements needed for optimal neck health. For instance, women of childbearing age may need more iron than men to account for losses during menstruation, while men may require more zinc for reproductive health.

Overall health is another significant factor in determining individual needs for nutritional supplements. Certain health conditions, such as autoimmune diseases or digestive disorders, can affect the body's ability to absorb and utilize nutrients, necessitating adjustments in supplementation. Additionally, individuals with chronic pain or inflammatory conditions may benefit from specific supplements that target inflammation and pain relief, such as curcumin or omega-3 fatty acids.

Specific nutritional deficiencies can also impact individual needs for supplementation. A healthcare professional can assess an individual's nutritional status through blood tests and dietary evaluations, identifying any deficiencies that may contribute to neck pain or other health issues. For example, a deficiency in vitamin D or magnesium may contribute to muscle weakness or spasms, potentially exacerbating neck pain. In such cases, targeted supplementation can help address the underlying deficiency and improve neck health.

Moreover, lifestyle factors can influence individual needs for nutritional supplements. Athletes or individuals with physically demanding occupations may require additional nutrients to support muscle repair and recovery, while sedentary individuals may need to focus on nutrients that support bone and joint health. Similarly, individuals who follow specific dietary patterns, such as vegans or those on a restricted calorie diet, may require supplementation to ensure adequate intake of essential nutrients.

Given the numerous factors that can influence individual needs for nutritional supplements, it is crucial to consult with a healthcare professional before starting any supplement regimen. A healthcare professional can help determine the appropriate supplements and dosages based on an individual's unique circumstances and provide guidance on potential interactions with medications or other supplements. By tailoring supplementation to individual needs, individuals can better support their neck health and overall well-being.

Ensuring the quality and safety of dietary supplements is a critical aspect of their effectiveness and potential benefits to neck health. With the vast array of supplement manufacturers and products on the market, it is crucial to carefully consider the source of the supplements and the standards by which they are produced.

One significant concern regarding the quality of dietary supplements is that they are not as strictly regulated as pharmaceutical drugs. The U.S. Food and Drug Administration (FDA) does not require pre-market approval for dietary supplements. As a result, manufacturers are responsible for ensuring the safety and efficacy of their products. This self-regulation can lead to inconsistencies in quality and potential risks to consumers.

To ensure that you are selecting high-quality supplements, it is essential to look for products from reputable manufacturers with a demonstrated commitment to quality and safety. Some ways to verify the quality of supplements include researching the company's manufacturing processes, sourcing of raw materials, and any certifications or seals of approval they have received.

Third-party testing is a valuable tool for verifying the quality and purity of dietary supplements. Independent laboratories can test supplements for the presence of contaminants, such as heavy metals, pesticides, and harmful bacteria, as well as confirm that the product contains the stated ingredients and amounts. Reputable supplement manufacturers often use third-party testing to validate their products and may display certification seals or logos on their packaging. Look for products that have been tested by organizations such as NSF International, United States Pharmacopeia (USP), or ConsumerLab.

In addition to selecting high-quality supplements, it is crucial to follow the recommended dosages provided by the manufacturer or a healthcare professional. Overconsumption of certain nutrients can lead to adverse effects, and in some cases, toxicity. It is also essential to consider any potential interactions between supplements and prescription medications, as well as the individual's overall health status.

Consulting with a healthcare professional before starting any supplement regimen is advisable, particularly for individuals with pre-existing medical conditions or who are taking prescription medications. Healthcare professionals can provide guidance on the appropriate supplements and dosages based on individual needs and help monitor for any potential adverse effects.

Ensuring the quality and safety of dietary supplements is critical for their effectiveness and potential benefits to neck health. By selecting products from reputable manufacturers that have been third-party tested for quality and purity, following the recommended dosages, and consulting with a healthcare professional, individuals can make informed decisions about incorporating supplements into their neck health regimen.

In conclusion, optimal nutrition plays a crucial role in maintaining neck health and managing neck pain. A well-balanced diet consisting of essential nutrients can support the musculoskeletal system and improve overall health. By incorporating proteins, carbohydrates, and healthy fats, individuals can provide the necessary building blocks for muscle, bone, and joint health. Additionally, vitamins and minerals such as vitamin D, calcium, and magnesium are essential for maintaining strong bones and supporting proper muscle and nerve function.

Furthermore, consuming foods rich in antioxidants, such as fruits and vegetables, can help reduce inflammation, which is often a contributing factor to neck pain. Specific compounds, such as curcumin found in turmeric and bromelain found in pineapple, have been shown to possess anti-inflammatory and pain-relieving properties. Including these natural compounds in one's diet or as supplements may offer additional benefits for those dealing with neck pain and inflammation.

When considering the use of supplements, it is essential to recognize that individual needs may vary due to factors such as age, sex, overall health, and specific nutritional deficiencies. Before starting any supplement regimen, it is crucial to consult with a healthcare professional who can assess individual needs and recommend the most appropriate supplements and dosages. This personalized approach can help ensure that individuals receive the necessary nutrients to support their neck health and manage pain effectively.

Moreover, it is vital to select high-quality, third-party tested supplements to ensure their safety and efficacy. The supplement industry is not tightly regulated, and the quality of products can vary widely. Choosing supplements from reputable manufacturers and those that have undergone third-party testing can help ensure that individuals receive safe and effective products.

Incorporating essential nutrients and targeted nutritional support into one's daily routine can have a significant impact on neck health and overall quality of life. By focusing on proper nutrition and, when necessary, supplementation, individuals can better manage neck pain, promote healing, and support the overall health of their musculoskeletal system. This holistic approach to neck health can not only alleviate current symptoms but also aid in the prevention of future issues, ultimately leading to improved well-being and a more active, pain-free lifestyle.

Chapter 19

Preventive Strategies for Neck Pain

Proactive Measures to Avoid Future Issues

Neck pain is a pervasive problem that affects people of all ages and backgrounds. It can significantly impact an individual's quality of life, limit mobility, and result in missed work or social activities. Prevention is key to avoiding the negative consequences associated with neck pain. This chapter will outline evidence-based preventive strategies that can be implemented to minimize the risk of developing neck pain, as well as proactive measures to manage existing neck pain and prevent it from worsening.

Physical risk factors for neck pain encompass a variety of elements, each of which can contribute to discomfort and strain in the neck. Gaining a deeper understanding of these risk factors can empower individuals to take appropriate steps to mitigate their impact on neck health.

Poor posture is a significant contributor to neck pain. Slouching, forward head posture, and rounded shoulders can place excessive strain on the neck muscles and cervical spine. Over time, this can lead to muscle imbalances, pain, and even degenerative changes in the spine. Proper posture involves maintaining the natural curves of the spine, with the head aligned over the shoulders, the chest open, and the shoulders relaxed and pulled back. By consciously practicing good posture throughout daily activities, individuals can minimize the risk of neck pain related to postural imbalances.

Muscle imbalances, another critical physical risk factor for neck pain, can result from a combination of weak and overactive muscles. For example, tight chest muscles and weak upper back muscles can contribute to rounded shoulders and increased neck strain. To address muscle imbalances, individuals should engage in a well-rounded exercise program that targets both strengthening and stretching exercises for the neck, shoulders, and upper back. This approach can help restore muscular balance, promote proper posture, and reduce the risk of neck pain.

Lack of exercise can also contribute to neck pain by weakening the muscles that support the cervical spine and reducing overall flexibility. A sedentary lifestyle can lead to stiff, weak muscles that are more susceptible to injury and strain. Engaging in regular physical activity, including aerobic exercise, resistance training, and flexibility exercises, can help maintain muscle strength, improve posture, and reduce the risk of neck pain. Moreover, exercise has been shown to have additional benefits, such as improved mental well-being and reduced stress, which can further contribute to preventing neck pain.

Repetitive strain is another physical risk factor that can contribute to neck pain. Activities that involve repeated neck movements or maintaining the neck in a fixed position for extended periods, such as working on a computer or using a smartphone, can lead to muscle fatigue and strain. To minimize the risk of neck pain associated with repetitive strain, individuals should take regular breaks from these activities, perform gentle neck stretches, and ensure their workspace is set up ergonomically to support proper posture.

Understanding and addressing physical risk factors for neck pain, such as poor posture, muscle imbalances, lack of exercise, and repetitive strain, are crucial for maintaining neck health. By implementing proactive strategies to mitigate these risk factors, individuals can reduce their likelihood of experiencing neck pain and improve their overall well-being.

Occupational risk factors for neck pain encompass a variety of work-related activities and conditions that can contribute to the development of neck pain. Understanding these factors is crucial for both workers and employers, as it enables them to implement appropriate preventive measures to reduce the risk of neck pain in the workplace.

Sedentary work, such as desk jobs that require prolonged sitting, is a significant occupational risk factor for neck pain. Extended periods of sitting can lead to poor posture, muscle imbalances, and increased strain on the neck and shoulders. Workers in sedentary occupations should be encouraged to take regular breaks to stand, walk, and stretch throughout the day. Employers can support this by providing adjustable workstations that allow for standing or sitting and encouraging short, frequent breaks for stretching and movement.

Heavy manual labor can also contribute to the risk of neck pain, as it often involves repetitive movements, heavy lifting, and awkward postures that can place strain on the neck and surrounding muscles. Workers in occupations that require heavy manual labor should be trained in proper lifting techniques, body mechanics, and ergonomics to minimize the risk of neck injury. Employers can also provide appropriate equipment, such as lifting aids, to assist workers in safely performing their duties and reducing strain on the neck.

Prolonged use of electronic devices, including computers and smartphones, is another significant occupational risk factor for neck pain. The repetitive motions and postures associated with these devices, such as tilting the head forward to view screens or cradling a phone between the ear and shoulder, can place excessive strain on the neck muscles and cervical spine. Workers should be encouraged to maintain proper posture while using electronic devices, positioning screens at eye level and using hands-free devices for phone calls. Employers can also provide ergonomic

377

accessories, such as monitor stands and headset devices, to support workers in maintaining proper posture while using electronic devices.

In addition to these specific risk factors, the overall work environment can play a role in the development of neck pain. High levels of stress, lack of social support, and limited opportunities for physical activity can all contribute to the risk of neck pain in the workplace. Employers can address these factors by fostering a supportive work culture, providing resources for stress management, and encouraging physical activity during breaks or after work hours.

By raising awareness of occupational risk factors for neck pain and implementing appropriate preventive measures, workers and employers can work together to create a healthier work environment and reduce the risk of neck pain associated with various occupational activities.

Psychological risk factors for neck pain are essential to address, as they can significantly impact the development or exacerbation of neck pain. Stress, anxiety, depression, and poor coping strategies are among the most common psychological risk factors. By understanding the role these factors play in neck pain and taking proactive steps to address them, individuals can improve their overall mental health and reduce their risk of neck pain.

Stress is a common psychological factor that contributes to neck pain. When an individual experiences stress, the body responds by releasing stress hormones, such as cortisol and adrenaline. These hormones can cause an increase in muscle tension, particularly in the neck and shoulders, leading to discomfort and pain. Prolonged stress can result in chronic muscle tension, which can exacerbate neck pain and contribute to the development of more severe conditions, such as cervical spine degeneration. Managing stress through relaxation techniques, time management, and social support can help reduce the impact of stress on neck pain.

Anxiety, like stress, can also contribute to neck pain. Individuals with anxiety disorders often experience muscle tension, as the body remains in a heightened state of arousal. This prolonged muscle tension can lead to neck pain and other musculoskeletal issues. Addressing anxiety through professional help, such as therapy or medication, can be a crucial step in reducing the impact of anxiety on neck pain. Additionally, incorporating relaxation techniques and regular exercise into daily routines can help alleviate anxiety and improve overall mental health.

Depression can also play a role in the development or exacerbation of neck pain. Individuals with depression may experience a range of physical symptoms, including muscle aches and pains. This can be due to increased muscle tension, as well as the impact of depression on an individual's ability to engage in regular exercise and self-care. Treating depression through therapy, medication, and lifestyle changes can help reduce the impact of depression on neck pain and improve overall well-being.

Poor coping strategies, such as negative self-talk, avoidance, and rumination, can contribute to the psychological factors that exacerbate neck pain. These maladaptive coping strategies can perpetuate a cycle of pain and psychological distress, making it difficult for individuals to manage their neck pain effectively. Developing healthy coping strategies, such as cognitive restructuring, problem-solving, and seeking social support, can help individuals better manage their psychological risk factors and reduce the impact of neck pain on their daily lives.

Addressing psychological risk factors for neck pain is essential for effective prevention and management. Stress, anxiety, depression, and poor coping strategies can all contribute to the development or exacerbation of neck pain. By recognizing and addressing these psychological factors, individuals can improve their mental health and reduce their risk of neck pain. Incorporating relaxation techniques, seeking professional help, and developing healthy coping strategies can all play a crucial role in mitigating the impact of psychological risk factors on neck pain.

Maintaining proper sitting posture is essential for preventing neck pain, particularly for individuals who spend long hours sitting at a desk. Proper sitting posture involves several key components that, when combined, help to support the natural curvature of the spine and reduce strain on the neck and surrounding muscles.

One important aspect of proper sitting posture is keeping the head aligned over the shoulders. This alignment helps to reduce the strain on the cervical spine and minimize the risk of developing neck pain. Frequently leaning forward or tilting the head to one side can cause muscle imbalances and strain, leading to discomfort and pain. To maintain proper head alignment, it is crucial to position the computer monitor at eye level, which allows the user to look straight ahead without tilting the head up or down.

In addition to proper head alignment, maintaining a neutral spine is another crucial component of proper sitting posture. A neutral spine refers to the natural curvature of the spine when it is not flexed or extended. This alignment provides optimal support for the head, neck, and back, minimizing strain and reducing the risk of neck pain. To maintain a neutral spine while sitting, it is important to use an ergonomic chair that offers adjustable lumbar support. This support should follow the natural curve of the lower back, providing additional support and preventing slouching or hunching.

Keeping the feet flat on the floor is also essential for maintaining proper sitting posture. This positioning helps to distribute body weight evenly and reduces the strain on the lower back and neck. When the feet are not flat on the floor, it can lead to an imbalance in weight distribution, causing additional stress on the spine and neck muscles. If necessary, a footrest can be used to ensure that the feet are adequately supported.

Another aspect of proper sitting posture is positioning the arms and shoulders correctly. The arms should be bent at a 90-degree angle, with the forearms resting on the desk or armrests. This positioning helps to minimize strain on the shoulders and neck by reducing the need for the muscles to support the weight of the arms. Additionally, the shoulders should be relaxed and not hunched or elevated, as this can contribute to muscle tension and neck pain.

Maintaining proper sitting posture is crucial for preventing neck pain, especially for individuals who spend long periods sitting at a desk. By focusing on key components, such as head alignment, neutral spine, foot placement, and arm positioning, individuals can significantly reduce the strain on their neck and surrounding muscles, minimizing the risk of developing neck pain. Ergonomic chairs with adjustable lumbar support and other workspace adjustments can also play a vital role in promoting proper sitting posture and preventing neck pain.

Adjusting the workspace to promote proper posture is a vital preventive measure for neck pain. A well-designed workspace can help individuals maintain correct body alignment, reducing strain on the neck and shoulders. When setting up a workspace, several factors should be considered, including the positioning of the computer monitor, the use of document holders, and the arrangement of frequently used items.

The positioning of the computer monitor plays a crucial role in maintaining proper head and neck posture. Ideally, the monitor should be placed at eye level, allowing the individual to maintain a neutral head position without tilting the head up or down. This positioning helps reduce strain on the cervical spine and the surrounding muscles. To achieve the appropriate height, monitor stands or adjustable monitor arms can be used. Additionally, the monitor should be placed at a comfortable viewing distance, generally around an arm's length away. This distance can help prevent eye strain and encourage proper posture.

Using a document holder can also aid in preventing neck pain by keeping paperwork at eye level, eliminating the need to constantly look down and strain the neck. Document holders come in various styles, such as freestanding holders, clip-on holders that attach to the side of the monitor, or inline holders that sit between the keyboard and the monitor. By selecting an appropriate document holder, individuals can maintain a neutral head and neck position while reading or referencing printed materials.

The arrangement of frequently used items in the workspace can also impact neck and shoulder strain. Placing essential items, such as the telephone, stapler, or reference materials, within easy reach can minimize the need for excessive reaching or twisting, which can strain the neck and shoulders. Additionally, using a headset or speakerphone for telephone calls can help prevent the habit of cradling the phone between the ear and shoulder, which can contribute to neck pain.

Other workspace adjustments can further reduce the risk of neck pain. For example, using an ergonomic keyboard and mouse can promote proper wrist and hand positioning, reducing strain on the upper extremities and, by extension, the neck and shoulders. Ensuring that the chair is properly adjusted with appropriate lumbar support can also contribute to maintaining a neutral spine and reducing the risk of neck pain.

Making purposeful workspace adjustments can significantly contribute to the prevention of neck pain. Ensuring the proper positioning of the computer monitor, utilizing document holders, and arranging frequently used items within easy reach can minimize strain on the neck and shoulders. By creating an ergonomic and well-organized workspace, individuals can promote proper posture, reduce muscle strain, and ultimately prevent neck pain.

In recent years, smartphone use has become an integral part of daily life for many people, but prolonged use has also been linked to increased neck pain. This is mainly due to the forward head posture typically adopted during smartphone use, which places significant strain on the neck muscles and cervical spine. When the head is tilted forward, even at a slight angle, the gravitational forces acting on the neck increase dramatically, leading to muscle strain, disc compression, and potential nerve irritation.

To minimize the risk of neck pain associated with smartphone use, it is essential to maintain proper posture while using these devices. Holding smartphones at eye level can help prevent the need to tilt the head forward, reducing the strain on the neck muscles and cervical spine. This might require adjusting arm positions or using smartphone stands or holders that elevate the device to a more suitable height.

Taking frequent breaks from smartphone use is another crucial preventive measure. By practicing the 20-20-20 rule, which involves looking at an object 20 feet away for 20 seconds every 20 minutes, individuals can give their neck muscles a chance to relax and recover from the strain caused by prolonged smartphone use. Additionally, setting time limits on smartphone use and engaging in other activities that do not require screen time can help maintain healthy neck posture.

Performing neck stretches throughout the day can also help alleviate the muscle tension and stiffness associated with prolonged smartphone use. Simple stretches, such as gently tilting the head side to side or rotating the head in a circular motion, can help maintain flexibility and relieve muscle tension in the neck. It is essential to perform these stretches slowly and gently to avoid causing further strain or injury.

Finally, incorporating strengthening exercises targeting the neck and upper back muscles into a regular workout routine can help build the muscular endurance necessary to maintain proper posture during smartphone use. By strengthening the muscles responsible for maintaining proper head and neck alignment, individuals can reduce the strain and fatigue that contribute to neck pain associated with prolonged smartphone use.

Adopting proper posture, taking breaks, performing neck stretches, and engaging in regular strengthening exercises are all essential strategies for preventing neck pain associated with smartphone use. By incorporating these practices into daily routines, individuals can reduce the risk of developing neck pain and promote overall neck health.

Performing regular strengthening exercises for the neck, shoulders, and upper back is crucial in preventing neck pain by improving muscle balance and posture. These exercises can help support the cervical spine, reducing strain and pressure on the neck structures. Furthermore, strengthening exercises can correct muscle imbalances, where certain muscles become overactive, and others become underactive, leading to poor posture and increased risk of injury.

Dumbbell shrugs are an effective exercise for targeting the upper trapezius muscles, which are essential for stabilizing the shoulder blades and supporting the neck. To perform dumbbell shrugs, hold a dumbbell in each hand with the arms hanging by your sides and your palms facing your body. Slowly lift your shoulders toward your ears, pause for a moment, and then lower your shoulders back down to the starting position. Maintaining proper form and control throughout the movement is essential to ensure the effectiveness of the exercise and prevent injury.

Lateral raises are another valuable resistance training exercise that targets the middle deltoids and helps strengthen the shoulder muscles, providing additional support to the neck. To perform lateral raises, hold a dumbbell in each hand with your arms by your sides and your palms facing your body. Keeping your elbows slightly bent, slowly raise your arms out to the sides until they are parallel to the floor, forming a T shape with your body. Pause for a moment at the top of the movement, and then slowly lower your arms back to the starting position.

Seated rows are an effective exercise for targeting the muscles in the upper back, including the rhomboids, latissimus dorsi, and middle trapezius. These muscles play a crucial role in maintaining proper posture and supporting the neck. To perform seated rows, sit on a rowing machine or use a cable machine with a horizontal bar attachment. Grasp the bar with an overhand grip, and pull the bar towards your chest while keeping your elbows close to your body. Squeeze your shoulder blades together at the end of the movement, and then slowly release the tension and return to the starting position.

In addition to these exercises, incorporating exercises that target the deep neck flexors, such as chin tucks and neck flexion exercises, can help improve neck stability and reduce the risk of neck pain. It is essential to perform these strengthening exercises regularly, ideally two to three times per week, and to progress the intensity and volume of the exercises gradually to ensure continued improvements in muscle strength and endurance.

It is also crucial to consult with a healthcare professional, such as a physical therapist or exercise physiologist, before beginning a strengthening program, particularly for individuals with existing neck pain or other health conditions. These professionals can provide personalized guidance on proper exercise technique and appropriate exercise progression to maximize the benefits of the strengthening program and minimize the risk of injury.

Incorporating regular flexibility exercises into a workout routine can contribute to the maintenance of a healthy range of motion in the neck, as well as the prevention of stiffness and pain. Flexibility exercises targeting the neck and surrounding muscles can help reduce muscle imbalances and alleviate tension, resulting in decreased discomfort and enhanced overall neck function.

Neck tilts are a simple yet effective exercise that can be performed to stretch the muscles on the sides of the neck. To perform a neck tilt, sit or stand with a straight posture and slowly tilt the head to one side, bringing the ear towards the shoulder. Hold this position for 15-30 seconds and then return to the starting position. Repeat the process on the other side. It is important to maintain a gentle stretch throughout the exercise and avoid forcing the head past its comfortable range of motion.

Neck rotations can help improve the flexibility of the neck by targeting the muscles responsible for turning the head. To perform a neck rotation, sit or stand with proper posture and slowly turn the head to one side, bringing the chin towards the shoulder. Hold this position for 15-30 seconds and then return to the starting position. Repeat the process on the opposite side. As with neck tilts, it is essential to maintain a gentle stretch and avoid forcing the head beyond its comfortable range of motion.

Shoulder rolls can help alleviate tension in the neck and upper back by targeting the trapezius and levator scapulae muscles. To perform shoulder rolls, sit or stand with proper posture and slowly roll the shoulders in a circular motion, moving them up, back, down, and forward. Perform 10-15 repetitions in one direction and then reverse the direction for another 10-15 repetitions. This exercise should be executed with control and smooth movements, avoiding any jerking or rapid motions that could strain the muscles.

Chin tucks are another useful flexibility exercise that can help strengthen and stretch the muscles responsible for maintaining proper neck alignment. To perform a chin tuck, sit or stand with a straight posture and gently pull the chin straight back, creating a double chin. Hold this position for 3-5 seconds and then return to the starting position. Repeat this process for 10-15 repetitions. Chin tucks can help improve posture by targeting the deep neck flexors, which are often weakened in individuals with neck pain.

In addition to these targeted exercises, incorporating general upper body stretches, such as chest openers and upper back stretches, can help improve overall flexibility and reduce muscle tension that contributes to neck pain. It is important to perform flexibility exercises with care and proper technique to avoid overstretching or straining the muscles. Consultation with a healthcare professional, such as a physical therapist, can help ensure that these exercises are executed safely and effectively for optimal neck health.

Aerobic exercise, also known as cardiovascular exercise, involves the use of large muscle groups in a rhythmic and continuous manner, which increases heart rate and improves oxygen consumption. Engaging in regular aerobic exercise has been shown to help prevent neck pain by promoting overall physical fitness, reducing stress, and improving muscle function.

Walking is a low-impact aerobic activity that is easily accessible and can be tailored to suit an individual's fitness level. Regular walking can help improve cardiovascular health, increase circulation, and promote muscle relaxation, which can aid in the prevention of neck pain. Moreover, walking encourages proper posture and alignment, reducing the risk of developing musculoskeletal issues that may contribute to neck pain.

Swimming is another low-impact aerobic exercise that can be particularly beneficial for those with neck pain or those looking to prevent it. As a full-body workout, swimming helps to strengthen muscles throughout the body, including those in the neck and upper back, which can provide support and stability to the cervical spine. The buoyancy of water also alleviates the impact on joints, making swimming an ideal exercise for individuals with joint issues or those recovering from injury.

Cycling, whether outdoors or on a stationary bike, offers an effective aerobic workout that can help prevent neck pain. Regular cycling can improve cardiovascular health, strengthen lower body muscles, and promote overall physical fitness. When cycling, it is important to maintain proper posture, with the neck in a neutral position and the shoulders relaxed, to minimize the risk of strain and discomfort. Additionally, adjusting the bike's seat and handlebars to the appropriate height can help maintain proper body alignment and reduce the risk of neck pain.

The incorporation of aerobic exercise into a regular fitness routine can also help alleviate stress and anxiety, which are known contributors to neck pain. Exercise stimulates the release of endorphins, the body's natural painkillers and mood elevators, which can help to reduce stress levels and promote relaxation. By effectively managing stress, individuals may experience a decrease in muscle tension in the neck and shoulders, reducing the likelihood of developing neck pain.

Aerobic exercise, such as walking, swimming, and cycling, plays a vital role in preventing neck pain by promoting overall physical fitness, reducing stress, and improving muscle function. To maximize the benefits of aerobic exercise, individuals should aim to engage in at least 150 minutes of moderate-intensity aerobic activity or 75 minutes of vigorous-intensity aerobic activity per week, as recommended by the American College of Sports Medicine and the American Heart Association. By incorporating aerobic exercise into a regular fitness routine, individuals can significantly reduce their risk of developing neck pain and improve their overall health and well-being.

Sleep position plays a crucial role in maintaining neck health, as the position we adopt while sleeping can either alleviate or exacerbate existing neck pain or contribute to the development of new pain. Optimal sleep positions aim to maintain the natural curve of the cervical spine, avoiding undue stress on the neck muscles, ligaments, and vertebrae.

Sleeping on the back, also known as the supine position, is considered one of the best sleep positions for promoting proper neck alignment. When lying in this position, a supportive pillow should be used to maintain the natural curve of the neck, without lifting the head too high or allowing it to drop too low. Memory foam pillows or cervical roll pillows can be particularly helpful for back sleepers, as they contour to the shape of the neck and provide consistent support throughout the night. Additionally, placing a small pillow under the knees can help maintain the natural curve of the lower back, promoting spinal alignment and reducing the risk of neck pain.

Side sleeping is another suitable sleep position for maintaining neck health. However, it is crucial to choose a pillow with the appropriate height and firmness to support the head and neck properly while sleeping on the side. The pillow should fill the gap between the shoulder and head, preventing the neck from tilting too far up or down. A contoured pillow or one with adjustable loft can be beneficial for side sleepers, ensuring proper support and alignment. Similar to back sleeping, placing a pillow between the knees can help align the hips and spine, reducing the risk of neck pain and discomfort.

Stomach sleeping should be avoided, as it forces the neck to rotate and extend to one side, placing strain on the muscles, ligaments, and vertebrae of the cervical spine. This unnatural position can lead to muscle imbalances, joint irritation, and nerve compression, increasing the risk of neck pain, stiffness, and discomfort. For individuals who struggle to change their sleep position, using a thin, low-loft pillow or no pillow at all can help minimize the strain on the neck while sleeping on the stomach. Placing a small pillow under the pelvis can also help maintain spinal alignment and reduce the risk of neck pain in stomach sleepers.

The sleep position plays a significant role in maintaining neck health and preventing neck pain. Adopting appropriate sleep positions, such as sleeping on the back or side, along with using a supportive pillow that maintains the natural curve of the neck, can significantly reduce the risk of developing neck pain and discomfort. Avoiding stomach sleeping and making necessary adjustments for those who struggle to change their sleep position can also contribute to better neck health and overall well-being.

Pillow selection plays a crucial role in promoting proper neck alignment and preventing neck pain during sleep. The ideal pillow should support the natural curve of the neck, maintain the spine's neutral alignment, and distribute pressure evenly across the head and neck. When selecting a pillow, individuals should consider their preferred sleep position, pillow materials, and the pillow's adjustability to ensure optimal support and comfort.

For back sleepers, it is essential to choose a pillow that supports the natural curve of the neck without causing the head to tilt too far forward or backward. A pillow that is too high or too low can lead to strain on the neck muscles and cervical spine, increasing the risk of neck pain. A contoured or cervical pillow with a lower central area and elevated sides can provide adequate support for the neck and maintain proper alignment. Memory foam or latex pillows that conform to the head and neck's shape can also be a good option for back sleepers, as they can help maintain the spine's neutral position.

Side sleepers require a pillow that fills the space between the head and the mattress while keeping the neck aligned with the spine. A higher pillow with a firm or medium-firm fill is typically recommended for side sleepers, as it can provide the necessary support and prevent the head from tilting downward. Memory foam, latex, or adjustable-fill pillows can be suitable options for side sleepers, as they can be shaped to provide optimal support for the neck and maintain proper spinal alignment.

Stomach sleepers should avoid using a thick or firm pillow, as this can force the neck into an unnatural position and increase the risk of neck pain. A thin or soft pillow, or no pillow at all, is recommended for stomach sleepers to minimize strain on the neck. However, stomach sleeping is not recommended in general, as it can lead to neck pain and other spinal issues.

Pillow materials can also impact neck support and comfort during sleep. Memory foam pillows are known for their ability to contour to the head and neck, providing customized support and pressure relief. Latex pillows offer similar contouring properties, with added durability and breathability. Down and feather pillows are soft and moldable but may require frequent fluffing to maintain their shape and support. Synthetic fill pillows, such as polyester, can be a more affordable option but may not provide the same level of support and durability as other materials.

Finally, adjustable-fill pillows, such as those filled with shredded memory foam, microbeads, or buckwheat hulls, can be customized to suit an individual's unique support and comfort preferences. By adding or removing fill, users can create the ideal pillow height and firmness to maintain proper neck alignment and prevent neck pain.

Selecting the right pillow is crucial for maintaining proper neck alignment during sleep and preventing neck pain. Individuals should consider their sleep position, pillow materials, and adjustability when choosing a pillow to ensure optimal support and comfort. A well-chosen pillow can contribute significantly to a restful night's sleep and promote overall neck health.

A supportive mattress that maintains proper spinal alignment is crucial for preventing neck pain. The ideal mattress should conform to the natural curves of the body, providing support to the head, neck, and spine, while also offering pressure relief for areas like the hips and shoulders. A medium-firm mattress is generally recommended for most individuals, as it provides the right balance of support and comfort. However, the optimal firmness level may vary depending on an individual's body type, sleep position, and personal preferences.

When selecting a mattress, it is essential to consider factors such as the mattress material, construction, and personal comfort preferences. Memory foam and latex mattresses are known for their contouring properties, which can help maintain proper spinal alignment by evenly distributing body weight and reducing pressure points. Innerspring mattresses, on the other hand, may provide more support but can sometimes create pressure points that lead to discomfort and poor sleep quality.

In addition to the mattress type, it is important to consider the overall construction and quality of the mattress. High-quality materials and craftsmanship can contribute to the longevity and support of a mattress. A well-constructed mattress will maintain its supportive qualities over time, whereas a poorly constructed mattress may quickly lose its shape and support, leading to increased neck pain and discomfort.

Regularly rotating and flipping a mattress, if applicable, can help maintain its supportive qualities by promoting even wear and preventing sagging. This can be particularly important for innerspring mattresses, which may be more prone to developing indentations and uneven wear over time. It is generally recommended to rotate a mattress every three to six months, although the frequency may vary depending on the mattress type and the manufacturer's recommendations.

Replacing a mattress when it no longer provides adequate support is another crucial aspect of maintaining proper spinal alignment and preventing neck pain. The lifespan of a mattress can vary depending on the type, quality, and use, but most mattresses should be replaced every 7-10 years. Signs that a mattress may need to be replaced include visible sagging, lumps or indentations, increased discomfort, and worsening sleep quality.

Selecting the right mattress is a crucial component of maintaining proper spinal alignment and preventing neck pain. The ideal mattress should provide a balance of support and comfort, conform to the natural curves of the body, and maintain its supportive qualities over time. By regularly rotating and replacing a mattress as needed, individuals can promote proper spinal alignment and minimize the risk of developing neck pain related to poor sleep posture and unsupportive sleep surfaces.

Relaxation techniques are essential tools in managing stress and preventing the muscle tension that contributes to neck pain. By incorporating these techniques into daily routines, individuals can promote relaxation and improve overall mental well-being, reducing the risk of stress-related neck pain. Various relaxation techniques can be employed, each with distinct benefits and approaches.

Deep breathing exercises are an effective method for promoting relaxation and reducing stress. These exercises involve slow, controlled breaths that help activate the body's relaxation response by stimulating the parasympathetic nervous system. One example of deep breathing is diaphragmatic breathing, where individuals focus on inhaling deeply through the nose, allowing the diaphragm to expand and the abdomen to rise, followed by exhaling slowly through the mouth. Practicing deep breathing exercises regularly can help reduce stress, lower heart rate, and decrease muscle tension, all of which can contribute to neck pain relief.

Progressive muscle relaxation (PMR) is another relaxation technique that focuses on systematically tensing and relaxing various muscle groups in the body. PMR can be particularly beneficial for individuals experiencing muscle tension and neck pain, as it helps increase awareness of muscle tension and teaches individuals how to release it effectively. To practice PMR, individuals start by tensing a specific muscle group, such as the muscles in the neck and shoulders, for a few seconds before releasing the tension and focusing on the sensation of relaxation. This process is repeated for various muscle groups throughout the body. Regular practice of PMR can lead to improved muscle relaxation and reduced neck pain.

Meditation is a mind-body practice that can help individuals cultivate a sense of relaxation, focus, and inner peace. There are various forms of meditation, such as mindfulness meditation, loving-kindness meditation, and body scan meditation, each with unique techniques and objectives. For example, mindfulness meditation involves focusing on the present moment non-judgmentally, observing thoughts and emotions as they arise and pass without becoming attached to them. Practicing meditation regularly has been shown to reduce stress, improve emotional well-being, and promote relaxation. By incorporating meditation into daily routines, individuals can better manage stress and reduce muscle tension, potentially alleviating neck pain.

In addition to these relaxation techniques, individuals can also explore other stress reduction practices such as yoga, tai chi, or guided imagery. These practices incorporate elements of both physical movement and mental focus, helping to relieve stress and promote relaxation. By exploring various relaxation techniques and incorporating them into daily routines, individuals can effectively manage stress and reduce the risk of stress-related neck pain.

Effective time management is essential in minimizing stress and reducing the risk of neck pain. By organizing tasks and efficiently allocating time, individuals can alleviate the physical and psychological strain that often results from long periods of focused work. Implementing various time management strategies can help in achieving a balanced workload and prevent stress-induced muscle tension in the neck.

One essential aspect of time management is setting priorities. By identifying the most important tasks and focusing on their completion, individuals can ensure that their time and energy are directed towards meaningful goals. This approach can help reduce feelings of overwhelm and anxiety, which often contribute to muscle tension in the neck and shoulders. Additionally, breaking larger tasks into smaller, manageable steps can provide a clear roadmap for achieving goals and prevent the stress associated with seemingly insurmountable tasks.

Establishing realistic goals is another crucial component of effective time management. Overcommitting and setting unrealistic expectations can lead to increased stress and frustration, which can exacerbate neck pain. By setting achievable goals and periodically reassessing progress, individuals can maintain motivation and reduce the risk of stress-related muscle tension. Recognizing personal limitations and seeking help when necessary can also contribute to better time management and overall well-being.

Taking regular breaks is an important time management strategy that can help prevent neck pain. Engaging in brief periods of rest and relaxation throughout the day allows individuals to recharge both physically and mentally. During breaks, incorporating gentle stretches and exercises targeting the neck and shoulders can help alleviate muscle tension and promote circulation. These breaks can also provide an opportunity to practice mindfulness techniques, such as deep breathing or meditation, which can further reduce stress and its impact on neck health.

Creating a structured daily routine can also be beneficial for managing time and preventing neck pain. By allocating specific time slots for work, exercise, relaxation, and sleep, individuals can establish a balanced lifestyle that promotes overall health and reduces the risk of stress-related neck pain. Maintaining a consistent routine can also help regulate the body's internal clock, improving sleep quality and further contributing to stress reduction.

Lastly, effective time management also involves learning to say no and setting boundaries. Taking on too many responsibilities or agreeing to unrealistic deadlines can contribute to increased stress and muscle tension in the neck. By establishing clear boundaries and learning to decline additional tasks when necessary, individuals can maintain a manageable workload and prevent the detrimental effects of stress on neck health.

A strong social support network plays a crucial role in managing stress and preventing neck pain. Social support refers to the emotional, practical, and informational assistance provided by friends, family, and colleagues. It can be instrumental in helping individuals navigate through difficult situations, reducing the negative impact of stress on physical and mental health.

Emotional support, which includes empathy, encouragement, and understanding, helps individuals feel validated and cared for during stressful periods. By sharing concerns and feelings with trusted friends and family members, individuals can experience relief from emotional distress and gain new perspectives on their situations. The reduction in stress brought about by emotional support can help alleviate muscle tension and prevent stress-related neck pain.

Practical support, such as assistance with daily tasks, can help individuals manage their workload and prevent the stress and muscle tension that often accompany long periods of focused work. By delegating tasks or seeking help with responsibilities, individuals can create a more balanced schedule, reducing the risk of stress-induced neck pain.

Informational support involves providing advice, guidance, or useful information to help individuals cope with stress. By seeking advice from friends, family, or professionals, individuals can gain new insights into their problems and develop more effective coping strategies. These coping strategies can help mitigate the effects of stress on the body, including the development of neck pain.

Engaging in enjoyable social activities can also be beneficial in managing stress and preventing neck pain. Participating in hobbies, sports, or cultural events with friends and family can help individuals take their minds off their worries and provide opportunities for relaxation and enjoyment. These positive experiences can help counteract the negative effects of stress on the body and reduce the risk of neck pain.

Research has shown that individuals with strong social support networks tend to have better overall health, including lower rates of chronic pain. By fostering connections with others, seeking help when needed, and actively participating in social activities, individuals can cultivate a supportive environment that promotes mental well-being and reduces the risk of stress-related neck pain.

Recognizing the early warning signs of neck pain is essential for taking proactive measures to prevent the problem from worsening. These warning signs can manifest in various ways, and individuals should be aware of the potential symptoms that may indicate the onset of neck pain.

Stiffness in the neck is a common early warning sign of neck pain. It may be accompanied by a limited range of motion and difficulty turning the head. Stiffness can be caused by muscle tension, poor posture, or strain from repetitive movements. When experiencing neck stiffness, it is crucial to address the underlying cause and implement self-care strategies, such as gentle stretching and improving posture, to prevent the issue from escalating.

Muscle tension is another early indicator of neck pain. It can result from physical factors, such as maintaining an awkward position for an extended period or engaging in activities that strain the neck muscles. Psychological factors, such as stress and anxiety, can also contribute to muscle tension. Identifying the cause of muscle tension and taking steps to alleviate it, such as practicing relaxation techniques or modifying activities, can help prevent the development of chronic neck pain.

Discomfort or mild pain in the neck region can signal the onset of neck pain. This discomfort may be localized or radiate to the shoulders or upper back. It is essential to pay attention to this warning sign and take appropriate measures to address the issue, such as adjusting ergonomics at work or incorporating targeted strengthening exercises to support the neck muscles.

Numbness or tingling in the arms or hands can also indicate potential neck problems, as these symptoms may be related to nerve compression in the cervical spine. If these symptoms are experienced, it is important to seek medical advice to determine the underlying cause and receive appropriate treatment recommendations.

Fatigue, particularly in the neck and shoulder muscles, may be another early warning sign of neck pain. This fatigue can result from poor posture, muscle imbalances, or overexertion during physical activities. Addressing the factors contributing to muscle fatigue and implementing strategies to improve muscle endurance, such as engaging in regular physical activity and maintaining proper posture, can help prevent the development of neck pain.

When individuals recognize these early warning signs of neck pain, it is crucial to take action to prevent the issue from worsening. Modifying activities that contribute to neck strain, seeking medical advice to identify the underlying cause, and implementing self-care strategies, such as stretching and strengthening exercises, can help manage pain and prevent further complications. By being vigilant and proactive in addressing these early warning signs, individuals can significantly reduce their risk of developing chronic neck pain and improve their overall quality of life.

Seeking professional help early in the course of neck pain is essential in preventing chronic pain and disability. A variety of medical professionals can be consulted to address neck pain, each offering different approaches and treatment options to effectively manage the issue and prevent future problems.

Physical therapists are trained healthcare professionals who specialize in diagnosing and treating musculoskeletal disorders. They can assess the underlying causes of neck pain, such as muscle imbalances, joint restrictions, or postural issues, and develop a tailored treatment plan to address these issues. Physical therapy interventions for neck pain may include manual therapy techniques, such as joint mobilizations or soft tissue massage, therapeutic exercises to strengthen and stretch the affected muscles, and postural education to promote proper body mechanics during daily activities. Additionally, physical therapists can provide recommendations for appropriate ergonomic adjustments to reduce strain on the neck during work or other activities.

Chiropractors are healthcare professionals who focus on the diagnosis and treatment of neuromusculoskeletal disorders, particularly those involving the spine. Chiropractic care for neck pain typically involves spinal manipulations or adjustments to correct misalignments and restore proper joint function. These adjustments can help alleviate pain, reduce muscle tension, and improve range of motion in the neck. Chiropractors may also recommend additional therapies, such as massage, electrical stimulation, or ultrasound, to supplement spinal adjustments and enhance the overall effectiveness of the treatment. Furthermore, chiropractors can provide education on proper posture, ergonomics, and self-care strategies to prevent future episodes of neck pain.

Physicians, including primary care providers and specialists such as orthopedic surgeons or neurologists, can play a crucial role in diagnosing and managing neck pain. They can help rule out underlying medical conditions that may be contributing to neck pain, such as degenerative disc disease, spinal stenosis, or nerve compression. Physicians may recommend a combination of conservative treatments, such as medication, physical therapy, or chiropractic care, to address neck pain. In some cases, when conservative treatments are not effective, or the underlying cause of neck pain is severe, physicians may consider surgical interventions to alleviate pain and restore function.

In addition to the above-mentioned professionals, other healthcare providers, such as massage therapists, occupational therapists, or acupuncturists, can also contribute to the management of neck pain. Massage therapists can provide targeted soft tissue manipulation to alleviate muscle tension and promote relaxation. Occupational therapists can help individuals adapt their daily activities and work environment to minimize strain on the neck and prevent the recurrence of neck pain. Acupuncturists can offer alternative treatment methods, such as needle insertion at specific points on the body, to help relieve neck pain and promote overall well-being.

Seeking professional help early in the course of neck pain is crucial for preventing chronic pain and disability. A multidisciplinary approach, involving various healthcare professionals, can provide a comprehensive and effective treatment plan to address the underlying causes of neck pain and prevent future problems.

Workplace training programs that focus on ergonomics, posture, and proper body mechanics are essential in creating a safe and healthy work environment, effectively helping prevent neck pain. These programs aim to educate employees on the best practices and techniques to maintain proper posture, minimize strain on the neck, and ultimately prevent neck pain from developing or worsening.

One crucial aspect of workplace training is the proper adjustment of workstations. Employees should be trained to set up their workstations in a way that promotes neutral body positioning, reduces strain on the neck and shoulders, and encourages natural movement throughout the day. This includes adjusting the height and position of computer monitors, keyboards, and chairs, as well as arranging frequently used items within easy reach to minimize unnecessary strain.

Additionally, workplace training should emphasize the importance of taking regular breaks and incorporating microbreaks into the workday. Microbreaks are short, frequent pauses taken during work activities to alleviate muscle tension and reduce the risk of developing repetitive strain injuries. During these breaks, employees can perform simple stretches and exercises targeting the neck, shoulders, and upper back, which can help maintain flexibility and prevent muscle stiffness.

397

Training programs should also address the hazards associated with prolonged use of electronic devices, such as smartphones and tablets. Employees should be educated on the risks associated with the forward head posture commonly seen during device usage and be encouraged to adopt healthier habits, such as holding devices at eye level, taking frequent breaks, and incorporating neck stretches into their daily routines.

Moreover, workplace training should cover the importance of physical fitness and exercise in maintaining neck health. Employees should be encouraged to engage in regular physical activity, including aerobic exercise, strength training, and flexibility exercises, to improve overall fitness, reduce stress, and maintain the health of the muscles and structures supporting the neck.

Workplace training should also address the psychological factors that can contribute to neck pain, such as stress and poor coping strategies. Employees should be provided with resources and strategies to manage stress effectively, including relaxation techniques, time management skills, and the importance of social support. By addressing these factors, workplace training can help employees better manage their stress and reduce the muscle tension that contributes to neck pain.

Finally, workplace training should emphasize the importance of early intervention when neck pain symptoms arise. Employees should be encouraged to seek professional help, such as consultations with physical therapists, chiropractors, or physicians, as soon as they experience discomfort or stiffness in the neck. Early intervention can help identify the underlying causes of neck pain, provide appropriate treatment recommendations, and prevent the issue from becoming chronic or leading to further complications.

Comprehensive workplace training programs that focus on ergonomics, posture, proper body mechanics, physical fitness, stress management, and early intervention can play a significant role in preventing neck pain and promoting a healthy work environment. By providing employees with the knowledge and tools necessary to maintain proper posture and minimize strain, these programs can effectively reduce the risk of neck pain and improve overall employee well-being.

Public health initiatives play a crucial role in reducing the prevalence of neck pain by raising awareness about risk factors and promoting preventive strategies. These initiatives often involve collaboration between governmental organizations, healthcare providers, and community stakeholders to develop and implement evidence-based programs and campaigns that address the root causes of neck pain and promote overall neck health.

One significant aspect of public health initiatives targeting neck pain is the promotion of physical activity and exercise. These programs aim to educate the public about the importance of regular exercise, particularly in strengthening and stretching the muscles that support the neck. By encouraging participation in activities such as swimming, yoga, Pilates, and resistance training, these initiatives can help individuals maintain muscle balance, flexibility, and overall neck health.

Another focus of public health initiatives is the promotion of proper posture and ergonomics. This can involve educating the public on maintaining proper posture while sitting, standing, and using electronic devices, as well as the importance of ergonomically designed workspaces. Workshops, seminars, and online resources can be employed to provide individuals with the necessary information and tools to evaluate their environments and make necessary adjustments to prevent neck strain.

Stress management is also a vital component of public health initiatives aimed at preventing neck pain. Programs that teach stress reduction techniques, such as mindfulness-based stress reduction, progressive muscle relaxation, and cognitive-behavioral therapy, can empower individuals to manage stress effectively and reduce the muscle tension that contributes to neck pain. These initiatives may also promote the importance of self-care, time management, and social support as integral components of stress management and overall neck health.

In addition to these targeted interventions, public health initiatives may also involve broader efforts to promote overall well-being and reduce the burden of chronic pain. This can include advocating for policies that support access to healthcare services, funding research on pain prevention and management, and providing resources for healthcare providers to improve their understanding of neck pain and its risk factors.

Public health initiatives that raise awareness about the risk factors for neck pain and promote preventive strategies are essential for reducing the prevalence of this common issue. By focusing on the importance of exercise, proper posture, and stress management, these initiatives can empower individuals to make informed decisions about their neck health and take proactive steps to prevent neck pain. Collaboration between governmental organizations, healthcare providers, and community stakeholders is vital to the development and implementation of evidence-based programs and campaigns that address neck pain and promote overall neck health.

In conclusion, preventive strategies for neck pain require a comprehensive approach that addresses the physical, occupational, and psychological risk factors contributing to the development and exacerbation of neck pain. By understanding and addressing these risk factors, individuals can take a proactive approach to maintain their neck health and significantly reduce the likelihood of developing neck pain.

Ergonomic adjustments, such as optimizing workspace layouts and practicing proper sitting posture, can help minimize the strain placed on the neck and shoulders during daily activities. Ensuring that the computer monitor is at eye level, using a document holder, and keeping frequently used items within easy reach can contribute to reducing neck pain associated with sedentary work environments.

Regular exercise, including strengthening, flexibility, and aerobic exercises, can help prevent neck pain by improving muscle balance, maintaining a healthy range of motion in the neck, and promoting overall physical fitness. In addition to preventing neck pain, engaging in regular physical activity can also improve mental health and well-being by reducing stress and anxiety levels.

Proper sleep hygiene, including selecting an appropriate pillow and mattress and adopting a sleep position that supports the natural curve of the neck, is crucial for preventing neck pain. A supportive sleep environment can help alleviate strain on the cervical spine, allowing the neck muscles to relax and recover during the night.

Managing stress through relaxation techniques, time management, and social support can play a significant role in preventing neck pain. Incorporating practices such as deep breathing, progressive muscle relaxation, and meditation into daily routines can help individuals better manage their stress levels and reduce the muscle tension that contributes to neck pain. Furthermore, effective time management and a strong social support network can assist in coping with stress, ultimately leading to a reduced risk of stress-related neck pain.

Early intervention is key to preventing the progression of neck pain and its potential impact on an individual's quality of life. Recognizing the early warning signs of neck pain and seeking professional help can ensure that appropriate treatment and preventive measures are implemented in a timely manner.

Public health initiatives and workplace training programs can play a critical role in raising awareness about the importance of neck pain prevention. By educating individuals about the risk factors for neck pain and promoting evidence-based preventive strategies, these initiatives can empower people to take control of their neck health and adopt proactive measures to avoid future issues.

In summary, a multifaceted approach to neck pain prevention, which addresses physical, occupational, and psychological risk factors, is essential for maintaining neck health and improving overall quality of life. By implementing ergonomic adjustments, engaging in regular exercise, maintaining proper sleep hygiene, managing stress, and seeking early intervention when necessary, individuals can significantly reduce their risk of developing neck pain and its associated complications.

402

Chapter 20

The Role of Technology in Neck Pain Management

Wearables, Telemedicine, and Remote Monitoring Solutions

Neck pain is a pervasive issue affecting millions of people worldwide. With the rapid advancement of technology, innovative solutions are being developed to assist in the management and treatment of neck pain. This chapter will explore the role of technology in neck pain management, focusing on wearables, telemedicine, and remote monitoring solutions. These technologies have the potential to revolutionize neck pain management, providing accessible and personalized care for individuals experiencing neck pain.

Poor posture is a significant contributor to neck pain, as it places undue stress on the muscles, ligaments, and spinal structures in the neck and upper back. Over time, this strain can lead to muscle imbalances, joint dysfunction, and increased pain. Wearable posture monitoring devices have emerged as a practical solution to help individuals maintain proper alignment and reduce neck pain. These devices leverage advanced technology to detect postural deviations and provide real-time feedback, promoting long-term improvements in posture and overall musculoskeletal health.

Wearable posture monitoring devices are available in various designs, with some devices worn on the upper back, attached to clothing, or even incorporated into clothing items such as shirts or bras. These devices use a combination of accelerometers, gyroscopes, and sometimes magnetometers to track the user's posture throughout the day. By measuring the orientation and movement of the body, these sensors can detect deviations from the optimal posture and provide feedback to the user accordingly.

Real-time feedback is a crucial component of posture monitoring devices, as it encourages immediate correction of postural deviations. Feedback mechanisms can vary depending on the device, but common methods include gentle vibrations, audible alerts, or visual cues displayed on a companion smartphone app. By providing instant reminders to correct their posture, users can develop increased body awareness and reinforce healthier postural habits.

In addition to real-time feedback, many posture monitoring devices are equipped with data tracking and analysis features. These features allow users to review their postural habits over time, set goals, and track progress towards improved posture. Some devices also offer personalized recommendations for exercises and stretches to address specific postural imbalances, further enhancing the user's ability to improve their posture and reduce neck pain.

It is important to note that while posture monitoring devices can be a valuable tool in promoting better posture and reducing neck pain, they should be used in conjunction with other interventions, such as physical therapy, ergonomic adjustments, and regular exercise. Additionally, it is essential for users to understand that posture monitoring devices are not a substitute for professional medical advice and should be used as a complement to a comprehensive neck pain management plan developed in consultation with a healthcare professional.

Posture monitoring devices offer a practical and innovative solution to help individuals maintain proper alignment and reduce neck pain. By leveraging advanced sensor technology and providing real-time feedback, these devices promote increased body awareness and healthier postural habits. When used in conjunction with other interventions and under the guidance of a healthcare professional, posture monitoring devices can be an effective component of a comprehensive neck pain management plan.

Smart textiles represent a promising frontier in the development of wearable technology for neck pain management. These innovative fabrics are embedded with sensors, actuators, and other electronic components, enabling them to monitor and respond to various physiological parameters, such as muscle tension, posture, and movement patterns. By providing real-time feedback, smart textiles have the potential to play a pivotal role in promoting healthier habits and alleviating neck pain.

One application of smart textiles in neck pain management is the development of neck braces or collars that incorporate sensor technology. These smart textile neck braces can continuously monitor muscle tension in the neck and provide feedback, such as gentle vibrations, visual signals, or audio cues, to encourage relaxation or proper positioning. This can help individuals become more aware of their posture and muscle tension, leading to improvements in neck pain symptoms over time.

Additionally, smart textiles can be integrated into pillows and bedding to monitor sleep posture and provide feedback to improve sleep quality. Poor sleep posture is a common contributor to neck pain, as it can place undue stress on the neck muscles and spinal structures. By incorporating sensors that detect head and neck position during sleep, smart textiles can help individuals identify and correct poor sleep posture. This can lead to improved sleep quality and reduced neck pain symptoms.

Smart textiles can also be integrated into clothing items, such as shirts and jackets, to monitor posture and movement patterns throughout the day. These garments can provide real-time feedback to users, reminding them to maintain proper posture and avoid potentially harmful movements that may exacerbate neck pain. By reinforcing healthy habits, smart textiles can contribute to the prevention and management of neck pain.

Despite the potential benefits of smart textiles in neck pain management, there are some challenges to consider. The integration of sensors and electronic components into fabrics must be done in a manner that is comfortable for the wearer and does not compromise the durability or washability of the textile. Additionally, the cost of producing and maintaining smart textile garments and accessories may be prohibitive for some individuals. Further research and development are needed to address these challenges and make smart textile technology more accessible and user-friendly.

Smart textiles offer an innovative and promising approach to neck pain management by providing real-time feedback on muscle tension, posture, and movement patterns. The integration of smart textiles into neck braces, pillows, bedding, and clothing items has the potential to revolutionize neck pain management and promote healthier habits. As research and development in this field continue to advance, it is anticipated that smart textiles will become an increasingly important tool in the prevention and treatment of neck pain.

Activity trackers, also known as fitness trackers or wearable devices, have gained popularity in recent years for their ability to monitor various aspects of physical activity and overall health. These devices typically utilize accelerometers, gyroscopes, and other sensors to track metrics such as steps taken, distance traveled, and calories burned. As neck pain is often associated with sedentary behavior and lack of physical activity, incorporating activity trackers into neck pain management strategies can provide numerous benefits.

Regular physical activity is essential for maintaining overall well-being, and it has been shown to reduce neck pain by improving muscle strength, flexibility, and posture. Activity trackers can encourage an active lifestyle by setting personalized daily goals and providing real-time feedback on progress. This feedback can serve as a powerful motivator for individuals to stay active and engage in regular exercise, which can, in turn, help alleviate neck pain.

Many activity trackers also offer features specifically tailored for neck pain management. For example, some devices are designed to detect periods of prolonged inactivity and provide reminders to take breaks, stretch, or perform neck exercises. These reminders can help individuals establish healthier habits and reduce the risk of developing neck pain associated with sedentary behavior.

In addition to tracking physical activity, some activity trackers also monitor sleep quality, which plays a crucial role in neck pain management. Poor sleep quality can exacerbate neck pain and contribute to a cycle of discomfort and fatigue. By providing insights into sleep patterns, activity trackers can help individuals identify potential issues and make necessary adjustments, such as improving sleep hygiene or adjusting their sleep environment.

Furthermore, some activity trackers offer integration with smartphone applications, allowing users to access additional resources and support for neck pain management. These applications may provide educational materials on proper posture, ergonomics, and exercises specifically targeted at alleviating neck pain. By incorporating these resources, individuals can develop a comprehensive neck pain management plan that combines physical activity, stretching, and posture correction.

It is important to note that while activity trackers can be a valuable tool in neck pain management, they should not replace professional medical advice and treatment. Individuals experiencing neck pain should consult with a healthcare professional to develop an appropriate treatment plan tailored to their specific needs.

Activity trackers can play a significant role in neck pain management by promoting regular physical activity, monitoring sleep quality, and providing personalized reminders and resources to address factors contributing to neck pain. By incorporating these devices into neck pain management strategies, individuals can take a proactive approach to improving their overall well-being and reducing neck pain.

Telemedicine, which involves the delivery of healthcare services using telecommunications technology, has become an increasingly popular solution for individuals seeking care for various health conditions, including neck pain. By leveraging videoconferencing and remote patient monitoring technologies, virtual consultations can provide individuals with access to healthcare professionals without the need for in-person appointments.

Virtual consultations can be particularly beneficial for those experiencing limited mobility, transportation challenges, or living in rural areas with limited access to healthcare providers. The convenience and flexibility offered by telemedicine allow patients to receive timely and appropriate care, regardless of their location or physical limitations.

During a virtual consultation, healthcare professionals can assess a patient's neck pain by asking targeted questions, observing the patient's posture and movements, and conducting a visual examination via video. The patient can also demonstrate any specific movements or positions that exacerbate their neck pain, allowing the healthcare professional to better understand the underlying causes and contributing factors.

Based on their assessment, healthcare professionals can provide recommendations for self-care, including advice on ergonomics, sleep positioning, and relaxation techniques, as well as prescribe exercises to improve strength, flexibility, and posture. In some cases, healthcare professionals may also prescribe medications or other treatments to alleviate neck pain, such as topical analgesics or muscle relaxants.

Telemedicine can facilitate interdisciplinary care by enabling healthcare providers from different disciplines to collaborate on a patient's care plan. For example, a primary care physician may consult with a physical therapist, chiropractor, or psychologist to address the various physical, biomechanical, and psychological factors contributing to the patient's neck pain. This collaborative approach ensures that the patient receives comprehensive and coordinated care, addressing all aspects of their condition.

Additionally, virtual consultations can help patients overcome barriers to care, such as long wait times or scheduling difficulties. Patients can often schedule virtual appointments more quickly than in-person appointments, allowing them to receive care sooner and potentially preventing the exacerbation of their neck pain. Telemedicine can also provide patients with access to healthcare professionals who specialize in neck pain management, regardless of their geographical location.

Virtual consultations have emerged as a valuable tool in the management of neck pain, providing individuals with convenient and accessible care tailored to their specific needs. By harnessing the power of telecommunications technology, telemedicine can overcome many barriers to care and facilitate interdisciplinary collaboration, ensuring that patients receive comprehensive and effective treatment for their neck pain.

Online rehabilitation programs have emerged as a valuable tool in the management of musculoskeletal conditions, including neck pain. These web-based platforms are designed to deliver personalized exercise and self-management programs tailored to the specific needs and limitations of each individual. By leveraging technology, online rehabilitation programs can provide accessible and cost-effective alternatives to traditional in-person therapy, while still offering the necessary guidance and support for patients to effectively manage their neck pain.

One of the key features of online rehabilitation programs is the availability of instructional videos, which demonstrate proper techniques and form for various exercises targeting neck pain. These videos often cover a range of exercises, from gentle stretches to more intensive strengthening exercises, providing patients with a comprehensive program to improve their neck function and reduce pain. By following the instructions in these videos, patients can ensure they are performing the exercises correctly, reducing the risk of injury and maximizing the benefits of their rehabilitation program.

Progress tracking is another essential component of online rehabilitation programs. These platforms often allow patients to log their exercises, monitor their symptoms, and track their overall progress. This information can be invaluable in motivating patients to adhere to their program and continue working towards their goals. Additionally, progress tracking enables healthcare professionals to remotely monitor their patients' progress, providing valuable insights into the effectiveness of the prescribed exercises and allowing for adjustments to be made as needed.

Remote support from healthcare professionals is a crucial aspect of online rehabilitation programs. Through video consultations, messaging systems, or online forums, patients can communicate directly with healthcare providers, such as physical therapists, chiropractors, or physicians. This support can help address any concerns or questions that may arise during the rehabilitation process, as well as provide encouragement and motivation for patients to stay committed to their program. Furthermore, remote support allows healthcare professionals to closely monitor their patients' progress and make necessary adjustments to their exercise program, ensuring it remains appropriate and effective for each individual's needs.

The convenience and cost-effectiveness of online rehabilitation programs make them an attractive option for many individuals experiencing neck pain. By allowing patients to complete exercises at their own pace and in the comfort of their own home, these programs can help overcome barriers related to transportation, scheduling, and financial limitations that may prevent some individuals from accessing traditional in-person therapy. Furthermore, online rehabilitation programs can provide patients with the tools and resources necessary to take an active role in their neck pain management, empowering them to make lasting improvements in their pain and overall quality of life.

Online rehabilitation programs offer a promising and innovative approach to neck pain management. By providing personalized exercise programs, progress tracking, and remote support from healthcare professionals, these web-based platforms can deliver effective and accessible care for individuals experiencing neck pain. As technology continues to advance and become more integrated into healthcare, online rehabilitation programs are likely to play an increasingly important role in the management of musculoskeletal conditions, including neck pain.

Virtual support groups have emerged as a valuable resource for individuals experiencing neck pain, offering a platform for connection, information sharing, and emotional support. These groups often utilize video conferencing, online forums, or social media platforms to facilitate communication among individuals facing similar challenges. By connecting with others who understand their experiences, individuals with neck pain can feel less isolated and more empowered to manage their condition.

One of the key benefits of virtual support groups is the ability to access them from anywhere, at any time. This flexibility makes it easier for individuals with busy schedules, limited mobility, or those living in remote areas to participate in support groups without the need for in-person attendance. Additionally, virtual support groups can cater to a diverse range of needs and preferences, with some groups focusing on specific types of neck pain, such as cervical spondylosis or whiplash, or addressing particular concerns, such as coping with chronic pain or navigating the healthcare system.

Virtual support groups can also provide a wealth of information, resources, and practical advice for managing neck pain. Group members often share their experiences with different treatments, self-care strategies, and lifestyle modifications, which can help individuals discover new approaches to managing their neck pain. Additionally, virtual support groups may feature guest speakers or educational content from healthcare professionals, providing evidence-based information and guidance on neck pain management.

Emotional support is another crucial aspect of virtual support groups. Living with neck pain can be challenging, and it can be helpful for individuals to share their feelings, frustrations, and successes with others who understand. The sense of camaraderie and shared experience in a virtual support group can help individuals feel more emotionally resilient and better equipped to cope with the challenges of neck pain.

Research has shown that participation in support groups can lead to improved self-efficacy, emotional well-being, and overall quality of life for individuals living with chronic pain. While more research is needed specifically on virtual support groups for neck pain, it is reasonable to assume that these benefits may extend to this population as well.

It is important to note that virtual support groups should not replace professional healthcare advice and treatment. Instead, they should be viewed as a complementary resource to help individuals better understand and manage their neck pain. To ensure the accuracy and reliability of information shared within virtual support groups, it is crucial for participants to verify information with healthcare professionals and seek evidence-based resources.

Virtual support groups offer a valuable platform for individuals with neck pain to connect, share information, and receive emotional support. The flexibility and accessibility of virtual support groups make them an appealing option for many individuals, and their potential benefits in terms of self-efficacy, emotional well-being, and overall quality of life make them an essential consideration in comprehensive neck pain management plans.

Home-based monitoring systems have gained traction in recent years as a convenient and effective method for collecting health-related data in a person's natural environment. These systems typically consist of various sensors and devices designed to gather information on an individual's health and well-being, with a particular focus on factors relevant to neck pain management. By tracking posture, sleep quality, and physical activity, these systems offer valuable insights into an individual's daily habits and routines that may contribute to neck pain.

One of the primary components of home-based monitoring systems for neck pain management is posture tracking. Advanced sensor technology, such as wearable sensors or cameras equipped with computer vision algorithms, can monitor an individual's posture throughout the day. By detecting and analyzing postural deviations, these systems can provide real-time feedback and reminders to correct posture, thereby reducing the risk of neck pain associated with poor alignment.

Another crucial aspect of home-based monitoring systems is sleep quality assessment. Sleep plays a vital role in overall health and well-being, and poor sleep quality can exacerbate neck pain. Home-based monitoring systems can include sensors integrated into mattresses, pillows, or wearable devices that track sleep patterns, body position, and movement during sleep. This data can help healthcare professionals identify sleep-related issues contributing to neck pain, such as improper sleep position or sleep disturbances, and recommend appropriate interventions, such as adjusting pillow height or practicing relaxation techniques before bedtime.

Physical activity monitoring is another essential component of home-based monitoring systems for neck pain management. Research has shown that regular physical activity can help reduce neck pain and improve overall health. Home-based monitoring systems can track an individual's daily activity levels using wearable devices, such as accelerometers or pedometers, or through motion sensors installed in the home environment. By collecting data on physical activity levels, healthcare professionals can identify sedentary behaviors or poor movement patterns that may contribute to neck pain and recommend appropriate exercise programs or lifestyle modifications.

The data collected by home-based monitoring systems can be securely transmitted to healthcare professionals for analysis and interpretation. By reviewing this information, healthcare providers can identify trends, detect potential risk factors, and develop personalized treatment plans tailored to an individual's specific needs. Moreover, home-based monitoring systems can facilitate remote patient monitoring, allowing healthcare professionals to track progress and adjust treatment plans as needed, without requiring frequent in-person appointments.

Home-based monitoring systems represent a promising approach to neck pain management by providing a comprehensive assessment of an individual's daily habits and routines. By monitoring posture, sleep quality, and physical activity, these systems can help healthcare professionals identify factors contributing to neck pain and develop personalized treatment plans to address these issues. As technology continues to advance, home-based monitoring systems are poised to play an increasingly important role in neck pain management and overall health care.

Mobile applications have emerged as a powerful tool in neck pain management, providing users with various resources to monitor their condition and implement necessary lifestyle changes. They offer a range of features designed to support individuals experiencing neck pain and improve their overall well-being.

One crucial feature of mobile applications for neck pain management is providing reminders for users to take breaks and stretch periodically throughout the day. These reminders can be particularly beneficial for individuals who have sedentary jobs or spend long hours in front of a computer. Regular breaks and stretching exercises can help alleviate muscle tension and promote better posture, reducing the risk of developing neck pain.

Another valuable feature of mobile applications for neck pain management is the inclusion of guided relaxation exercises. These exercises may involve deep breathing, progressive muscle relaxation, or visualization techniques that help users manage stress and anxiety, both of which can contribute to neck pain. Regular practice of these relaxation exercises can lead to improved mental well-being and a reduction in muscle tension in the neck.

Instructional videos on proper posture and ergonomics are also an essential component of mobile applications for neck pain management. These videos provide users with visual guidance on maintaining correct body alignment while sitting, standing, and performing various tasks. They may also offer recommendations on setting up a workspace that supports proper posture, such as adjusting chair height, monitor placement, and keyboard positioning. By following these guidelines, users can reduce strain on their neck muscles and minimize the risk of developing neck pain.

In addition to these features, some mobile applications can sync with wearable devices or home-based monitoring systems to track and analyze data related to neck pain management. This integration allows users to monitor their progress and receive personalized feedback based on their specific needs and goals. For example, a mobile application may analyze data from a wearable posture monitor to provide tailored recommendations on improving posture or identifying patterns of muscle tension. By leveraging this data, users can gain valuable insights into their condition and make informed decisions on managing their neck pain.

Moreover, mobile applications for neck pain management can provide users with access to educational resources and support networks. This may include articles on neck pain causes, treatment options, and prevention strategies, as well as forums where users can connect with others experiencing similar issues. Access to these resources can empower users to take an active role in managing their neck pain and promote a sense of community and support.

Mobile applications play a significant role in neck pain management by offering a range of features designed to support users in monitoring their condition and making necessary lifestyle changes. These features include reminders to take breaks and stretch, guided relaxation exercises, instructional videos on proper posture and ergonomics, and integration with wearable devices or home-based monitoring systems for data tracking and analysis. By leveraging the power of mobile technology, individuals experiencing neck pain can take a proactive approach to manage their condition and improve their overall well-being.

Artificial intelligence (AI) and machine learning are powerful tools with the potential to revolutionize neck pain management by analyzing large amounts of data and identifying patterns and trends that contribute to neck pain. These advanced technologies can process data from various sources, including wearable devices, home-based monitoring systems, and electronic health records, to create personalized treatment plans tailored to an individual's unique needs and preferences.

One application of AI in neck pain management involves the analysis of data from wearable devices and home-based monitoring systems. By tracking posture, movement, and muscle tension, AI algorithms can identify patterns that contribute to neck pain and provide targeted recommendations for adjustments, such as ergonomic improvements or exercise routines. This personalized approach to neck pain management ensures that interventions are tailored to address the specific factors contributing to an individual's pain, increasing the likelihood of successful treatment outcomes.

Machine learning can also play a vital role in developing predictive models to identify individuals at risk of developing neck pain. By analyzing large datasets containing information on demographics, lifestyle factors, and medical history, machine learning algorithms can identify patterns and trends associated with neck pain risk. This information can be used to develop targeted prevention strategies and early interventions for individuals identified as being at high risk, potentially preventing the development of chronic neck pain and associated complications.

Furthermore, AI and machine learning technologies can be used to optimize telemedicine and online rehabilitation programs for neck pain management. By continuously monitoring patient progress and adapting treatment plans based on individual needs, AI-powered systems can provide real-time feedback and support, enhancing the effectiveness of these programs. For example, AI algorithms can analyze data on exercise adherence, pain levels, and functional improvements to identify areas where patients may need additional support or modifications to their treatment plan. This adaptive approach ensures that patients receive the most appropriate care, maximizing the potential for positive outcomes.

AI and machine learning can also be employed in the development of virtual assistants for neck pain management. These virtual assistants can provide patients with personalized exercise routines, ergonomic recommendations, and pain management strategies based on their specific needs and progress. By utilizing natural language processing and machine learning algorithms, these virtual assistants can engage in dynamic conversations with patients, answering questions and providing tailored advice to help manage neck pain more effectively.

Despite the potential benefits of AI and machine learning in neck pain management, several challenges must be addressed to ensure the successful implementation of these technologies. Ensuring data privacy and security is paramount, as sensitive health information must be protected from unauthorized access. Additionally, the development of AI algorithms requires large, high-quality datasets to ensure accurate and reliable predictions. Collaborative efforts between healthcare providers, technology developers, and researchers are necessary to address these challenges and fully realize the potential of AI and machine learning in neck pain management.

The integration of wearables, telemedicine, and remote monitoring solutions is essential for a more comprehensive and coordinated approach to neck pain management. As technologies continue to advance, there is an increasing need for interconnected systems that allow for seamless data sharing and communication among healthcare professionals, patients, and caregivers.

One aspect of technology integration involves the development of platforms that aggregate data from various sources, such as wearables, mobile applications, and home-based monitoring systems. These platforms can enable healthcare professionals to access and analyze information more efficiently, providing a holistic view of an individual's condition and progress. By consolidating data in a centralized platform, healthcare providers can more easily identify patterns, track trends, and make informed decisions regarding treatment plans.

In addition to data aggregation, technology integration can also facilitate interdisciplinary care by improving communication between healthcare providers from different disciplines. For instance, a physical therapist, chiropractor, and psychologist could collaborate on a patient's care plan by sharing information and insights through a shared platform. This interdisciplinary approach ensures that all relevant aspects of an individual's neck pain management are considered, leading to more effective and personalized treatment plans.

Furthermore, integrating technology can help bridge communication gaps between healthcare providers, patients, and caregivers. For example, a telemedicine platform could allow patients to communicate with their healthcare providers in real-time, ask questions, and receive guidance on managing their neck pain. Likewise, caregivers could access the platform to stay informed about the patient's progress, receive updates on treatment plans, and learn about strategies for supporting their loved one's neck pain management.

Integrating technologies also has the potential to improve patient engagement and self-management. Patients can use wearables and mobile applications to track their progress and receive personalized feedback on their posture, physical activity, and sleep habits. This real-time feedback can empower individuals to take an active role in their neck pain management, leading to better adherence to treatment plans and improved outcomes.

However, integrating various technologies also poses challenges related to data privacy, security, and interoperability. Healthcare providers, technology developers, and regulatory bodies must work together to establish guidelines and best practices to ensure that data is shared securely and ethically. Additionally, overcoming technical barriers, such as ensuring compatibility between different devices and platforms, is crucial for seamless integration and effective communication.

The integration of wearables, telemedicine, and remote monitoring solutions is a critical component of advancing neck pain management. By creating interconnected systems that facilitate data sharing, interdisciplinary care, and improved communication, healthcare providers can develop more comprehensive and personalized treatment plans for individuals experiencing neck pain. As technology continues to evolve, it is essential to address the challenges and barriers associated with integration to harness the full potential of these innovative solutions.

As the use of technology in neck pain management continues to grow, concerns regarding data privacy and security must be addressed. The collection, storage, and sharing of sensitive health information require strict protocols and safeguards to protect patient privacy and prevent unauthorized access. Healthcare providers, technology developers, and regulatory bodies must work together to establish guidelines and best practices to ensure the safe and ethical use of technology in neck pain management.

One of the primary concerns in data privacy and security is the risk of unauthorized access to sensitive health information. This risk can arise from various sources, including hackers, data breaches, and insider threats. To mitigate this risk, healthcare providers and technology developers should implement robust security measures such as encryption, secure data storage, and strict access controls. These measures can help protect sensitive information from unauthorized access and ensure that only authorized personnel can access patient data.

Another concern related to data privacy and security is the potential misuse of health data by third parties, such as insurance companies or employers. The collection and storage of sensitive health information can expose individuals to potential discrimination or stigmatization based on their health conditions. To address this issue, regulatory bodies must establish strict guidelines for the sharing and use of health data. These guidelines should ensure that health data is only used for the intended purpose of providing care and improving patient outcomes, and not for unauthorized purposes that could harm individuals.

Informed consent is another crucial aspect of data privacy and security in neck pain management technology. Patients should be fully informed about the collection, storage, and sharing of their health data and should have the opportunity to provide or withhold consent for these activities. This requires healthcare providers and technology developers to develop

418

clear and concise privacy policies and consent forms that outline how patient data will be used and shared. Additionally, patients should have the right to access, review, and correct their health data, as well as the option to withdraw their consent at any time.

Continuous monitoring and auditing of data privacy and security practices are essential to ensure compliance with established guidelines and best practices. Healthcare providers and technology developers should regularly review and update their data protection measures to keep up with the rapidly evolving cybersecurity landscape. This can involve conducting risk assessments, implementing security updates, and providing ongoing training for personnel on data privacy and security best practices.

Collaboration between healthcare providers, technology developers, and regulatory bodies is crucial to ensure the safe and ethical use of technology in neck pain management. By working together to establish guidelines, best practices, and robust security measures, these stakeholders can protect patient privacy, prevent unauthorized access to sensitive health data, and foster trust in the use of technology for neck pain management.

While technology has the potential to improve access to care for individuals experiencing neck pain, barriers related to cost and accessibility must be considered. Wearable devices, telemedicine services, and remote monitoring solutions can be expensive, which may limit their availability to individuals with limited financial resources. High upfront costs for devices or ongoing fees for telemedicine services can create significant barriers for those who could benefit from these technologies.

Additionally, individuals living in rural areas or those with limited access to technology may face challenges in utilizing these services. In rural communities, reliable high-speed internet connections may be scarce or expensive, making it difficult for patients to access telemedicine services or use remote monitoring solutions effectively. Moreover, these populations may also lack access to local healthcare providers who are familiar with or able to prescribe and support the use of technology-based neck pain management solutions.

To address these barriers, several strategies can be employed. One approach is to implement subsidies or sliding-scale payment models, which can help ensure that technology-based neck pain management solutions are accessible to all who need them. These financial assistance programs can be sponsored by governments, healthcare providers, or device manufacturers and could provide financial support to individuals who might otherwise be unable to afford the necessary technology.

Another strategy involves the development and promotion of low-cost alternatives to expensive wearables and telemedicine services. For example, free or low-cost mobile applications that provide guidance on neck exercises, posture correction, and self-care strategies can be a valuable resource for individuals with limited financial resources. Healthcare providers can also develop and share educational materials online, which can help make information about neck pain management more widely available.

In terms of addressing the challenges faced by rural populations, investment in digital infrastructure, such as expanding high-speed internet access, can help improve the availability of telemedicine services and remote monitoring solutions. Furthermore, training and education programs for healthcare providers in rural areas can ensure that they are well-equipped to prescribe and support the use of technology-based neck pain management solutions.

Collaborative efforts between government agencies, healthcare providers, technology developers, and community organizations can help bridge the gap in accessibility and cost. By working together, these stakeholders can develop innovative solutions that ensure individuals experiencing neck pain have access to the technology-based care they need, regardless of their financial situation or geographical location.

In conclusion, technology has emerged as a vital component in the management of neck pain, offering groundbreaking solutions to enhance the evaluation, treatment, and prevention of this common condition. Wearables, telemedicine, and remote monitoring solutions equip individuals with the necessary tools to track their condition, consult healthcare professionals, and implement lifestyle modifications to alleviate neck pain. The effective utilization of technology can lead to significant improvements in the quality of life for those experiencing neck pain while simultaneously contributing to a more efficient and accessible healthcare system.

The continuous advancement of technology in neck pain management necessitates a focus on integration, data privacy and security, and accessibility. Seamless integration of wearables, telemedicine, and remote monitoring solutions can result in comprehensive and coordinated care, allowing healthcare providers to access and analyze information more effectively. This integration can also foster interdisciplinary care and enhance communication between healthcare providers, patients, and caregivers.

As technology becomes more deeply embedded in neck pain management, addressing data privacy and security concerns is of utmost importance. The collection, storage, and sharing of sensitive health information require stringent protocols and safeguards to protect patient privacy and prevent unauthorized access. Collaboration among healthcare providers, technology developers, and regulatory bodies is essential in establishing guidelines and best practices for the safe and ethical use of technology in neck pain management.

Accessibility and cost are additional factors that must be considered to ensure equitable access to technology-based neck pain management solutions. Wearable devices, telemedicine services, and remote monitoring solutions can be expensive, potentially limiting their availability to individuals with constrained financial resources. Moreover, individuals residing in rural areas or those with limited access to technology may encounter challenges in utilizing these services. Strategies to address these barriers, such as subsidies or sliding-scale payment models, can help guarantee that technology-based neck pain management solutions are accessible to all who need them.

By embracing the potential of technology, healthcare providers and patients can collaborate in developing comprehensive and personalized care plans that cater to the unique needs and preferences of individuals experiencing neck pain. In the future, technology is poised to play an increasingly significant role in neck pain management, leading to better patient outcomes and an overall improvement in the healthcare landscape.

Chapter 21

Navigating the Future of Neck Pain Treatment

Emerging Therapies and Innovations in Pain Management

Neck pain is a prevalent condition that affects a significant portion of the global population. Despite advances in diagnosis and treatment, neck pain remains a challenging condition to manage for both patients and healthcare professionals. As researchers and clinicians continue to explore new methods and technologies to address neck pain, a variety of emerging therapies and innovations hold promise for improving pain management in the future. This chapter will discuss the latest developments in neck pain treatment and explore the potential implications of these advancements on the future of pain management.

Cell-based therapies are an emerging approach to treating neck pain, harnessing the body's natural regenerative capabilities to promote healing and reduce inflammation. Two primary types of cell-based therapies are currently being investigated for their potential in neck pain treatment: stem cell injections and platelet-rich plasma (PRP) therapy.

Stem cell injections involve the use of multipotent cells that have the ability to differentiate into various types of specialized cells. In the context of neck pain, stem cells may be derived from sources such as adipose (fat) tissue, bone marrow, or umbilical cord blood. These cells are harvested, processed, and then injected into the affected area, where they can potentially stimulate tissue repair and regeneration. The regenerative properties of stem cells make them an attractive option for treating degenerative conditions such as cervical disc degeneration, facet joint arthritis, and other musculoskeletal disorders that can contribute to neck pain.

Platelet-rich plasma (PRP) therapy, on the other hand, involves the use of a concentrated solution of platelets obtained from the patient's own blood. Platelets are essential components of the blood clotting process and contain a multitude of growth factors that can stimulate tissue repair and regeneration. During PRP therapy, a sample of the patient's blood is drawn and centrifuged to separate the platelets from the other blood components. The resulting PRP solution is then injected into the affected area to promote healing and reduce inflammation. PRP therapy has been used to treat a variety of musculoskeletal conditions, including tendon injuries, muscle strains, and joint inflammation.

Initial studies have shown promising results for the use of stem cell injections and PRP therapy in treating various musculoskeletal conditions, including neck pain. In some cases, patients have reported significant improvements in pain, function, and overall quality of life. However, it is important to note that these studies are often small in scale, and results can vary greatly between individuals.

As cell-based therapies are still relatively new in the field of pain management, more extensive research is needed to determine the long-term safety and efficacy of these treatments for neck pain. In particular, future studies should focus on identifying the optimal sources and types of stem cells, refining PRP preparation techniques, and establishing standardized treatment protocols. Additionally, research should explore potential risks and complications associated with these therapies, such as infection, tissue damage, or the development of tumors. As more evidence becomes available, cell-based therapies may become a valuable addition to the array of treatment options available for neck pain management.

Gene therapy is a groundbreaking approach that has the potential to revolutionize the treatment of various medical conditions, including those related to neck pain. The concept of gene therapy involves the delivery of genetic material into cells to correct or replace faulty genes, thereby addressing the underlying cause of a disease or disorder. In the context of neck pain, researchers are investigating the use of gene therapy to target specific genes involved in inflammation and pain signaling pathways, which are critical factors in the development and persistence of pain.

One potential application of gene therapy in neck pain treatment is the modulation of genes responsible for the production of pro-inflammatory cytokines. These cytokines, such as tumor necrosis factor-alpha (TNF-alpha) and interleukin-6 (IL-6), play a crucial role in the inflammatory response that can contribute to neck pain. By using gene therapy to suppress the expression of these pro-inflammatory genes, it may be possible to reduce inflammation and alleviate pain in affected individuals. Initial studies in animal models have shown promising results, with reduced inflammation and pain observed following the administration of gene therapy targeting these pro-inflammatory cytokines.

Another potential application of gene therapy in neck pain treatment involves targeting genes associated with pain signaling pathways, such as the nerve growth factor (NGF) gene. NGF is a protein that plays a key role in the survival, development, and maintenance of nerve cells, including those involved in the transmission of pain signals. Researchers are exploring the use of gene therapy to inhibit the expression of the NGF gene, potentially reducing pain signaling and providing relief for individuals with neck pain. Early research in this area has shown promise, with animal studies demonstrating decreased pain sensitivity following NGF gene silencing.

Despite the potential benefits of gene therapy in neck pain treatment, there are several challenges and considerations that must be addressed before this approach can be widely adopted. One of the primary challenges is the development of safe and effective gene delivery methods. Current gene therapy techniques involve the use of viral vectors, which can efficiently deliver genetic material into cells but may also pose risks related to immune reactions and potential off-target effects. To overcome these challenges, researchers are investigating alternative gene delivery methods, such as non-viral vectors and CRISPR/Cas9-based gene editing techniques, which may offer improved safety and specificity.

Another consideration in the development of gene therapy for neck pain is the need for rigorous clinical trials to establish the safety, efficacy, and long-term effects of these treatments. To date, most research in this area has been conducted in preclinical animal models, and further studies are needed to determine the optimal dosing, timing, and delivery methods for gene therapy in human subjects. As research in this area progresses, it is essential for healthcare professionals and patients alike to stay informed about the latest developments in gene therapy for neck pain treatment and consider the potential benefits and risks of this innovative approach.

Gene therapy holds significant promise for the future of neck pain treatment. By targeting specific genes involved in inflammation and pain signaling pathways, it may be possible to address the underlying causes of pain and promote healing more effectively. While still in the early stages of development, continued research and advancements in gene therapy technology could pave the way for a new era of personalized and targeted pain management strategies.

Targeted drug delivery systems have become a focal point of research in pain management due to their potential to enhance the effectiveness of pain medications while minimizing side effects. By delivering medications directly to the site of pain, these systems can reduce the amount of medication needed, which in turn can lead to fewer systemic side effects and improved patient outcomes.

One example of a targeted drug delivery system is the implantable drug delivery device, which can be placed in the affected spinal structures. These devices are designed to release pain-relieving medications in a controlled manner, providing targeted pain relief to individuals with neck pain. Implantable drug delivery systems can be filled with various medications, such as opioids or nonsteroidal anti-inflammatory drugs (NSAIDs), to address different types and levels of pain.

Another approach to targeted drug delivery is the use of drug-loaded nanoparticles, which can be engineered to release medication at specific sites within the body. These nanoparticles can be designed to target inflamed or damaged tissues, such as those associated with neck pain, and release their therapeutic payload upon reaching the target site. This approach has the potential to maximize the pain-relieving effects of medications while minimizing the risk of systemic side effects.

In addition to implantable devices and nanoparticles, researchers are also exploring the use of hydrogels and other biocompatible materials for targeted drug delivery. These materials can be designed to release medication in response to specific triggers, such as changes in pH or temperature, or in response to specific biological markers associated with inflammation or tissue damage. By incorporating these stimuli-responsive materials into drug delivery systems, researchers can create targeted treatments that only release medication when and where it is needed.

While targeted drug delivery systems hold significant promise for the future of neck pain treatment, there are still challenges to overcome. One of the main challenges is developing drug delivery systems that can effectively penetrate the complex and highly regulated environment of the spinal structures. Additionally, long-term safety and efficacy data are needed to ensure these systems are both safe and effective for use in patients with neck pain.

Targeted drug delivery systems have the potential to revolutionize the treatment of neck pain by providing more effective and safer pain management options. As research in this field progresses, it is likely that we will see the development of increasingly sophisticated drug delivery systems that can be tailored to individual patient needs, paving the way for more personalized and targeted pain management strategies.

Transcranial magnetic stimulation (TMS) is a non-invasive, FDA-approved technique that utilizes electromagnetic induction to stimulate specific regions of the brain. By placing a coil near the scalp, TMS generates rapidly changing magnetic fields that can induce electrical currents in the underlying neural tissue. These currents can modulate the activity of nerve cells, influencing the brain's overall function.

While TMS has primarily been employed as a treatment for mental health conditions such as major depressive disorder and obsessive-compulsive disorder, recent research has begun to explore its potential in managing chronic pain, including neck pain. The application of TMS in pain management is based on the understanding that chronic pain involves alterations in the central nervous system, particularly in areas of the brain responsible for pain processing and modulation. By targeting these specific brain regions, TMS aims to normalize neural activity, resulting in a reduction of pain perception.

There are several ways that TMS might help alleviate neck pain. One mechanism is by targeting the primary motor cortex (M1), which is involved in motor function and sensory processing. By stimulating the M1 region, TMS has been shown to induce analgesic effects through the activation of pain inhibitory systems and modulation of the sensory-discriminative aspect of pain. Another approach focuses on the dorsolateral prefrontal cortex (DLPFC), a region associated with cognitive and emotional aspects of pain. Stimulation of the DLPFC has been linked to improvements in pain-related mood and anxiety, as well as enhanced descending pain inhibition.

Recent clinical trials investigating the use of TMS for neck pain have shown promising results, with some studies reporting significant reductions in pain intensity, improved function, and enhanced quality of life. However, further research is required to determine the most effective treatment protocols, including the optimal stimulation frequency, intensity, and duration. Additionally, identifying specific patient populations that may benefit most from TMS therapy is crucial to maximizing its potential in neck pain management.

It is also important to note that TMS is generally considered a safe and well-tolerated treatment, with minimal side effects. The most common side effects include mild discomfort or pain at the stimulation site and transient headaches. However, there is a rare risk of seizure associated with TMS, particularly in individuals with a history of epilepsy or other seizure disorders. Therefore, a thorough evaluation of a patient's medical history and potential contraindications is essential before initiating TMS therapy for neck pain management.

Transcranial magnetic stimulation is an emerging, non-invasive treatment option with the potential to address chronic neck pain by targeting specific brain regions involved in pain processing and modulation. While initial research findings are promising, further investigation is needed to optimize treatment parameters and identify the patients most likely to benefit from TMS therapy. As our understanding of TMS and its applications in pain management continues to grow, it may become an increasingly important tool in the comprehensive treatment of neck pain.

Wearable technologies have been gaining attention as a promising means of pain management, particularly for those suffering from neck pain. These devices, which include smart clothing and biofeedback gadgets, offer a non-invasive, personalized approach to monitoring and addressing factors that contribute to neck pain.

Smart clothing, for example, incorporates sensors and other electronic components directly into garments, providing a discreet and comfortable means of tracking a wearer's posture, muscle tension, and movement. These garments can be designed to provide real-time feedback to users, alerting them when their posture is suboptimal, and helping them make necessary adjustments. Over time, this type of feedback may train the user to adopt healthier postural habits, ultimately reducing neck pain.

Biofeedback devices, on the other hand, are designed to monitor various physiological parameters such as muscle tension, heart rate, and skin conductance. When combined with wearable technology, these devices can offer valuable insights into the physical factors that contribute to neck pain. For example, a wearable biofeedback device may detect when a user's neck muscles are excessively tense and prompt the individual to perform a relaxation exercise or change their position to alleviate the tension. By fostering greater self-awareness and promoting proactive pain management strategies, wearable biofeedback devices have the potential to significantly reduce neck pain.

Another potential application of wearable technologies in neck pain management is the integration of virtual and augmented reality systems.

These immersive technologies, when combined with wearable devices, can provide users with personalized exercise programs, guided stretching routines, and real-time feedback on their posture and muscle activation patterns. This fusion of technology can create engaging and interactive experiences that support users in developing healthier habits and reducing their neck pain.

Furthermore, advancements in sensor technology and data analytics have the potential to enhance the efficacy of wearable devices for pain management. For example, machine learning algorithms could analyze data collected from wearable devices to identify patterns and correlations between specific behaviors and pain levels. This information could then be used to develop personalized recommendations for users, such as targeted exercise programs or ergonomic adjustments.

Wearable technologies offer a promising avenue for addressing neck pain through real-time feedback, personalized interventions, and improved self-awareness. As technology continues to advance, it is likely that we will see the development of increasingly sophisticated wearable devices specifically tailored for pain management. This emerging field has the potential to transform the way we approach neck pain treatment, providing individuals with the tools and knowledge they need to take control of their pain and improve their overall quality of life.

Virtual reality (VR) and augmented reality (AR) technologies have emerged as promising tools in the field of pain management, particularly in the context of neck pain. These immersive technologies have the potential to revolutionize the way individuals manage their pain by offering novel, engaging, and interactive experiences.

One of the key applications of VR in pain management is distraction therapy. Distraction therapy has been shown to be effective in reducing pain perception by drawing the patient's attention away from their pain and towards an immersive virtual environment. In the case of neck pain, patients may be guided through calming and engaging virtual scenarios, such as nature walks or underwater explorations, that can help alleviate pain perception by diverting focus from their discomfort. Research has shown that VR distraction therapy can be particularly effective for acute pain, and it may also provide benefits for those with chronic neck pain.

Additionally, VR and AR technologies can be utilized to provide biofeedback and guided exercise programs for individuals with neck pain. By combining real-time information about the patient's posture, muscle activation, and range of motion with immersive virtual environments, these technologies can help patients develop better body awareness and improve their posture. For example, patients can wear AR-enabled glasses or use a VR headset to receive visual cues and feedback on their posture and movement, allowing them to make adjustments in real-time. This can help individuals learn to maintain proper alignment, reducing strain on the neck muscles and spinal structures.

Furthermore, VR and AR can be used to deliver customized exercise programs designed to strengthen the muscles that support the neck and improve overall function. Patients can follow along with virtual trainers or therapists, who demonstrate specific exercises and stretches tailored to the individual's needs. This approach not only increases patient engagement but also ensures that exercises are performed correctly, reducing the risk of injury and maximizing the therapeutic benefits.

As VR and AR technologies continue to advance, it is likely that they will be integrated more extensively into pain management strategies. For instance, virtual support groups and therapy sessions could be developed to provide patients with neck pain an opportunity to connect with others experiencing similar challenges, fostering a sense of community and support. Additionally, the development of more sophisticated biofeedback systems that utilize machine learning algorithms could lead to highly personalized treatment plans that adapt to the patient's progress and needs.

Virtual reality and augmented reality technologies offer significant potential in the management of neck pain. Through distraction therapy, biofeedback, guided exercise programs, and the possibility of future applications such as virtual support groups, VR and AR technologies can provide engaging, interactive, and effective tools for individuals suffering from neck pain. As research continues and these technologies become more refined, it is likely that they will play an increasingly important role in the landscape of pain management.

431

Telehealth and remote rehabilitation have gained popularity in recent years, particularly due to the COVID-19 pandemic, which necessitated a shift towards remote healthcare delivery. These technologies enable healthcare professionals to provide care and support to patients remotely, overcoming geographical barriers and increasing accessibility to specialized care. This is particularly significant for patients with neck pain, as it allows them to access expert care that may not be available in their local area.

In the context of neck pain, remote rehabilitation programs can take various forms. Video consultations allow healthcare providers to assess patients, monitor their progress, and provide guidance and support through a virtual platform. This approach can be particularly helpful for individuals who have difficulty traveling to in-person appointments or live in rural areas with limited access to specialized care.

Online exercise programs tailored to neck pain management can also play a significant role in remote rehabilitation. These programs often include video demonstrations, written instructions, and progress tracking features that help patients follow a personalized exercise regimen to alleviate neck pain. The exercises may focus on strengthening neck and shoulder muscles, improving posture, and promoting flexibility. This approach enables patients to engage in self-directed rehabilitation at their own pace and in the comfort of their homes.

Wearable devices that provide real-time feedback are another emerging technology with potential applications in remote rehabilitation for neck pain management. These devices can monitor posture, muscle tension, and other factors that contribute to pain. By providing real-time feedback, wearable technologies can help individuals make adjustments to their behavior and environment, potentially reducing neck pain and promoting better pain management. For example, a wearable device could alert a user when they are slouching or engaging in other behaviors that may exacerbate neck pain. This feedback could serve as a valuable tool for reinforcing positive habits and promoting long-term pain relief.

As telehealth technology continues to advance, it is likely that remote rehabilitation will play an increasingly important role in the management of neck pain and other musculoskeletal conditions. Remote monitoring systems may become more sophisticated, allowing healthcare providers to track patients' progress more accurately and make data-driven decisions regarding their care. Additionally, the integration of artificial intelligence and machine learning algorithms into telehealth platforms could enable the development of personalized treatment plans that are tailored to the specific needs of each patient.

Telehealth and remote rehabilitation represent a significant advancement in the management of neck pain. By overcoming geographical barriers and increasing accessibility to specialized care, these technologies have the potential to improve patient outcomes and promote better pain management. As technology continues to advance and become more integrated into healthcare delivery, remote rehabilitation will likely become an increasingly important aspect of neck pain treatment.

Minimally invasive spine surgery (MISS) is an emerging surgical approach that aims to minimize tissue damage and reduce recovery time compared to traditional open surgery. This innovative method has gained significant interest in recent years due to the potential benefits it offers for patients suffering from various spine-related conditions, including neck pain.

One of the key advantages of MISS techniques is the utilization of smaller incisions. By making smaller incisions, there is less disruption to the muscles, ligaments, and other soft tissues surrounding the spine. This reduction in tissue trauma can lead to decreased postoperative pain, reduced blood loss, and a lower risk of infection. Moreover, patients typically experience less scarring and improved cosmetic outcomes with MISS techniques compared to traditional open surgery.

MISS procedures also involve the use of specialized instruments designed specifically for these minimally invasive techniques. These instruments, such as tubular retractors and endoscopes, allow surgeons to access the spine through small incisions while preserving the surrounding tissues. Tubular retractors create a working channel through which surgeons can perform various spinal procedures, while endoscopes provide enhanced visualization of the surgical field. This combination of specialized instruments enables surgeons to perform complex spine surgeries with greater precision and control.

Advanced imaging technology plays a crucial role in MISS by providing real-time, high-resolution images of the surgical area. Intraoperative imaging techniques, such as fluoroscopy and computer-assisted navigation, help guide surgeons during the procedure and minimize the risk of complications. These technologies allow for more accurate placement of implants, such as screws and rods, reducing the likelihood of nerve or tissue damage.

One notable advantage of MISS is the potential for shorter hospital stays and quicker return to daily activities. As patients experience less postoperative pain and tissue damage, they often require less pain medication and have a faster recovery period. This accelerated recovery can lead to cost savings for both patients and healthcare systems, as well as reduced reliance on postoperative rehabilitation services.

Despite these advantages, it is important to note that MISS is not suitable for all patients or all types of spinal conditions. Patient selection is crucial for the success of MISS, and factors such as the patient's overall health, the specific spinal condition, and the surgeon's experience with MISS techniques must be considered. Additionally, MISS procedures can be technically demanding, requiring specialized training and expertise on the part of the surgeon.

As MISS techniques continue to evolve and more research is conducted, it is expected that the range of conditions for which MISS can be applied will expand. This growth in the adoption of MISS has the potential to transform the management of neck pain and other spinal conditions, leading to better patient outcomes and improved quality of life for those affected by these conditions.

Artificial disc replacement (ADR) is an innovative surgical procedure that involves replacing a damaged intervertebral disc with a synthetic implant. This advanced technique has emerged as a viable alternative to spinal fusion surgery for certain patients with neck pain caused by degenerative disc disease, particularly in cases where conservative treatments have proven to be ineffective. ADR aims to preserve spinal motion and biomechanics while providing pain relief and improved function.

The primary goal of ADR is to maintain spinal motion, thereby reducing the risk of adjacent segment degeneration – a potential complication of spinal fusion surgery. Spinal fusion involves fusing two or more adjacent vertebrae, which can result in the loss of spinal mobility and increased stress on the adjacent segments. This increased stress may contribute to the degeneration of the adjacent intervertebral discs and facet joints, leading to the development of pain and potential need for additional surgeries.

ADR procedures utilize a variety of synthetic implant designs, including those made from metal, plastic, or a combination of materials. These implants are designed to mimic the natural motion of the intervertebral disc, allowing for flexion, extension, and rotation of the spine. The choice of implant material and design depends on factors such as the patient's anatomy, the extent of disc damage, and the surgeon's preference.

While ADR is still a relatively new procedure, early results have been promising. Studies have shown that many patients experience reduced pain and improved function following ADR surgery. Furthermore, some studies have demonstrated that ADR patients tend to have shorter hospital stays and faster recovery times compared to those who undergo spinal fusion surgery.

However, it is essential to note that ADR may not be suitable for all patients with neck pain. Specific conditions, such as spinal instability, severe facet joint degeneration, or spinal infections, may contraindicate the use of ADR. A thorough evaluation by a spine specialist is necessary to determine if ADR is an appropriate treatment option for an individual patient.

As technology advances and long-term data become available, ADR is expected to become a more common treatment option for individuals with neck pain caused by degenerative disc disease. Further research and development of implant materials and designs, along with advancements in surgical techniques and imaging technology, will likely improve the safety and efficacy of ADR procedures in the future. This progress has the potential to offer patients a more effective, motion-preserving alternative to spinal fusion surgery, ultimately enhancing their quality of life.

Artificial intelligence (AI) and machine learning algorithms are revolutionizing various aspects of healthcare, including pain management. Predictive analytics and personalized medicine are two interconnected areas where AI can make a significant impact on the treatment of neck pain. By analyzing large datasets of patient information, AI algorithms can identify patterns and relationships that may not be apparent to human clinicians, allowing for more accurate prediction of individual patient outcomes and the development of tailored treatment plans.

One of the key applications of AI in predictive analytics for neck pain management is the identification of patient subgroups that may respond better to specific treatment modalities. By analyzing data from clinical trials and real-world patient populations, machine learning algorithms can help identify subgroups of patients with similar characteristics, such as age, medical history, underlying cause of pain, and genetic factors. This information can be used to develop personalized treatment plans that target the unique needs of each patient, potentially leading to improved outcomes and a reduction in unnecessary treatments.

Another application of AI in personalized medicine for neck pain is the development of predictive models to estimate treatment response and prognosis. These models can incorporate a wide range of variables, such as demographic information, clinical measurements, imaging data, and genetic markers, to predict the likelihood of a successful treatment outcome for a given patient. By identifying patients who are more likely to benefit from specific interventions, healthcare professionals can allocate resources more efficiently and avoid treatments that may have a low chance of success.

Furthermore, AI can play a role in optimizing the timing and sequencing of treatments for neck pain. Machine learning algorithms can analyze longitudinal patient data to determine the optimal order and timing of interventions, such as physical therapy, medication, and surgery. This information can help clinicians develop treatment plans that maximize the likelihood of a successful outcome and minimize the risk of complications.

In addition to improving the effectiveness of existing treatments, AI can also facilitate the discovery of novel therapeutic approaches for neck pain. For example, machine learning algorithms can be used to analyze large-scale molecular data, such as gene expression profiles and protein interactions, to identify potential drug targets and biomarkers associated with neck pain. This information can be used to guide the development of new medications and diagnostic tools, ultimately leading to more effective and targeted treatments for neck pain.

As AI technology continues to advance, it is essential for healthcare professionals and researchers to collaborate in the development and implementation of these tools in clinical practice. By leveraging the power of AI and machine learning, it is possible to move towards a future of personalized pain management strategies that improve the quality of life for individuals suffering from neck pain.

Robotic-assisted surgery represents a significant advancement in the field of pain management, with the potential to revolutionize the treatment of neck pain and other musculoskeletal conditions. By incorporating AI and machine learning technologies, robotic systems can help surgeons perform complex procedures with a level of precision and control that would be difficult or impossible to achieve manually. This increased accuracy can lead to improved patient outcomes, reduced postoperative complications, and shorter recovery times.

In the context of neck pain, robotic-assisted surgery is especially relevant for minimally invasive spine surgery, such as microdiscectomy or laminectomy, and artificial disc replacement procedures. These surgeries require a high degree of precision to minimize the risk of damaging surrounding tissues, nerves, and blood vessels. Robotic systems can provide enhanced visualization, improved dexterity, and increased stability during these delicate procedures, making it easier for surgeons to navigate the complex anatomy of the cervical spine.

One of the key advantages of robotic-assisted surgery is the ability to create detailed, patient-specific surgical plans using advanced imaging techniques like computed tomography (CT) or magnetic resonance imaging (MRI). These images can be used to create a three-dimensional model of the patient's spine, which can then be integrated with the robotic system. This integration allows the surgeon to visualize the patient's unique anatomy in real-time during the procedure, enabling more precise and targeted surgical interventions.

Moreover, AI and machine learning technologies can be integrated into robotic-assisted surgery systems to analyze vast amounts of data, such as patient outcomes and surgical techniques, to optimize surgical procedures continually. This ongoing analysis can help identify best practices and refine surgical techniques, further improving patient outcomes and reducing the risk of complications.

Despite the potential benefits of robotic-assisted surgery for neck pain treatment, it is important to acknowledge the limitations and challenges associated with this technology. High costs, limited availability, and the need for specialized training may present barriers to widespread adoption. Additionally, long-term data on patient outcomes following robotic-assisted spine surgery is still limited, and further research is needed to determine the true benefits and potential risks associated with these procedures.

Robotic-assisted surgery, with the integration of AI and machine learning technologies, offers promising advancements in the treatment of neck pain and other musculoskeletal conditions. By providing surgeons with enhanced precision, control, and real-time visualization, this innovative approach has the potential to improve patient outcomes and redefine the standard of care for spinal surgery. As research continues and technology advances, it is likely that robotic-assisted surgery will become an increasingly common and integral component of neck pain treatment and management.

The future landscape of neck pain treatment is rapidly evolving, with numerous emerging therapies and innovations in pain management showing considerable promise for improving the lives of individuals suffering from neck pain. Novel therapeutic approaches such as cell-based therapies, including stem cell injections and platelet-rich plasma therapy, and gene therapy have the potential to address the underlying causes of neck pain and promote healing more effectively than traditional treatment methods.

In addition to these groundbreaking therapies, advancements in non-invasive pain management techniques, such as transcranial magnetic stimulation (TMS), virtual reality (VR), and augmented reality (AR) applications, are poised to offer patients innovative ways to cope with and alleviate their pain. These cutting-edge technologies provide patients with the tools to manage their pain in more accessible, engaging, and effective ways, ultimately improving their overall quality of life.

Furthermore, the field of neck pain treatment is witnessing significant advancements in surgical techniques, such as minimally invasive spine surgery (MISS) and artificial disc replacement (ADR), which offer the potential for better patient outcomes and reduced recovery times. These state-of-the-art surgical approaches provide patients with less invasive options for addressing the root causes of their neck pain, resulting in less postoperative discomfort and quicker return to daily activities.

The integration of artificial intelligence (AI) and machine learning into pain management strategies is also poised to revolutionize the field, enabling more personalized, targeted treatments for neck pain sufferers. AI-driven predictive analytics can help healthcare professionals better understand individual patient needs and tailor treatment plans accordingly, while robotic-assisted surgery offers greater precision and control in surgical procedures, ultimately leading to improved patient outcomes.

As these emerging therapies and innovations continue to be researched and refined, it is of paramount importance for healthcare professionals and patients alike to stay informed about the latest developments in neck pain treatment. This knowledge empowers both parties to make informed decisions about the most appropriate and effective treatment options available. By embracing these new technologies and approaches, we can move towards a future of more effective, targeted, and personalized pain management strategies, ultimately improving the quality of life for individuals suffering from neck pain. This future will require collaboration among researchers, healthcare professionals, patients, and technology developers to ensure that these innovative solutions are both safe and effective in addressing the complex and multifaceted nature of neck pain.

About the Author

Jeffery J. Rowe, MD

Dr. Jeffery Rowe completed two years of General Surgery residency at the Medical College of Pennsylvania/Hahnemann University. After two years, he began his Physical Medicine and Rehabilitation residency at the University of Pennsylvania. Following his residency, he was fellowship trained in Interventional Spine and Pain Medicine. He became board certified in Physical Medicine & Rehabilitation in 2004 and became board certified in Pain Medicine in 2005.

Dr. Rowe has more than eight years of experience in Burn Surgery and Critical Care and more than twenty years of surgical experience. His extensive surgical background and management of critically injured burn patients combined with his extensive experience and specialty training in the performance of diagnostic and therapeutic injections in the spine gives him a unique ability to perform minimally invasive procedures including both trial and surgically implanted spinal cord stimulators, Dorsal Root Ganglion Stimulators. He also performs minimally invasive lumbar decompression, SI joint fusions, implants interspinous spacer and fusion devices and intrathecal pumps.

Dr. Rowe has gained international recognition for his many contributions to the study and treatment of pain and his dedication to furthering the field, particularly pain syndromes considered the most difficult to manage. Dr. Rowe is considered a key opinion leader in the pain management field, providing lectures and training throughout the country to other physicians and medical practices.

As a consultant Dr. Rowe is contracted to educate for some of the largest neuromodulation companies. Dr. Rowe trains physicians to surgically implant Spinal Cord Stimulators (SCS), Dorsal Root Ganglion Stimulators (DRG), Peripheral Nerve Stimulators (PNS), interspinous spacer devices and posterior non-pedicle fusion devices.

Dr. Rowe also performs minimally invasive lumbar decompression and intradiscal allograft injections that rehydrate discs for patients that have lumbar degenerative disc disease. In addition, Dr. Rowe treats axial low back pain associated with degenerative changes in the spine with a basivertebral nerve ablative procedure.

www.ingramcontent.com/pod-product-compliance
Lightning Source LLC
Chambersburg PA
CBHW052118270326
41930CB00012B/2670